BASIC
RADIOLOGY

BASIC RADIOLOGY

EDITORS

Michael Y. M. Chen, M.D.

Associate Professor of Radiology
Department of Radiology
Bowman Gray School of Medicine
Wake Forest University
Winston-Salem, North Carolina

Thomas L. Pope, Jr., M.D.

Professor of Radiology
Department of Radiology
Bowman Gray School of Medicine
Wake Forest University
Winston-Salem, North Carolina

David J. Ott, M.D.

Professor of Radiology
Department of Radiology
Bowman Gray School of Medicine
Wake Forest University
Winston-Salem, North Carolina

McGraw-Hill
HEALTH PROFESSIONS DIVISION

New York   St. Louis   San Francisco   Auckland   Bogotá   Caracas   Lisbon   London   Madrid
Mexico City   Milan   Montreal   New Delhi   San Juan   Singapore   Sydney   Tokyo   Toronto

McGraw-Hill

*A Division of The **McGraw·Hill** Companies*

BASIC RADIOLOGY

Copyright ©1996 by *The **McGraw-Hill** Companies,* Inc. All rights
reserved. Printed in the United States of America. Except as permitted
under the United States Copyright Act of 1976, no part of this publication
may be reproduced or distributed in any form or by any means, or stored
in a data base or retrieval system, without the prior written permission of
the publisher.

1234567890 KGP KGP 98765

ISBN 0-07-011148-0

This book was set in Times Roman by Compset, Inc.

The editors were Martin J. Wonsiewicz and Steven Melvin; the
production supervisor was Clare Stanley.

Quebecor/Kingsport was printer and binder.

This book is printed on acid-free paper.

Library of Congress Cataloging-in-Publication Data

Basic radiology / editors, Michael Y. Chen, Thomas L. Pope, David J.
    Ott.
        p.   cm.
    Includes index.
    ISBN 0-07-011148-0 (alk. paper)
    1. Radiography, Medical.   2. Diagnostic imaging.   I. Chen,
Michael Y. M.   II. Ott, David J. (David James) .
    [DNLM: 1. Radiography.   WN 180 B311 1995]
RC78.B34   1995
616.07'57—dc20
DNLM/DLC
for Library of Congress   95-19434

To the memory of my mother
M. Y. M. C.

To Lou, David, and Jason, to my mom and to the memory of my dad
T. L. P., Jr.

To my family
D. J. O.

CONTENTS

CONTRIBUTORS

Sam T. Auringer, M.D.

Associate Professor, Department of Radiology, Bowman Gray School of Medicine, Wake Forest University, Winston-Salem, North Carolina [6]

Robert E. Bechtold, M.D.

Associate Professor, Department of Radiology, Bowman Gray School of Medicine, Wake Forest University, Winston-Salem, North Carolina [11]

Michael Y. M. Chen, M.D.

Associate Professor of Radiology, Department of Radiology, Bowman Gray School of Medicine, Wake Forest University, Winston-Salem, North Carolina [1, 8]

Caroline Chiles, M.D.

Associate Professor, Department of Radiology, Bowman Gray School of Medicine, Wake Forest University, Winston-Salem, North Carolina [4]

Robert H. Choplin, M.D.

Professor, Department of Radiology, Bowman Gray School of Medicine, Wake Forest University, Winston-Salem, North Carolina [4]

Robert L. Dixon, Ph.D.

Professor, Department of Radiology, Bowman Gray School of Medicine, Wake Forest University, Winston-Salem, North Carolina [2]

Mary Gena Frederick, M.D.

Assistant Professor, Department of Radiology, Duke University Medical Center, Durham, North Carolina [1]

Rita I. Freimanis, M.D.

Assistant Professor, Department of Radiology, Bowman Gray School of Medicine, Wake Forest University, Winston-Salem, North Carolina [5]

Lawrence E. Ginsberg, M.D.

Assistant Professor of Radiology, University of Texas, M.D. Anderson Cancer Center, Houston, Texas [13]

Tamara Miner Haygood, M.D.

Assistant Professor, Department of Radiology, Bowman Gray School of Medicine, Wake Forest University, Winston-Salem, North Carolina [6]

Dalane W. Kitzman, M.D.

Assistant Professor, Department of Internal Medicine, Bowman Gray School of Medicine, Wake Forest University, Winston-Salem, North Carolina [3]

Johnny U. V. Monu, M.D.

Assistant Professor, Department of Radiology, Bowman Gray School of Medicine, Wake Forest University, Winston-Salem, North Carolina [6, 7]

David J. Ott, M.D.

Professor of Radiology, Department of Radiology, Bowman Gray School of Medicine, Wake Forest University, Winston-Salem, North Carolina [10]

Thomas L. Pope, Jr., M.D.

Professor of Radiology, Department of Radiology, Bowman Gray School of Medicine, Wake Forest University, Winston-Salem, North Carolina [3, 7]

Daniel W. Williams III, M.D.

Associate Professor, Department of Radiology, Bowman Gray School of Medicine, Wake Forest University, Winston-Salem, North Carolina [12]

Ronald J. Zagoria, M.D.

Associate Professor, Department of Radiology, Bowman Gray School of Medicine, Wake Forest University, Winston-Salem, North Carolina [9]

Numbers in brackets refer to chapters written or cowritten by the contributor.

PREFACE

Our main goal in writing this book was to produce a concise text on current radiologic imaging for senior medical students and all residents interested in radiology. After the introductory chapters, the book follows an organ-system approach. Applicable imaging techniques and their use and indication are included in each organ-related chapter. Also present are question-oriented exercises that cover common pathologic conditions for each organ system.

The first chapter describes the various diagnostic imaging techniques that are available: conventional radiography, nuclear medicine, ultrasonography, computed tomography, and magnetic resonance imaging. The second chapter provides an introduction to the physics of radiation and its related biological effects. The remaining chapters focus on individual organ systems, including the heart, lungs, breast, bones, joints, abdomen, urinary tract, alimentary tract, liver, biliary system, pancreas, brain, and spine. All of these chapters are organized in essentially the same way. Each begins with a brief description of recent developments in radiologic imaging of the organ system under discussion. This description is followed by a review of imaging techniques that are applicable in evaluating each organ and then by illustrations of normal anatomy. The next section covers technique selection and emphasizes proper ordering of various imaging examinations on the basis of clinical presentation, patient preparation (if applicable), and potential conflicts between techniques. The last section consists of questions based on imaging exercises. Each exercise is made up of one to five cases, with appropriate images and related questions that focus on common diseases or specific symptoms for that organ system. At the end of each chapter is a short list of suggested readings selected from general references.

We hope that this book will help medical students and residents in areas other than radiology to better understand the many imaging modalities available and how to select appropriate techniques for examination of their patients. Our further hope is that the exercises will provide a stimulating interactive approach that will familiarize readers with the more common diseases that can be shown with current imaging methods.

ACKNOWLEDGMENTS

We are indebted to our many contributors who kindly provided chapters for this book in their areas of expertise, and to other colleagues who supplied additional figures. We also wish to thank C. Douglas Maynard, M.D., Director of the Division of Radiological Sciences and Professor and Chairman of the Department of Radiology of the Bowman Gray School of Medicine, who has provided us with the supportive environment needed to complete this endeavor.

We express our gratitude to Donna S. Garrison, Ph.D., and Nancy A. Ragland for their help in editing and proofreading many of the chapters in the text. We also thank our many secretaries, Julianne R. Berckman, Judith F. Cornelius, Peggy T. Inch, Sandrae S. Johnston, Sharon R. Meister, Betty J. Metcalf, Dese H. Simpson, and Miriam L. Vernon for their assistance in preparing the manuscripts. In addition, we appreciate the able skills of our audiovisual personnel, Ellen E. Henson and Joyce Goodman.

Finally, this book would not have been possible without the able support of Dr. Jane E. Pennington, Martin J. Wonsiewicz, Steven Melvin, Clare Stanley and their fine associates at McGraw-Hill.

Michael Y. M. Chen, M.D.

Thomas L. Pope, Jr., M.D.

David J. Ott, M.D.

BASIC
RADIOLOGY

PART 1

INTRODUCTION

1

SCOPE OF DIAGNOSTIC IMAGING

Mary Gena Frederick
Michael Y. M. Chen

CONVENTIONAL RADIOGRAPHY
   Contrast Studies
   Computed Tomography

NUCLEAR MEDICINE

ULTRASONOGRAPHY

MAGNETIC RESONANCE IMAGING

The field of diagnostic radiology has undergone tremendous growth in the past several decades. Angiography developed in the 1950s, nuclear medicine in the 1960s, ultrasound and computed tomography (CT) in the 1970s, magnetic resonance (MR) imaging and interventional radiology in the 1980s, and positron emission tomography (PET) in the early 1990s. It is increasingly difficult for clinicians and medical students to stay abreast of the new techniques available for diagnosis and management of disease. Subspecialty fields in radiology include pediatric, musculoskeletal, breast, interventional, neurologic, abdominal, thoracic, gastrointestinal, genitourinary, nuclear medicine, and ultrasound imaging. As this list shows, radiologic subspecialties can be organ-oriented or modality-oriented. Radiologists interact with members of virtually every clinical specialty as consultants for film interpretation, management considerations, and interventional procedures. The purpose of this textbook is to provide medical students or house officers with an overview of diagnostic radiology that will help to guide both consultations with colleagues and selection of radiologic studies to ensure the best possible patient care.

Since Professor Wilhelm Conrad Roentgen's discovery of x-rays in 1895, diagnostic imaging has progressed to encompass four primary technologies: (1) ionizing radiation transmitted through the body after bombardment of a tungsten target with an electron beam (x-rays), (2) ionizing radiation emitted after injection or ingestion of a radioactive pharmaceutical (nuclear medicine), (3) sound waves directed into the body and measurement of their reflected echoes (ultrasound), and (4) radiofrequencies ap-

plied while the patient is stationed in a large-bore magnet, causing movement of the hydrogen ions in tissues (MR imaging). Specific indications for the use of each of these modalities in evaluating various organ systems are described in subsequent chapters.

The most current concern in radiology, as in all medical fields, is the issue of health care reform, which stresses proper use of diagnostic studies to contain costs. The clinician-radiologist relationship will assume even greater importance as the two work together to tailor the examinations for each patient to be certain that all studies contain useful information that can influence treatment and outcome.

CONVENTIONAL RADIOGRAPHY

Although new techniques have assumed a major role in most areas of diagnostic radiology, the plain film remains fundamental, particularly in the evaluation of chest disease, breast tissues, bone trauma, and abdominal disease. Plain-film radiography relies heavily on the natural contrast between radiographic densities of air, fat, soft tissue, and bone. Therefore, this technique is most advantageous in parts of the body with inherently high contrast, e.g., the lungs and the heart (Fig. 1-1). Modifications of plain-film radiography are fluoroscopy, tomography, and mammography.

Fluoroscopy uses the x-ray beam in a continuous manner and thereby differs from the snapshot method of radiographs. With fluoroscopy, the physician can evaluate

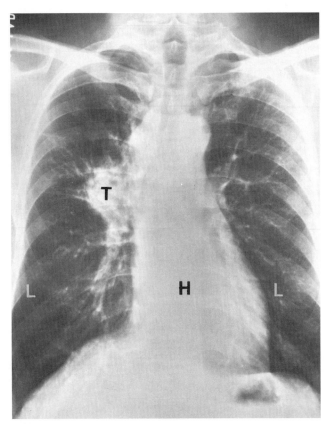

FIG. 1-1 Standard posteroanterior chest radiograph demonstrates the striking contrast between the heart (H) and lungs (L). A tumor (T) is seen at the right hilum.

dynamic processes such as diaphragmatic excursion or bowel peristalsis; can watch contrast medium in the blood vessels, bowel, kidneys, or joint spaces; and can follow the path of an opaque object such as a feeding tube or an intravascular catheter. The fluoroscopic image is usually projected on a television monitor from a high-resolution camera, and the background of fluoroscopic light is amplified with image intensifiers. The image viewed on the screen may be transferred to hard-copy film or video recorder. The fluoroscopic image is opposite to that of plain film. For instance, bones are white on a plain film but black on fluoroscopy, and the lung is black on the standard film but white on fluoroscopy. Although fluoroscopy is vital to many fields, such as gastrointestinal and interventional radiology, minimizing fluoroscopy to reduce radiation exposure to the patient should be a constant consideration.

Tomography produces an image on which one plane of the body is in sharp focus and the structures on both sides of this plane are intentionally blurred. This technique reduces the number of confusing superimposed shadows. To achieve this, the x-ray tube and the film move at the same time. More complex motions of the x-ray tube other than simple linear tomography allow for less streaking and

better blurring and thus improve image quality. Tomography is particularly useful in evaluation of the kidneys, bronchi, and skeleton.

Mammography is a plain-film study that uses specially designed equipment with low voltages and a film-screen combination to evaluate breast tissue and calcification with high contrast resolution for detail at a low radiation dose. Breast compression is important during mammography to reduce radiation exposure and improve image quality. The American Cancer Society has established screening guidelines for mammography to optimize detection of occult breast cancer.

Contrast Studies

To examine structures that do not inherently contrast with surrounding tissues, a number of different contrast media are used. Most contrast studies are used for evaluation of the gastrointestinal tract, the urinary tract, the vascular system, and the spinal canal. Less common uses include studies of the lymph nodes and lymph channels for malignancies (lymphangiography), the uterine cavity and fallopian tubes for tubal patency or uterine anomalies (hysterosalpingography), the sinus tracts for abscesses and cavities (fistulography), the salivary glands for obstruction or tumor (sialography), the joints for cartilage or ligamentous tears (arthrography), the gallbladder for gallstones (oral cholecystography), and the biliary tree for obstruction or cancer (cholangiography). In addition, use of contrast media assists the interventional radiologist in placing percutaneous nephrostomy tubes, abscess catheters, biliary drainage catheters, gastrostomy tubes, or intravascular stents.

The contrast agent most commonly used in the gastrointestinal tract is barium. A high-density compound suspended in water, barium provides excellent radiographic contrast and is safe for introduction into the gut. The most common studies are the antegrade upper gastrointestinal series and the retrograde colonic enema. Contrast material can be administered orally or rectally, and single- or double-contrast technique can be used. In a single-contrast study (Fig. 1-2), the barium suspension is administered alone. In a double-contrast study, it is administered with air or effervescent agents.

Water-soluble contrast agents, such as Gastrografin (Schering AG, Berlin, Germany), are used in the gastrointestinal tract in an antegrade or retrograde fashion to evaluate a suspected perforation or postoperative complication. Water-soluble contrast agents may be absorbed by the peritoneum if they leak, whereas a barium suspension cannot be absorbed or cleaned from the peritoneal cavity. However, water-soluble agents cost more and create a lower contrast density in comparison with barium suspensions. In addition, a major disadvantage of Gastrografin is hypertonicity, which draws fluid into the gastrointestinal tract and causes a cathartic effect or circulatory hypovolemia.

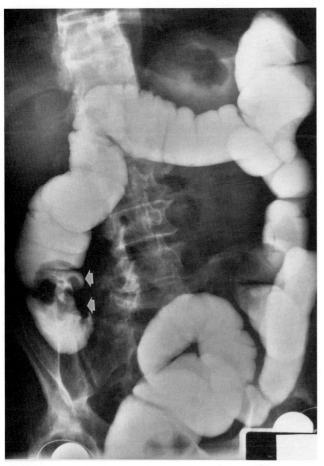

FIG. 1-2 A single-contrast retrograde colonic enema in the left posterior oblique view demonstrates an annular lesion representing a cecal carcinoma (*arrows*). Bilateral hip prostheses are an incidental observation.

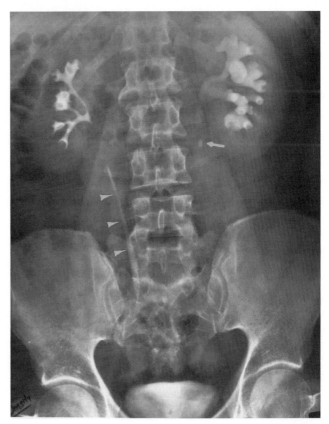

FIG. 1-3 An anteroposterior film from an intravenous urogram was taken at 10 min in a patient with a proximal left ureteral calculus (*arrow*) and associated left collecting system dilatation. The right collecting system is normal, and the right ureter (*arrowheads*) and bladder are visualized.

Therefore, water-soluble agents should be used with caution in the dehydrated, malnourished, or debilitated patient.

For urography (studies of the urinary tract), the most common contrast materials are ionic or nonionic water-soluble agents. Contrast material is injected into a peripheral vein, after which the kidneys are filmed as they concentrate the iodinated contrast material. Next, the ureters and bladder are filmed as the contrast medium is excreted. This type of study, usually combined with tomography, is commonly referred to as *intravenous urography* (IVU) (Fig. 1-3). The predominant indication of IVU is stone disease or hematuria of an unknown cause. To perform a retrograde study of the urethra, urinary bladder, or ureters, water-soluble contrast material is instilled directly. These studies are used to evaluate vesicoureteral reflux, tumor, or calculi.

Angiography, the study of the vascular system, uses water-soluble agents for intravascular visualization. The agent is introduced intraarterially or intravenously through a catheter that is placed percutaneously under fluoroscopic control. Radiographs are exposed in a series while the contrast material travels through the blood vessels (Fig. 1-4). Digital radiography is a means of acquiring, storing, and manipulating images electronically. Commonly used in the field of vascular radiology, it has the advantage of increased contrast resolution at the expense of spatial resolution and therefore requires a lower dose of contrast material. Arterial angiography is performed primarily for evaluation of atherosclerotic disease, aneurysm, or dissection. Venous angiography is performed prior to interventional procedures, such as placement of an inferior vena cava filter, to evaluate vessel size and thrombus. It is also used in diagnostic studies such as pulmonary angiography to exclude thrombus.

Myelography, the study of the spinal roots and canal, is performed by placing a needle between the spinous processes and introducing a small volume of nonionic contrast material into the subarachnoid space. After gravity distributes the contrast material in the subarachnoid space, various oblique standard radiographs are acquired and a CT examination is typically performed. The most common

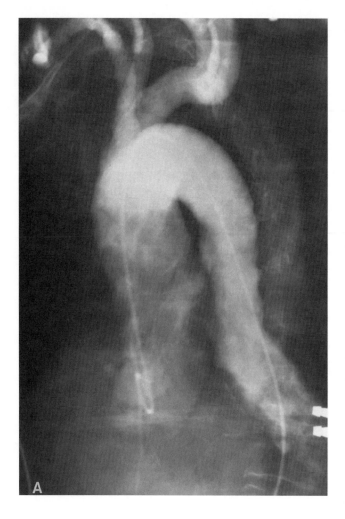

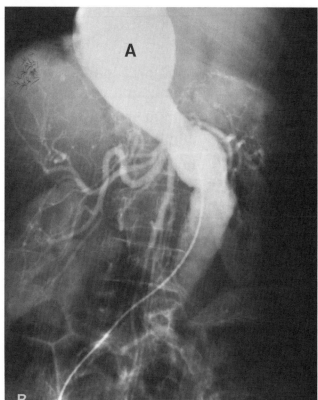

FIG. 1-4 (*A*) An aortogram with the pigtail catheter situated in the proximal ascending aorta demonstrates tortuosity of the descending thoracic aorta. (*B*) The aortogram of the same patient shows aneurysmal dilatation (A) of the lower thoracic/upper abdominal aorta, as well as the ectactic course as seen by the meandering course of the catheter. (*Courtesy of Vincent J. D'Souza, M.D., Winston-Salem, N.C.*)

indication for myelography is a herniated nucleus pulposus from a lumbar vertebral disk.

Computed Tomography

On plain radiographs, all tissues and organs have an appearance identical to that of water density, but the high contrast resolution of CT allows further differentiation between various tissues. With CT, an x-ray beam and a detector system move through an arc of 360 degrees, irradiating the subject with a highly collimated beam. The detector system measures the intensity of radiation passing through the subject, and a computer reconstructs the image by assigning shades of gray to the structures according to the attenuation of the x-ray beam. The information is displayed on a television screen, where the visual intensities can be altered. To enhance blood vessels, organs, or vascular neoplasms, contrast material is injected intravenously. The contrast agent is identical to that used in urography or arteriography. In addition, oral contrast material is administered for bowel visualization. Artifacts are produced by motion and high-density materials. Spiral CT or helical CT

is a new technology in which the x-ray source rotation and the patient advancement occur continuously and simultaneously. The image can be obtained during one breath hold. The predominant advantage is in minimizing the possibility of missing small lesions that may change position when the patient breathes during scanning, as may happen with conventional CT.

Neuroimaging is performed for the evaluation of a variety of neurologic findings. This type of study is particularly useful in defining and localizing brain tumors and strokes and in evaluating patients with neurologic emergencies such as intracerebral hemorrhage or hematoma. Although it is still performed occasionally, CT of the spine has been largely replaced by MR imaging.

Abdominal and pelvic studies are particularly useful in the evaluation of visceral neoplasms (Fig. 1-5), infections, inflammatory disease, trauma, and in staging lymphoma. CT of the chest is most useful for staging lung cancer and other neoplasms, evaluating metastases, and characterizing pulmonary nodules. The musculoskeletal system can be evaluated for a variety of bone and soft-tissue disorders such as fractures, tumors, and infections.

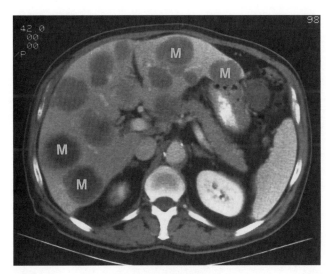

FIG. 1-5 Contrast-enhanced CT image of the upper abdomen demonstrates multiple low-attenuation areas confirmed as multiple liver metastases (M) from colon carcinoma.

NUCLEAR MEDICINE

The principles of nuclear imaging depend on the selective uptake of certain compounds by different organs of the body. These compounds must be normally involved in the physiologic metabolism of the organ to be imaged. They are labeled with a radioactive substance of sufficient energy level to be detected from outside the body with the aid of special devices such as a gamma camera. The carrier mechanisms include compartmental localization, physiologic incorporation, phagocytosis, capillary blockage, and cell sequestration. Radionuclide bone imaging is used widely to evaluate benign and malignant disorders and skeletal trauma (Fig. 1-6). Cardiac nuclear medicine concentrates on identification of viable myocardium and analysis of ventricular function. The most common pulmonary study is the ventilation-perfusion study to evaluate pulmonary emboli. Less common studies include renal imaging for evaluating blood flow and function, thyroid imaging for nodules, hepatobiliary imaging for gallbladder disease, brain imaging for blood flow, and more recently, dynamic cerebral (metabolism) imaging with positron emission tomography (PET). The unique advantage of nuclear medicine is in the evaluation of physiologic function, but morphologic resolution with this technique is inferior to that of other radiographic procedures.

ULTRASONOGRAPHY

Diagnostic ultrasound is a noninvasive imaging technique that uses sound waves in the frequency range of 1 to 10 MHz, which is above the normal human ear response of 20 to 20,000 Hz. Sound waves are directed into the body and reflected by various body structures. The time needed for

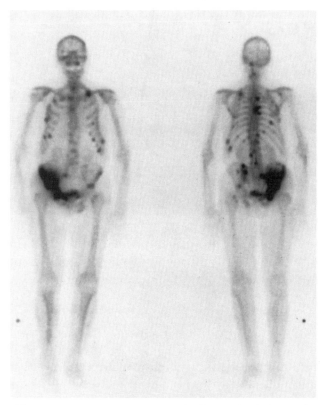

FIG. 1-6 A ^{99m}Tc-MDP bone scan in the anterior and posterior projections demonstrates multiple foci of increased radiopharmaceutical accumulation (spine, ribs, pelvis, and left clavicle) with the typical appearance of bone metastases. (*Courtesy of Robert J. Cowan, M.D., Winston-Salem, N.C.*)

the reflected waves to return determines the depth of the structures, and the amount of beam absorption determines the intensity of the returning wave. Echoes or reflections of the ultrasound beam from interfaces between tissues with different acoustic properties yield information on the size, shape, and internal structure of organs and masses. Static ultrasound imaging is no longer used. Real-time ultrasound techniques are used in dynamic imaging. Ultrasound has many common applications, including imaging of the abdomen for kidney, gallbladder, liver, and pancreas diseases (Fig. 1-7); the pelvis for ovarian or endometrial abnormalities; the fetus for anomalies; the vascular system for thrombosis, atherosclerotic disease, or arterial-venous communications; the testicles for tumor, infection, or torsion; the chest for size and location of pleural fluid collections; and the pediatric brain for hemorrhage or congenital defects. The advantages are the portability, lack of ionizing radiation, and ability to scan the body in any plane. Disadvantages are operator dependency and limited usage for imaging the lungs and skeleton because of the inability of the sound waves to penetrate gas or bone.

Doppler ultrasound uses the frequency shift in the reflected beam to detect and monitor moving substances such as blood. With color Doppler ultrasound, color in the

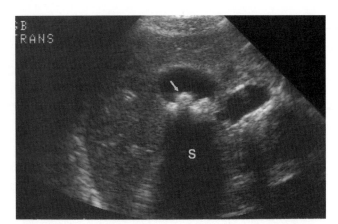

FIG. 1-7 A transverse ultrasound image of the gallbladder demonstrates a gallstone (*arrow*) with the characteristic distal acoustic shadowing (S) because sound waves cannot penetrate the gallstones.

vessels is assigned according to the direction and velocity of flow. Endoscopic sonography, which was developed in the 1980s, employs a sonographic head installed in the head of the endoscope to enable the endoscopist to assess the depth of invasion of a lesion, particularly in the esophagus or colon.

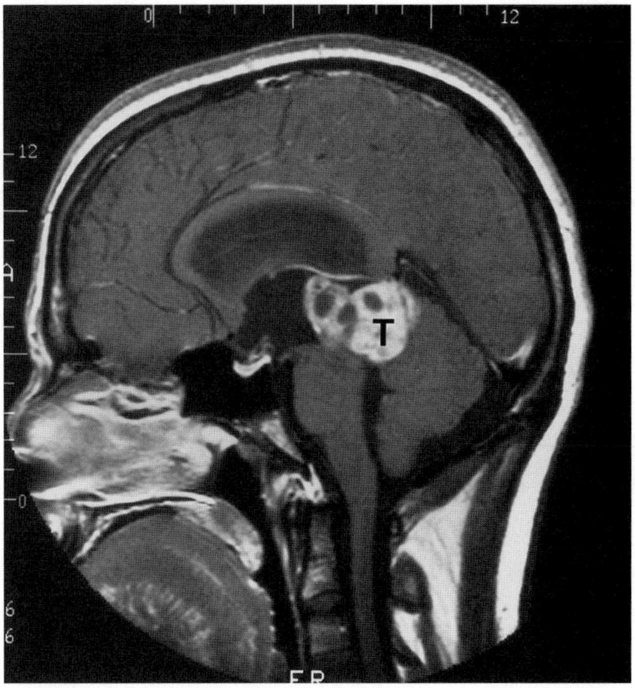

FIG. 1-8 A midline sagittal T_1-weighted contrast-enhanced MR image depicts a large tumor (T) in the region of the pineal gland. (*Courtesy of Daniel W. Williams, III, M.D., Winston-Salem, N.C.*)

MAGNETIC RESONANCE IMAGING

In MR imaging, a sequence of radiofrequency pulses passes through the body of a patient who is positioned in a large-bore magnet. Each pulse causes hydrogen ions in the patient to alter their alignment, thereby producing a responding pulse that is emitted from the patient and detected by receiving coils. It is then recorded with the aid of computers. Although many nuclei may be used for MR imaging, the most common is hydrogen because of its abundance in tissue and its sensitivity to the phenomenon of magnetic resonance. The emitted signal strength depends on several factors such as hydrogen density, flow, and magnetic relaxation times. A discussion of basic MR imaging physics appears in the next chapter.

Like CT, MR imaging displays structures in a transverse or axial fashion. However, MR imaging has the additional advantage of multiplanar imaging; axial, sagittal, and coronal planes are the most common. A further advantage of MR imaging is that it highlights the pathologic changes in different tissues by altering the pattern of radiofrequency pulses and thus the signal generated as a result of inherent contrast in the tissue. Other advantages of MR imaging include its superb contrast resolution and lack of ionizing radiation. MR imaging was first employed almost exclusively in brain and spine studies. Most brain MR imaging studies are performed to evaluate tumors, strokes, and infections (Fig. 1-8); most spine MR imaging studies are for herniated disks, infection, metastases, and spinal stenosis. MR imaging is now also used for musculoskeletal, vascular, abdominal, pelvic, and breast studies. The most common musculoskeletal applications are knee studies for torn menisci or ligaments and shoulder studies for torn rotator cuffs. Less common MR imaging examinations include liver studies for metastases, vascular studies for slow flow or thrombus, breast studies for ruptured implants, and cardiac studies for aortic dissections, aneurysms, or congenital anomalies.

BIBLIOGRAPHY

Eisenberg RL: *Radiology: An Illustrated History.* St. Louis, Mosby–Year Book, 1992.

Goldberg BB (ed): *Textbook of Abdominal Ultrasound.* Baltimore, Williams & Wilkins, 1993.

Gottschalk A et al (eds): *Diagnostic Nuclear Medicine,* 2d ed. Baltimore, Williams & Wilkins, 1988.

Lee JKT et al (eds): *Computed Body Tomography with MRI Correlation,* 2d ed. New York, Raven Press, 1989.

McClennan BL: Ionic and nonionic iodinated contrasted media: Evolution and strategies for use. *AJR* 155:225, 1990.

Mittelstaedt CA (ed): *General Ultrasound.* New York, Churchill-Livingstone, 1992.

Moss AA et al (eds): *Computed Tomography of the Body: With Magnetic Resonance Imaging,* 2d ed. Philadelphia, Saunders, 1992.

Thrall JH (ed): *Current Practice of Radiology.* Philadelphia, BC Decker, 1993.

2

THE PHYSICAL BASIS OF DIAGNOSTIC IMAGING

Robert L. Dixon

IMAGING WITH X-RAYS

What Is an X-Ray?

An x-ray is a discrete bundle of electromagnetic energy called a *photon.* In this regard, it is similar to other forms of electromagnetic energy such as light, infrared, ultraviolet, radio waves, or gamma rays. The associated electromagnetic energy can be thought of as oscillating electric and magnetic fields propagating through space at the "speed of light." The various forms of electromagnetic energy differ only in frequency (or wavelength). Since the energy carried by each photon is proportional to the frequency (the proportionality constant is called *Planck's constant*), the higher-frequency x-ray or gamma-ray photons are much more energetic than, for example, light photons and can readily ionize the atoms in materials on which they impinge. The energy of a light photon is on the order of 1 eV, whereas the average energy of an x-ray photon in a diagnostic x-ray beam is on the order of 30 keV and its wavelength is smaller than the diameter of an atom (10^{-8} cm).

   In summary, an x-ray beam can be thought of as a swarm of photons traveling at the speed of light, each photon representing a bundle of electromagnetic energy.

Production of X-Rays

Electromagnetic radiation may be produced in a variety of ways. One method is the acceleration or deceleration of electrons. For example, a radio transmitter is merely a source of high-frequency alternating current that causes electrons in an antenna wire to which it is connected to oscillate (accelerate and decelerate), thereby producing radio waves (photons) at the transmitter frequency. In an x-ray tube, electrons boiled off from a hot filament (Fig. 2-1) are

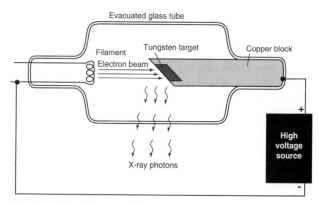

FIG. 2-1   Simple x-ray tube.

accelerated toward a tungsten anode by a high voltage on the order of 100 kV. Just before hitting the anode, the electrons will have a kinetic energy in kiloelectronvolts equal in magnitude to the kilovoltage (e.g., if the voltage across the x-ray tube is 100 kV, the electron energy is 100 keV). When the electrons smash into the tungsten anode, most of them hit other electrons, and their energy is dissipated in the form of heat. In fact, the anode may become white hot during an x-ray exposure, which is one reason for choosing an anode made of tungsten, with a very high melting point. The electrons penetrate the anode to a depth of less than 0.1 mm. A small fraction of the electrons, however, may have a close encounter with a tungsten nucleus, which, due to its large positive charge, exerts a large attractive force on the electron, giving the electron a hard jerk (acceleration) of sufficient magnitude to produce an x-ray photon. The energy of the x-ray photon, which is derived from the energy of the incident electron, depends on the magnitude of the acceleration imparted to the electron. The magnitude of the acceleration, in turn, depends on how close the electron passes by the nucleus. If one imagines a target consisting of a series of concentric circles, such as a dart board, with the bull's-eye centered on the nucleus, more electrons clearly will impinge at larger distances than in the bull's-eye, and hence a variety of x-ray photon energies will be produced at a given tube voltage (kV) up to a maximum equal to the tube voltage (a hit in the bull's-eye), where the electron gives up all its energy to the x-ray photon. Increasing the voltage will shift the x-ray photon spectrum to higher energies, and higher-energy photons are more penetrating. The radiation produced in this manner is called *Bremsstrahlung* ("braking radiation") and represents only about 1 percent of the electron energy dumped into the anode by the electron beam; the other 99 percent goes into heat. The other reason for using tungsten is that it is a heavy element with a large positive charge in the nucleus that can provide enough acceleration to the electron to produce an x-ray photon.

The electron current from filament to anode in the x-ray tube is called the mA, since it is measured in milliamperes. The mA is simply a measure of the number of electrons per second making the trip across the x-ray tube from filament to anode. The rate of x-ray production (number of x-rays produced per second) is proportional to the product of milliamperage and kilovoltage squared. The quantity of x-rays produced in an exposure of duration s (in seconds) is proportional to the product of mA and time and is called the mAs. The quantity of x-rays at a given point is generally measured in terms of the amount of ionization per cubic centimeter of air produced at that point by the x-rays and is measured in roentgens (R) or in coulombs per kilogram of air. This quantity is called *exposure,* and 1 R of exposure results in 2×10^9 ionizations per cubic centimeter of air.

The electron beam is made to impinge on a small area of the anode on the order of 1 mm in diameter in order to approximate a point source of x-rays. Since a radiograph is a shadow picture, the smaller the focal spot, the sharper is the image. By analogy, a shadow picture on the wall (such as a rabbit made with one's hand) will be much sharper if a point source of light such as a candle is used rather than an extended light source such as a fluorescent tube. The penumbra (or unsharpness) of the shadow will depend not only on the source size but also on the magnification, as can be illustrated by making a shadow of one's hand on a piece of paper using a small light source such as a single light bulb. The closer your hand is brought to the paper (the smaller the magnification), the sharper are the edges of the shadow. Similarly, magnification of the x-ray image produced by the point source is less, the closer the patient is to the film and the further the source is from the film. The *magnification factor M* is defined as the ratio of image size to object size and is equal to the ratio of the focal-to-film distance divided by the focal-to-object distance ($M \geq 1$, and $M = 1$ means no magnification is produced; i.e., either the object is right against the film, or the focal spot is infinitely far away). The penumbra, blurring, or unsharpness Δx produced on an otherwise perfectly sharp edge of an object and due to the finite focal spot size of dimension a is expressed by the equation

$$\Delta x = a(M - 1)$$

Unfortunately, the smaller the focal spot, the more likely the anode will melt. The power (energy per second) dumped into the anode is equal to the product of the kilovoltage and the milliamperage; i.e., at 100 kV and 500 mA, 50,000 W of heat energy is deposited into an area on the order of a few square millimeters (imagine a 50,000-W light bulb to get an idea of the heat generated).

Interaction of X-Rays with Matter

X-rays primarily interact with matter through interaction of their oscillating electric field with the atomic electrons in the material. Having no electric charge, the x-rays are more penetrating than other types of ionizing radiation (such as alpha or beta particles) and are therefore useful for imaging the human body. The x-rays may be absorbed or scattered by the atomic electrons. In the absorption process (photoelectric absorption), the x-ray is completely absorbed, giving all its energy to an inner-shell atomic electron, which is then ejected from the atom and goes on to ionize other atoms in the immediate vicinity of the initial interaction. In the scattering process (compton scattering), the x-ray ricochets off an atomic electron, losing some of its energy and changing its direction. The recoiling electron also goes on to ionize hundreds of atoms in the vicinity. Electrons from both processes go on to ionize many other atoms and are responsible for the biologic damage produced by x-rays.

The attenuation of the x-ray intensity with thickness of material follows an exponential law due to the random hit-or-miss nature of the interaction. The process is similar to firing a volley of rifle bullets into a forest, where the bullets may either stick in a tree (be absorbed) or ricochet off a tree (scatter). The deeper you go into the forest, the fewer bullets there are; however, a bullet still has a chance of traveling through the forest without hitting a tree. Likewise, an x-ray can make it all the way through a patient's body without touching anything and remain unchanged, as if it had passed through a vacuum instead. These are called *primary x-rays.* Typically, only about 1 percent of the incident x-rays penetrate the patient, and only about a third of these are primary x-rays; the rest are *scattered x-rays* that do not contribute to the anatomic image. An x-ray image is a shadow or projection image, which assumes that x-rays reaching the film have traveled in a straight line from the source, but this is true only for primary x-rays. As Fig. 2-2A shows, the film density (blackness) at point *P* on the film is related to the anatomy along line *FP.* The scattered photon reaches the film along the path *FSP* and is relaying information about the anatomy at the random point *S* to point *P* on the film. Scatter simply produces a uniform gray background; it does not contribute to the image. Because scatter reduces image contrast, it is desirable that the scatter be removed. This task is accomplished by use of an antiscatter grid (Fig. 2-2B). This grid consists of a series of narrow lead strips with radiolucent (low-attenuation) interspace material to remove some of the scatter. With the grid, the scattered photon shown in the figure can no longer reach the film, but the primary x-rays can. More of the scatter than primary x-rays are eliminated by the grid; hence image contrast increases, but at the cost of an increase of a factor of 2 to 3 in patient dose. This increase occurs because the scatter, which was previously blackening the film, has been reduced, and therefore, higher x-ray exposure to the front of the patient is necessary to get the requisite number of x-rays through the grid to blacken the film. The grid is usually made to move a few interspaces during the exposure by a motor drive in order to wash out the grid lines.

The absorption process is more prevalent at lower kilovoltages and in materials with higher atomic numbers. Bones appear white on an x-ray film because photoelectric absorption of x-rays is greater in bone than in soft tissue due to the higher atomic number of bone. Lead is a useful shielding material for x-rays due to its high atomic number. The probability of the absorption process decreases rapidly with photon energy (as $1/E^3$), and the scattering process decreases slowly (as $1/E$); hence the x-ray beam becomes more penetrating as kilovoltage increases. The scattering process is roughly independent of the atomic number of the attenuating material (all electrons look alike to the photon for the scattering process), whereas the absorption process is more probable for tightly bound electrons such as the inner electrons in heavier elements.

Increasing the kilovoltage is therefore beneficial to the patient in that it reduces the radiation dose; i.e., fewer x-rays into the front side of the patient are needed to get the requisite number out of the backside to blacken the film; however, an increase in kilovoltage will reduce image contrast because the absorption process, which is sensitive to atomic number, will decrease and the scattering process is independent of the atomic number of the materials. Even with materials of the same atomic number, contrast improves at lower kilovoltage settings due to higher attenuation, which results in greater differential attenuation between different thicknesses of the same material. Thus there is a tradeoff between image quality (contrast) and patient dose that must be weighed in the selection of kilovoltage.

The Radiographic Image

For production of radiographic images, the x-ray film is placed in a cassette and sandwiched between two fluorescent screens that glow under x-ray exposure, and it is primarily the light from these fluorescent screens that blackens the film. Although x-ray film, which is quite similar to ordinary photographic film, can be blackened by direct x-ray exposure, the film does not absorb the penetrating x-rays very efficiently, since the emulsion consists of silver halide crystals embedded in a low atomic number gelatin base. The fluorescent screens, called *intensifying screens,* are made of high atomic number materials, which therefore absorb x-rays very efficiently and also emit hundreds of light photons per x-ray absorbed. These light photons, in turn, are efficiently absorbed by the film. As a result, x-ray exposure to the patient is reduced by a factor on the order of 100 compared with direct x-ray exposure of the film. The screens do produce a loss of sharpness of the image due to the spreading out of the light from the point of x-ray absorption before the light reaches the film. This effect can be reduced by making the screen thinner; however, it then

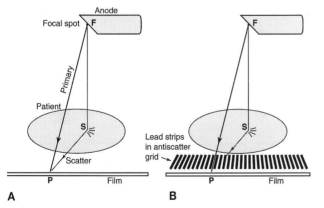

FIG. 2-2 (*A*) Scattered and primary x-ray photons reaching the same point *P* on film. (*B*) Scattered photon is removed by antiscatter grid, while primary photon gets through.

absorbs a smaller fraction of the incident x-rays and therefore results in a "slower" system (more patient exposure is required).

Recall that the quantity of x-rays produced during an exposure is proportional to

$$mAs \cdot kV^2$$

However, because the beam is more penetrating at high kilovoltage, the x-ray exposure that reaches the film through a patient is roughly proportional to

$$mAs \cdot kV^4$$

That is, it depends very strongly on kilovoltage. The exposure time required to blacken the film is thus proportional to

$$s \approx \frac{1}{mA \cdot kV^4}$$

The heat deposited in the anode is proportional to the product of kV and mAs.

Choice of an exposure technique is generally made by first selecting the kilovoltage. A lower kilovoltage gives greater image contrast but also higher patient exposure and requires a longer exposure time at a given milliampere setting because the x-ray beam is less penetrating and x-ray production is lower at the lower kilovoltages. Thus, for thick body parts, care must be taken not to choose too low a kilovoltage.

Generally, x-ray tubes have two focal spot sizes produced by two different (selectable) filament sizes. That is, they have a large and a small focal spot (e.g., 1.25 and 0.6 mm). With the small focal spot, however, the electron energy is deposited in a smaller area, thereby creating a higher anode temperature; hence, at a given kilovoltage, the maximum milliamperage that can be used without melting the anode is limited to a lower value, thereby resulting in a longer exposure time. The small focal spot will result in a sharper image; however, if the longer exposure time required by its selection does not "stop" patient motion, then motion of the patient during the exposure may blur out any sharpness gain realized by use of the small focal spot. In any case, the small focal spot is useful only for looking at fine detail, such as bony detail, and its use does not significantly improve, for instance, an abdominal radiograph in which soft-tissue contrast is the objective. The small focal spot might be used for radiographs of the skull or extremities. The exposure time selected should be short enough to stop the motion of the anatomic part being radiographed. A very short time would be required for the heart and somewhat longer times for the abdomen or chest. Exposure time is less critical for the head or extremities, which are not subject to motion in most cases.

Having selected the kilovoltage and exposure time, one must then select the milliamperage so that the milliampere-seconds (the product of milliamperage and time) is large enough to blacken the film suitably. If the milliamperage required is above 200 to 300 mA, a small focal spot generally cannot be used, because it will not allow this high a value of milliamperage without melting the anode.

On many x-ray units, a phototimer sensor (automatic exposure control) is used to automatically terminate the x-ray exposure when a given x-ray exposure has been accumulated at the cassette position. In this way, the film is blackened sufficiently regardless of patient thickness and kilovoltage selection. When using this feature, however, the operator loses control of the exposure time, and choosing the highest milliamperage allowable by the tube will ensure the minimum exposure time.

Fluoroscopy

If, instead of using the light from a fluorescent screen to blacken a film, one viewed the fluorescent screen directly with the naked eye, then one would be performing fluoroscopy as it was done in the early days of medical x-ray use. Unfortunately, the image made in this fashion was very dim, even at a high exposure rate to the patient, so modern fluoroscopy uses an image intensifier that amplifies the light from a fluorescent screen. A typical fluoroscopic imaging system is shown in Fig. 2-3. The image-intensifier tube is an evacuated glass or metal tube with a fluorescent screen (input phosphor) that glows with the image produced by the x-ray pattern that exits the patient. The light from the input phosphor causes ejection of electrons from a photoelectric material adjacent to the input phosphor. These electrons are accelerated via a high voltage (30 kV), as well as being focused to preserve the image

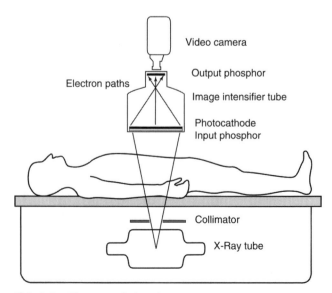

FIG. 2-3 Fluoroscopic imaging system.

onto a small (1-in-diameter) screen (the output phosphor), which glows with the image due to the energy deposited by the impact of the accelerated electrons. The output phosphor glows much brighter than the input phosphor (about 3000 times) due to the energy gain provided by acceleration of the electrons and also due to minification of the image on the output phosphor. The image on the output phosphor can be viewed with the naked eye, usually with a series of lenses and mirrors, but the image is more commonly viewed by focusing a video camera onto the output phosphor and viewing the image on a TV monitor via a closed-circuit TV system. The fluoroscopic image generally has less contrast and less resolution of fine detail than a radiographic image; however, it is clearly convenient to view the image in real time—particularly when observing the flow of radiopaque contrast agents ingested or injected into the body. (These contrast materials, such as iodine or barium compounds, have a higher atomic number than soft tissue and hence absorb more x-rays). During fluoroscopic examinations, the x-ray tube is typically operated below 100 kV and below 3 mA tube current. Even so, entrance exposure rates (at the point where the x-ray beam enters the patient) are about 2 to 5 R/min, depending on patient thickness; hence fluoroscopic examinations generally result in significantly higher patient exposures than do radiographic examinations.

Fluoroscopic systems generally have an automatic brightness control in which the brightness of the output phosphor is sensed by using a light detector. The brightness signal from this detector is compared with a reference level, and the difference signal is used to instruct the x-ray generator to vary milliamperage or kilovoltage (or both) in order to maintain a constant brightness at the output phosphor. For example, after ingestion of barium in a barium-swallow examination, the barium absorbs significantly more x-rays, and the image would tend to go dark without such a system; however, as the brightness falls below the reference level, the automatic brightness control causes the x-ray generator to increase the milliamperage or kilovoltage to maintain a constant brightness on the monitor.

Recording of Fluoroscopic Images

Fluoroscopic images can be recorded for later viewing by several methods. The TV image can be recorded using a videotape recorder or a videodisc recorder, the latter having the advantage of allowing viewing of one frame at a time as well as providing random access rather than the sequential viewing required by videotape.

In addition, some systems have the capability of digitizing the electric signal from a TV frame and storing it in computer memory chips. These systems often have a "last image hold" capability that holds the last TV frame on the monitor. This method is also used in digital subtraction angiography (DSA); that is, the analog signal from the TV camera is digitized and stored frame by frame in a computer memory in a 512 ×512 or 1024 ×1024 image matrix. A short radiographic x-ray pulse is usually used for making the image. Images made just before and after injection of contrast material into the arteries can be subtracted digitally so that only the vascular system appears in the subtracted image.

Spot-Film Devices

The aforementioned image-recording methods merely store the image recorded by the TV camera, which is of lower quality than a radiographic image and has even poorer resolution than the image appearing on the output phosphor of the image-intensifier tube due to the limitations of the TV imaging process. In order to record higher-quality images during a fluoroscopic examination, spot-film devices are used. The most common device transports a conventional radiographic screen/film cassette to a position in front of the image intensifier at the push of a button on the fluoroscopic carriage. The x-ray tube is then switched into a radiographic mode (i.e., the milliamperage is increased from a low mA to 200 to 400 mA to shorten exposure time), and a conventional radiographic image is obtained on film. An alternative system is a photospot camera, which is typically a 105-mm roll-film camera that photographs the output phosphor image produced by a radiographic pulse from the x-ray tube. A 100-mm cut-film camera also may be used as a photospot camera. Photospot films are smaller and have lower resolution, a smaller field of view of the patient, and a grainier appearance than conventional spot films using a cassette, but they have the advantage of greater convenience as well as reduced exposure time due to the high gain provided by the image-intensifier tube.

Computed Tomography

In radiography or fluoroscopy one is creating a shadow picture or a projection of the attenuation properties of the human body onto a plane. Thus each ray from the source to a given point on the film, such as ray *FP* in Fig. 2-2, conveys information about the sum of the attenuation along a line in the body; i.e., anatomic structures are piled on top of each other and flattened into the radiographic image. In an attempt to give a different perspective, one may obtain projections from two different directions (e.g., a lateral and an anteroposterior radiograph) so that the structures that are piled on top of each other differ in each projection. In the late 1960s, a British engineer, Goeffry Hounsfield, concluded that if one obtained projection data from a sufficient number of different angles, one could reconstruct the attenuation properties of each volume element in the body and display these as a cross-sectional image. This required the computational power of a computer to accomplish, and the basic idea is illustrated in Fig. 2-4. The x-rays from a source are detected by a series of individual detectors

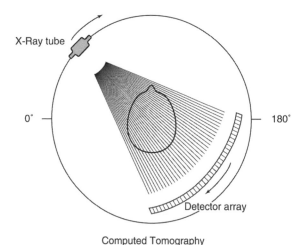

Computed Tomography

FIG. 2-4 Computed tomographic (CT) scanning geometry. A single projection of the head is illustrated.

(rather than film) after penetrating the body, and each detector defines a ray from the source through the body, thereby creating a projection. The width of the x-ray beam in the dimension perpendicular to the page is only about 10 mm; hence only one slice of the body in the longitudinal direction is imaged at a time.

   The x-ray tube and the detector bank are rotated 360 degrees about the patient to obtain, for example, 720 projections at 1/2-degree intervals. The computer is then able to reconstruct a cross-sectional image of the slice of the body by dividing the slice into an imaginary matrix. In a matrix of 512×512 pixels in the transverse plane, each pixel represents an area of about 0.5×0.5 mm in a 25-cm-diameter body. The computer assigns a numerical value to each pixel, which represents the amount of attenuation contributed by the volume element of the body represented by that pixel, and these numbers are converted into a gray-scale image for viewing. After one slice is completed, the patient is advanced via a motorized couch by 10 mm in order to image the adjacent slice, and up to 30 slices (images) may be done to reconstruct the anatomy over a 30-cm length of the patient.

MAGNETIC RESONANCE IMAGING

The technique called *nuclear magnetic resonance,* developed by physicists in the 1940s, was first used for imaging the human body in the late 1970s. The nuclei of some atoms (notably hydrogen nuclei in the body) have a fundamental angular momentum called *spin,* which causes them to behave like tiny spinning magnets. When placed in a uniform external magnetic field and excited by a radio pulse tuned to a resonant frequency that is proportional to the externally applied magnetic field strength (Larmor frequency), the axis of rotation of the nuclei will precess

around the applied magnetic field direction in a similar fashion to the precession of a leaning gyroscope or top about the gravitational field direction (Fig. 2-5). This precession can be detected, since the collection of precessing magnets (protons in the body) induces an oscillatory voltage in a pickup or receiver coil. This oscillation at the Larmor frequency can be detected by connecting the pickup coil to a radio receiver, and one could therefore, in effect,

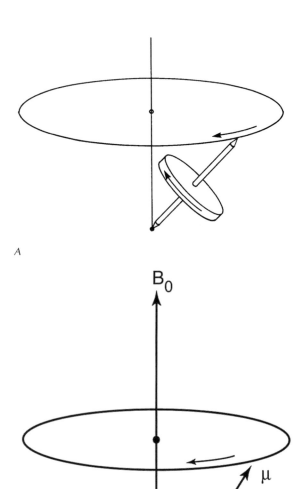

FIG. 2-5 (*A*) Precession of a gyroscope about the earth's gravitational field. (*B*) Precession of the spin axis of a proton of magnetic moment μ about an applied magnetic field B_0

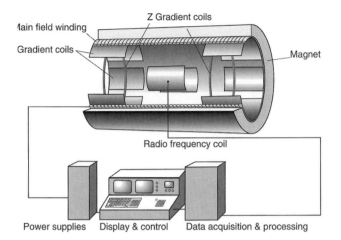

FIG. 2-6 Magnetic resonance imaging hardware.

hear the protons "singing" in unison into the coil at the Larmor frequency. This provides no imaging information; however, if the external magnetic field is made nonuniform in space in a known fashion (i.e., a magnetic field gradient is utilized), then protons at different locations will precess at different frequencies, thereby creating a relationship between location in the body and precessional frequency. With application of such a gradient, the protons no longer sing in unison but at different frequencies depending on their location, as in a chorus; i.e., the sopranos would be located where the magnetic field was largest and the baritones where it was smallest. By listening to different frequencies, one could deduce from the signal strength at a given frequency how many protons were present at the location corresponding to that frequency. This method of imaging allows one to map the density of protons in the body in three dimensions; however, most images are obtained and displayed as planar cross-sectional images similar to those in CT scans and having a slice thickness of 10 mm and a matrix size that is typically 128 $\times$ 256. For greater contrast, the proton-density images also may be weighted by the relaxation times (T1, T2), which are measures of the realignment times of protons with respect to the magnetic field direction. This weighing is typically accomplished by varying the radiofrequency pulse durations and spacings in a variety of pulse sequences, the spin-echo pulse sequence being the most commonly used.

The hardware of a (nuclear) magnetic resonance imaging machine (Fig. 2-6) consists typically of a cylindrical superconducting coil surrounding the patient to generate a large, static magnetic field; auxiliary coils for generating the magnetic field gradients; radio transmitter/receiver coils in close proximity to the patient; electronics for radiofrequency transmitting and receiving; and a computer to orchestrate the events and to reconstruct the spatial image from the frequency spectra.

ULTRASOUND IMAGING

Sound (or pressure) waves in the 3- to 10-MHz frequency range are used for imaging the body by detecting the intensity of the reflected waves from various organs and displaying this reflected intensity as a gray-scale (or color) image. The sound waves are generated by applying an electrical pulse to a piezoelectric crystal. This crystal also acts as a receiver of the reflected waves after the transmitter pulse is terminated. A typical ultrasound transducer contains a linear array of such crystals, which can be fired in sequence or operated as a phased array to cause the ultrasound beam to rapidly scan across an area 5 to 10 cm in width for real-time imaging. The useful imaging depth is determined by the frequency; the higher frequencies (shorter wavelengths) have less penetrability. For example, at 10 MHz, the imaging depth is limited to a few centimeters. Unfortunately, the lower the frequency, the poorer is the axial resolution, since objects that are closer together than a wavelength cannot be separated. Hence there is a tradeoff between axial resolution and penetration depth. Since ultrasound radiation is nonionizing, no adverse biologic effects have been observed at diagnostic power levels.

BIOLOGIC EFFECTS OF X-RAYS

The biologic effects of x-irradiation are due to the recoiling electrons produced by the absorption or scattering of the incident x-rays, these electrons having enough kinetic energy to ionize hundreds of atoms along their trajectory. These electrons may damage DNA molecules directly or produce free radicals that can chemically damage genetic material; either effect may result in cell death or mutation. Magnetic resonance (MR) imaging and ultrasonic imaging do not utilize ionizing radiation, and there is no significant evidence that any biologic damage results from these imaging modalities.

Effect on the Patient

The primary risk to patients undergoing medical x-ray examinations is radiation-induced cancer, primarily leukemia, thyroid, breast, lung, and gastrointestinal cancer. These relative risks are considered to be related to radiation dose and effective dose, which is essentially the exposure to various critical organs multiplied by an organ-weighting factor (the units of radiation dose or exposure—a rem, a rad, and a roentgen—are essentially equivalent for x-ray and gamma-ray irradiation). Table 2-1 lists typical effective doses in millirem for various examinations and the resulting relative increase in cancer risk per million persons. For example, if 1 million persons received lumbar spine examinations, there would be 51 additional (ran-

**TABLE 2-1   TYPICAL EFFECTIVE DOSES AND RESULTING INCREASED RISK
OF FATAL CANCER FOR VARIOUS X-RAY EXAMINATIONS**

X-Ray Examination	Typical Effective Dose, mrem	Lifetime Risk of Fatal Cancer per Million Persons
Lumbar spine	127	51
Upper gastrointestinal tract	244	98
Abdomen (KUB)	56	22
Pelvis	44	18
Chest	8	3

domly occurring) cases of cancer (above that occurring naturally) in this population over their lifetime.

The Pregnant Patient

The fetus consists of rapidly dividing cells and hence is more sensitive to radiation, particularly in the first trimester. The principal risks to the fetus from in utero irradiation are cancer induction, malformation (e.g., small head size), or mental retardation.

Every fertile female patient should be asked if she might be pregnant; if so, the relative risks of the diagnostic x-ray procedure versus the expected benefit should be weighed before the procedure is performed, or alternate imaging procedures such as MR imaging or ultrasound should be considered. It should be noted, however, that the added risk from diagnostic x-ray procedures is generally negligible compared with the normal risks of pregnancy,

since fetal doses are typically below 5 rad in these procedures.

The National Council on Radiation Protection (NCRP) in its report NCRP 54 states:

> The risk (to the fetus) is considered to be negligible at 5 rad or less when compared to the other risks of pregnancy, and the risk of malformations is significantly increased above control levels only at doses above 15 rad. Therefore, exposure of the fetus to radiation arising from diagnostic procedures would rarely be cause, by itself, for terminating a pregnancy.

If the x-ray examination involves the abdomen in such a way that the fetus is in the direct x-ray beam, then fetal doses are typically in the 1- to 4-rad range depending on the number of films and fluoroscopic time (if any). If the examination does not involve the abdomen and the fetus receives only scatter radiation, the fetal dose is generally small (typically well below 1 rad).

PART 2

CHEST

3

IMAGING OF THE HEART AND GREAT VESSELS

Thomas L. Pope, Jr.
Dalane W. Kitzman

The heart and great vessels are complex structures that are critically important to human function. They serve as the "pump" and major proximal "pipes" distributing blood and nutrients to the body. This chapter describes the normal radiographic appearance of the heart, pericardium, and great vessels (aorta and pulmonary vessels) and briefly outlines some of the more common pathologic entities in this organ system. Critical evaluation of the findings on the imaging examinations of this region is not possible without paying attention to the lung fields, since these two organ systems mirror changes in each other. The most common abnormalities encountered in this organ system are hypertension, pulmonary arterial hypertension (usually secondary to chronic pulmonary disease), congestive heart failure, atherosclerotic arterial disease, and cardiac valvular disease. Less common cardiac and great vessel diseases such as congenital heart disease and diseases of the pericardium are described in less detail. The last topic—monitoring devices and postoperative changes—is one with which students should be familiar.

We are assuming that the student understands the basic normal anatomy of this organ system from the basic science and clinical years. At the completion of this chapter the student should have an understanding of the wide range of imaging modalities used to evaluate the heart and great vessels, an appreciation for the potential yield from these examinations, a basic knowledge of the normal imaging anatomy on the plain film, and a familiarity with some of the more common postoperative alterations and the monitoring devices used in this organ system.

TECHNIQUES AND NORMAL ANATOMY

A number of techniques have been developed to evaluate the heart and great vessels (Table 3-1). In this section we briefly describe the major tests used in imaging this system.

Plain Film

The most common imaging test for evaluating the heart and great vessels is the so-called plain film (or chest radiograph), which consists of an upright posteroanterior (PA) and a left lateral (LAT) projection. The terms *posteroanterior* and *left lateral* refer to the direction the x-ray beam takes through the body before it reaches the film. Chest radiographs are usually obtained with high kilovoltage and milliamperage to minimize exposure time and cardiac motion. When possible, the distance between the x-ray tube source and the film is at least 6 ft to minimize magnification and distortion.

TABLE 3-1   IMAGING TESTS FOR HEART, GREAT VESSELS, AND PERICARDIUM

Plain radiographs

    Posteroanterior (PA) and lateral

    Oblique

Fluoroscopy without contrast

Fluoroscopy with contrast

    Barium swallow

Echocardiography

Radionuclide imaging

Computed tomography (CT)

Angiography

    Angiocardiography

    Coronary arteriography

    Great vessel (aortography)

    Pulmonary

Magnetic resonance imaging (MRI)

Positron emission tomography

The examination is performed ideally with the patient at maximal inspiration. A good rule of thumb for estimating adequate inspiration is to be able to count 9 to 10 posterior ribs or 5 to 6 anterior ribs from the lung apices to the hemidiaphragms through the aerated lungs (Fig. 3-1). If the chest radiograph is exposed in the expiratory phase of respiration, the film may artifactually show increased heart size, extreme vascular congestion, and bilateral ill-defined pulmonary radiopacities mimicking diffuse lung disease (Fig. 3-2). After bronchoscopy, percutaneous lung biopsy, and some other procedures, an expiratory-phase film may be obtained for the purpose of excluding pneumothorax, a potential complication of these procedures.

In severely ill, debilitated patients or patients who cannot be transported to the radiology department, the chest radiograph must be obtained in the supine position. In addition, patients in the intensive care unit (ICU) who have intravascular catheters or who are undergoing mechanical ventilation routinely have daily chest radiographs to monitor for complications that may not be revealed by physical examination or laboratory data. These examinations are done with the film cassette behind the patient in bed and are therefore anteroposterior (AP) projections. The technical factors, which are controlled by the technologist at the time of the examination, vary with the size of the patient and the distance of the film from the x-ray source (or

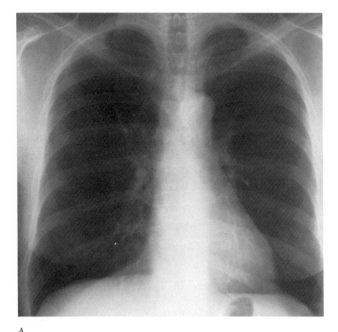

A

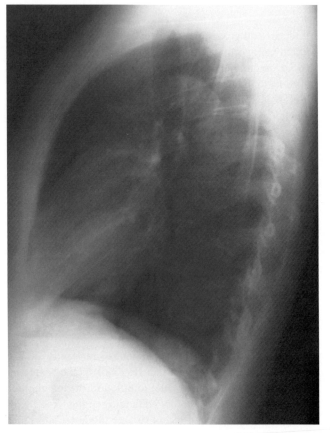

B

FIG. 3-1 Normal PA (*A*) and lateral (*B*) films of a 45-year-old woman. Note the normal heart size and clear lung fields. There is adequate inspiration because 8 anterior ribs and 10 posterior ribs are identified through the aerated lungs. (*Courtesy of Herbert Pope, M.D., White Sulphur Springs, W.V.*)

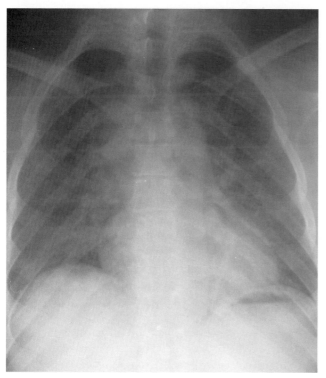

FIG. 3-2 Expiratory phase of a respiration chest film shows low lung volume, crowded bronchovascular markings, and apparent increased heart size. If the degree of inspiration is not noted, the interpreter may incorrectly diagnose a disease the patient does not have. (*Courtesy of Robert H. Choplin, M.D., Winston-Salem, N.C*).

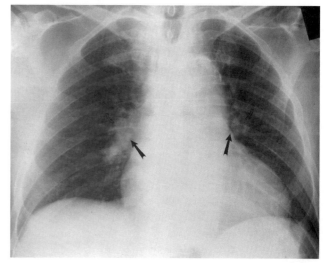

FIG. 3-3 Supine AP chest radiograph showing apparent increase in heart size and prominent bronchovascular markings (*arrows*).

machine). An attempt is still made to obtain the examination during maximum inspiration, but this objective may be difficult to achieve in some patients, especially those who have dyspnea.

With the patient in the supine position, there is normally a slight redistribution of the pulmonary vascular markings to the upper lobes, and the heart may appear enlarged relative to its appearance on the upright PA film because it is farther from the film and is therefore magnified (Fig. 3-3). Some patients are able to sit for their examinations, and others may be radiographed in a semiupright position. The technologist should mark the exact position of the patient when the radiograph is obtained, and the date and time of the examination should be recorded in all cases.

The routine chest radiograph, whether it is obtained in the upright, semiupright, sitting, or supine position, should always be the initial screening examination in the evaluation of this organ system. Because it is the baseline screening study, the information derived from it is coupled with the clinical symptoms and physical examination to help decide whether other imaging tests are needed and which ones will potentially give the best yield. Decisions regarding further imaging tests also depend on the potential for treatment of any abnormality that may be discovered by

further imaging, the cost of the next examination, the availability of the technique, and the availability or expertise of the interpreting imager.

The plain film is an excellent screening test for the patient suspected of having diseases of the heart and great vessels because the anatomy of these areas is so nicely demonstrated. Initially, the demographic data on the patient should be evaluated, and comparison studies, if any, should be obtained. The comparison film has often been called "the radiologist's best friend."

The size of the normal cardiac silhouette is determined by the *cardiothoracic ratio* (CT ratio) from the PA view. This measurement is made by comparing the cardiac diameter from its right and left lateral borders inferiorly and dividing this number by the widest diameter of the chest measured from the inner aspect of the lung fields near the hemidiaphragms. The average normal value for this ratio in adults is 0.45, although the rule of thumb is that a ratio of less than 50 percent is normal (Fig. 3-4). Any measurement over 50 percent is usually considered abnormal in an upright inspiratory-phase PA film. The AP film distorts this measurement, and the CT ratio cannot be used reliably for this projection (see Fig. 3-3). The size of the patient and the degree of lung expansion also should be considered. For instance, in a small person with a petite frame and a small thoracic cage, the heart size may be slightly over the 50 percent cardiothoracic ratio and still be normal. Furthermore, if the patient has chronic obstructive pulmonary disease (COPD) with emphysema causing overexpansion of the lung fields, the heart may be enlarged, but because of the overexpansion of the chest cavity, the cardiothoracic ratio may still be normal (Fig. 3-5). In actual practice, the CT ratio is not measured on every patient but is estimated visually.

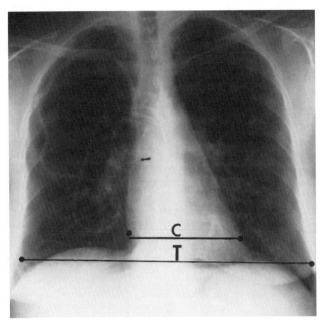

FIG. 3-4 Upright PA chest film in a patient with leukemia shows normal cardio- (C) thoracic (T) ratio and how it is measured. Incidentally noted is the tip of an internal jugular triple-lumen catheter in the superior vena cava (*arrow*).

The configuration or contour of the heart, mediastinum, and great vessels on the PA view should be evaluated next (Fig. 3-6). A reasonable approach is to begin in the upper right side of the mediastinum just lateral to the spine and below the right clavicle. The curved soft-tissue shadow represents the right border of the superior vena cava (SVC). Below the SVC is the right cardiac border formed by the right atrium. The inferior heart border, or base of the heart, is the area situated just above the diaphragm; its border is composed primarily of the shadow of the right ventricle, although there is some contribution from the left ventricular shadow. The left ventricle makes up the majority of the shadow of the apex of the heart to the left of the spine. The right and left pulmonary arteries are generally well demarcated on the normal PA film as they emerge from the mediastinum. Their most prominent and recognizable component, the right descending pulmonary artery (RDPA), originates just to the right of the superior cardiac border and descends inferiorly. It usually can be followed easily until it branches. The left main pulmonary artery is less well defined, but its origin usually can be seen well just before it branches. The aortic shadow (aortic arch) originates in the upper right portion of the heart border just below the RDPA and courses obliquely across the mediastinum to descend down the chest on the left side of the thoracic vertebrae. In the normal person it has smooth

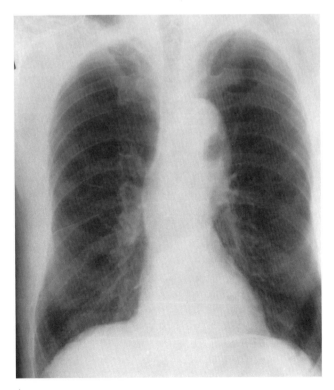

A

FIG. 3-5 Upright PA (*A*) and lateral (*B*) films of a patient with a long history of smoking and cardiomegaly by ECG. The chest film shows a normal heart size by the CT ratio, but the emphysema and overexpansion of the lungs distort this relationship. In part *B* note the markedly ectatic aorta (*arrowheads*). (*Courtesy of Herbert Pope, M.D., White Sulphur Springs, W.V.*)

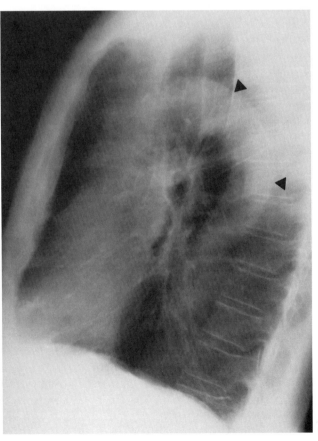

B

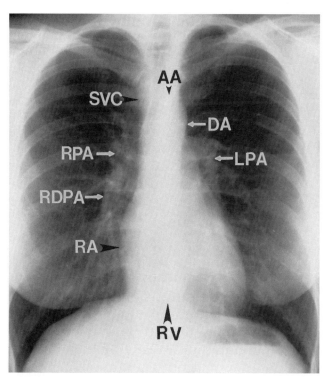

FIG. 3-6   PA view of normal chest (RA = right atrium; RDPA = right descending pulmonary artery; RPA = right main pulmonary artery; SVC = superior vena cava; AA = aortic arch; DA = proximal descending thoracic aorta; LPA = left pulmonary artery; and RV = right ventricle).

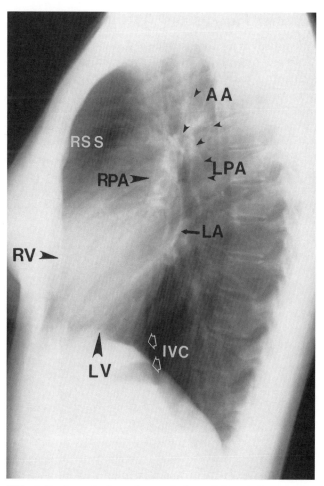

FIG. 3-7   Lateral view of normal chest (RV = right ventricle; RSS = retrosternal clear space; AA = ascending aorta; LPA = left pulmonary artery; RPA = right pulmonary artery en face; IVC = inferior vena cava; LA = left atrium; and LV = left ventricle).

contours and no calcification. Dilatation or ectasia, localized bulges, and calcification may occur within the aorta, and all are abnormal. Of course, the spine, ribs, adjacent soft tissues, and upper abdominal contents should all be scrutinized. The left atrium, because of its posterior location, is not usually seen as a discrete structure on the normal PA view. If it is enlarged, it appears as an extra opacity adjacent to the right atrium, as will be discussed later.

The lateral view of the chest also can give important information about the normal and pathologic cardiac contour and is a film that is often misunderstood by clinicians (Fig. 3-7). Just behind the sternum there is normally a radiolucent area called the *retrosternal clear space* (RSS). The anterior border of the cardiac shadow is composed primarily of the anteriorly located right ventricular wall and the anterobasal segment of the right ventricle (RV). The posterobasal margin of the cardiac silhouette is formed by the left ventricle (LV). The posterior and inferior linear soft-tissue shadow leading into the heart is formed by the inferior vena cava (IVC). Note the intersection of the IVC and right atrial shadows (open arrow). The left atrial (LA) shadow forms the upper part of the cardiac contour posteriorly. The arch of the aorta (AA) usually can be discerned on the normal lateral chest films as a smooth curving

shadow originating anteriorly, crossing the mediastinum in a semilunar fashion, and then descending down the posterior mediastinum as a linear shadow superimposed over the vertebral bodies. The left pulmonary artery (LPA) usually can be seen just below the aortic arch before it branches, and the right pulmonary artery (RPA) is seen en face down its lumen as an oval soft-tissue structure crossing the mediastinum just in front of the carina and slightly below and in front of the left pulmonary artery.

Oblique Films

Oblique films of the chest are sometimes obtained to clarify a radiographic finding seen on the upright AP, PA, or lateral projections. The right and left oblique projections are often obtained at the same time. However, these views are rarely used or needed in most clinical settings and are mentioned here mainly for historical interest.

Cardiac Fluoroscopy (Without Contrast)

Fluoroscopy is a technique whereby an x-ray machine creates a real-time gray-scale image on an intensifying screen similar to a television. Prior to the advent of angiography (with injection of contrast material into vessels), the major indications for fluoroscopy were suspected abnormal cardiac motion or suspected cardiac or great vessel calcifications. These calcifications occur mainly in the coronary arteries, cardiac valves, or great vessels, particularly the aorta. Today, cardiac fluoroscopy without the injection of contrast material is used mainly to monitor the placement of catheters and pacemakers, as described in the final section.

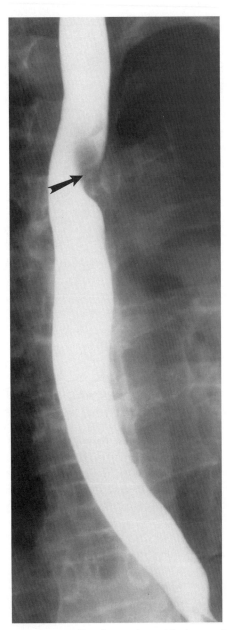

FIG. 3-8 Barium swallow in a patient with aberrant left subclavian artery shows extrinsic compression of the esophagus by the aberrant vessel (*arrow*).

Barium Swallow

Prior to the advent of computed tomography (CT) and magnetic resonance (MR) imaging, the barium swallow examination was used to evaluate suspected cardiac chamber enlargement, particularly left atrial enlargement, or aberrant vascular anatomy, such as an aberrant left subclavian artery. The radiologist observes as the patient drinks barium under fluoroscopy and takes appropriate pictures to document pertinent findings. The characteristic extrinsic impression of the aberrant subclavian artery on the esophagus is one of the more recognizable abnormalities (Fig. 3-8). Left atrial enlargement historically was diagnosed in this manner, but the technique is rarely used today because other axial imaging modalities are available.

Echocardiography

Echocardiography uses high-frequency ultrasound to evaluate the heart and great vessels. The major indications for the technique are listed in Table 3-2. The examination provides a dynamic rendition of cardiac great vessel anatomy and, when combined with the Doppler technique, yields information regarding cardiac and great vessel blood flow (hemodynamics) as well. Because of the high frame rates inherent in ultrasonography, echocardiography can image the heart in a dynamic real-time fashion so that the motion of cardiac structures can be evaluated reliably. Echocardiography is useful in assessing ventricular function, valvular heart disease, myocardial disease, pericardial disease, intracardiac masses, and aortic abnormalities. With Doppler technology, cardiac chamber function, valvular function, and intracardiac shunts frequently seen in congenital heart disease can be assessed. Combined Doppler echocardiography is a commonly performed procedure because it is relatively inexpensive and widely available, provides a wealth of information, is noninvasive and involves no risk of ionizing radiation, and can be performed promptly at the bedside in critically ill patients. Furthermore, the results are available immediately with no special postexamination

TABLE 3-2   MAJOR INDICATIONS FOR ECHOCARDIOGRAPHY

Ventricular function

Congenital heart disease

Valvular heart disease

Cardiac/great vessel blood flow

Cardiomyopathy versus pericardial effusion

Suspected cardiac masses

Aortic disease (proximally)

image processing required. However, this technique is technically challenging and requires a great deal of operator expertise. Also, a small percentage of patients have poor acoustic "windows" that can severely degrade image quality. The latter disadvantage can be obviated by placing the sonographic probe in the esophagus, a procedure called *transesophageal echocardiography* (TEE). TEE yields consistently excellent images of the heart and great vessels but involves a small amount of discomfort and risk to the patient. More recently, echocardiography has been combined with stress-testing modalities to assess inducible myocardial ischemia in patients with chest pain syndromes using wall motion analysis of left ventricular function (Figs. 3-9 and 3-10).

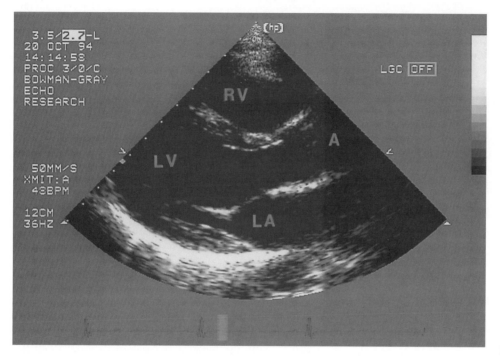

A

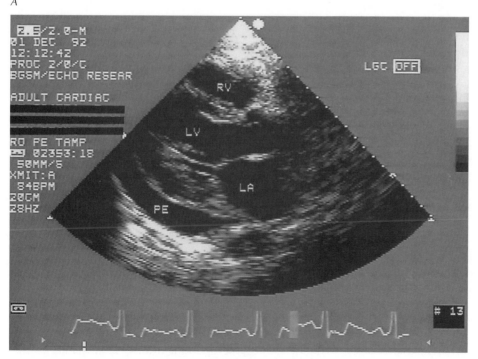

B

FIG. 3-9 (*A*) Normal transthoracic two-dimensional echocardiogram from a healthy subject. Views are taken from the left midparasternal region through an intercostal space. The structure closest to the apex of the screen is the chest wall. The mitral valve, separating the left atrium and left ventricle, is partially open in this image from early systole (A = aorta; LA = left atrium; LV = left ventricle; and RV = right ventricle). (*B*) Transthoracic two-dimensional echocardiogram, left parasternal view, from a patient with a moderate-sized posterior pericardial effusion (PE), visualized as an echolucent space (echodensity similar to blood seen in the cardiac chambers) between the epicardium and pericardium (RV = right ventricle; LV = left ventricle; and LA = left atrium).

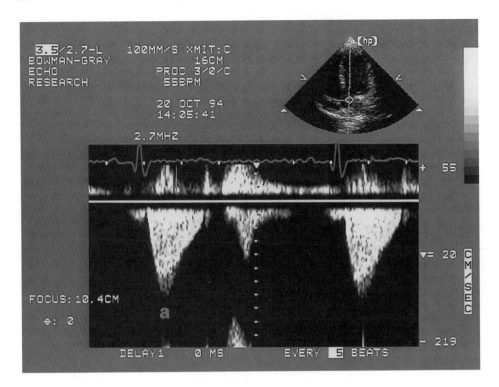

FIG. 3-10 Transthoracic cardiac spectral Doppler tracing taken from an intercostal space over the cardiac apex. The Doppler sample is placed in line with the left ventricular outflow and aorta (shown in miniature two-dimensional echocardiogram image at top left of picture). Velocity of flow is denoted along left edge of tracing in centimeters per second. The Doppler tracing shows that aortic peak velocity (a) is normal (140 cm/s). This technique can reliably assess the presence of and quantitate the severity of aortic stenosis.

Radionuclide Imaging (Nuclear Medicine)

Cardiac radionuclide imaging, used primarily for the patient with suspected myocardial ischemia or infarction, requires an intravenous injection of radioactively labeled compounds that have an affinity for the myocardium. These compounds localize within the myocardium in diseased or damaged areas, and their distribution can be imaged by a radioactivity detector such as a gamma camera. These tests are used most commonly in the evaluation of patients with angina and atypical chest pain (Fig. 3-11).

Computed Tomography

Computed tomography (CT) renders axial imaging by using traditional x-ray tubes arranged in a circular configuration. The standard CT scanner provides static axial images of the heart and great vessels, whereas the newer techniques such as spiral and ultrafast CT can provide images with volumetric data that can be reconstructed in different planes. An in-depth discussion of these techniques is beyond the scope of this textbook, but the Bibliography may be consulted for additional information. Contrast administration also can be helpful if diseases of the vascular tree are suggested on the plain film. The major indications for CT are to characterize or confirm a suspected mediastinal or pulmonary mass seen on the standard PA and lateral chest radiograph, to evaluate patients suspected of having an aortic abnormality, and, rarely, to evaluate pericardial effusion prior to pericardiocentesis (Fig. 3-12).

Angiography

Coronary angiography is one of the most commonly performed imaging tests for evaluating the heart and great vessels. After the introduction of a catheter into a peripheral vessel, usually the femoral or axillary vein or artery, the angiographer, under direct fluoroscopic visualization, "floats" the catheter intravascularly to the region of interest, injects contrast material to confirm the location of the catheter, and then injects larger amounts of contrast material for diagnostic purposes. This injection of contrast material can be either videotaped, filmed with standard or digital films, or stored digitally so that it can be reviewed later. There are four major types of angiography: angiocardiography (heart), coronary arteriography (coronary arteries), aortography (aorta), and pulmonary angiography (pulmonary arteries and lungs). Technical references can be consulted for more in-depth discussion.

Angiocardiography is used primarily to evaluate ventricular contractility and wall motion and cardiac output in patients with suspected myocardial dysfunction. It is also used for patients in whom murmurs are detected at physical examination to evaluate cardiac valve function. The purpose of coronary arteriography is to define the degree of coronary artery obstruction, usually caused by atherosclerosis. In this procedure, a catheter is generally placed into the origin of each coronary artery orifice, and contrast material is injected into the arteries during videotaping or filming, as described above (Fig. 3-13). Coronary angiography also can be performed in the acute setting of suspected coronary occlusion, and a balloon catheter or

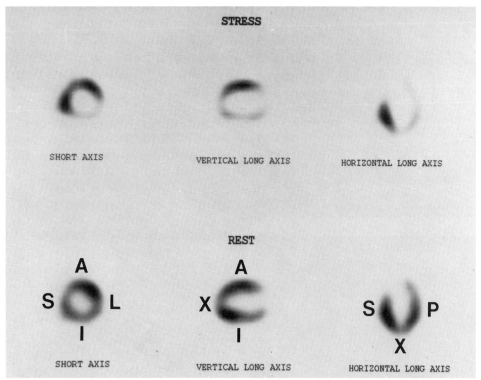

FIG. 3-11 Thallium myocardial perfusion images. Images obtained with the patient at peak stress (*top row*) are compared with those obtained during rest (*bottom row*). The wall segments are labeled on the resting images (*bottom row*). Seen in the short-axis views (*left*) are the anterior wall segment (A), lateral wall (L), inferior wall (I), and septum (S). In the vertical long-axis views (*center*), the anterior wall, inferior wall, and apex (X) can be seen. Seen in the horizontal long-axis views (*right*) are the posterolateral wall (P), septum, and apex. In normal persons, perfusion is homogeneous in all segments, and stress and resting images appear similar. In patients with obstructive coronary artery disease, relative lack of perfusion is seen during stress in wall segments supplied by the obstructed arteries. The rest perfusion images in this patient are normal. However in the stress images, the inferior, lateral, and posterolateral walls show "dropout," consistent with reduced perfusion in these wall segments relative to adjacent normal segments. The patient subsequently underwent coronary arteriography, which showed a high-grade obstruction in the left circumflex coronary artery. (*Courtesy of Robert J. Cowan, M.D., Winston-Salem, N.C.*)

thrombolytic agent can be placed through the catheter in an attempt to relieve the coronary artery thrombosis.

Aortography is used primarily to evaluate suspected aortic valvular regurgitation or suspected aortic dissection. Aortic dissection can be demonstrated with a high sensitivity and specificity by this technique (Fig. 3-14). Pulmonary angiography is indicated in patients who are suspected of having pulmonary emboli and whose nuclear medicine ventilation-perfusion scan results are equivocal. It is also useful in patients who have equivocal nuclear medicine scans and who have a contraindication to anticoagulation therapy. Pulmonary angiography is also used to measure the pressures within the pulmonary arteries in patients suspected of having pulmonary arterial hypertension (Fig. 3-15).

Magnetic Resonance Imaging

Magnetic resonance (MR) imaging is an exciting imaging technique that can be used for cardiac and great vessel evaluation. Using high-field-strength magnets to generate images by radiofrequency pulse manipulation of hydrogen atoms, MR imaging offers superb soft-tissue differentiation, is noninvasive, and usually requires no contrast material administration. Sophisticated MR imaging techniques can show the overall cardiac morphology and can measure cardiac and great vessel output and pressures. The major indications for MR imaging are congenital heart disease and suspected intracardiac masses, valvular dysfunction, and aortic abnormality (in particular, aortic dissection) (Fig. 3-16). MR imaging also has shown some promise in diagnosing pulmonary embolism and in measuring the degree of damage from coronary artery atherosclerosis. This exciting technique now supplements invasive tests such as angiography but has the potential to replace most of these other diagnostic examinations in the future. At the present time, however, it is quite expensive, and the most appropriate MR imaging sequences and techniques to evaluate the heart and great vessels are still being developed (Fig. 3-17).

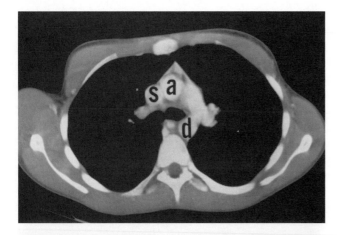

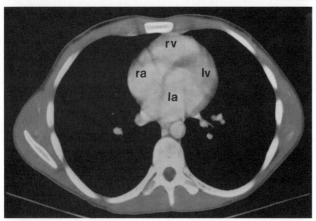

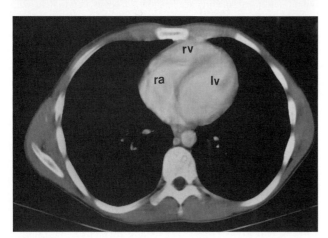

FIG. 3-12 Three axial CT images in the superoinferior direction show the superior vena cava (s), ascending aorta (a), descending aorta (d), right ventricle (rv), right atrium (ra), left atrium (la), and left ventricle (lv).

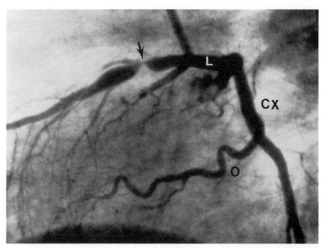

A

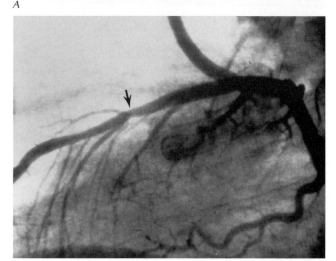

B

FIG. 3-13 (*A*) Coronary arteriogram. Images were obtained from the left lateral projection with contrast injection into the left main coronary artery. The left anterior descending (L), left circumflex (CX), and first obtuse marginal (O) branches are visualized. Severe stenosis is seen in the midportion of the left anterior descending artery (*arrow*) in this patient, who had unstable angina pectoris. (*Courtesy of Gregory Braden, M.D., Winston-Salem, N.C.*) (*B*) Coronary arteriogram, same projection and patient, obtained 1 day later. The stenosis in the left anterior descending coronary artery (*arrow*) has been reduced after percutaneous balloon angioplasty. (*Courtesy of Gregory Braden, M.D., Winston-Salem, N.C.*)

Positron Emission Tomography

The latest high-technology imaging technique for evaluating the heart and great vessels is positron emission tomography (PET). PET is a very expensive and complex test that uses a combination of a cyclotron and radionuclide imaging. Its major drawbacks are its expense and its low spatial resolution. An investigational tool at the present time, it has shown promise in assessing myocardial viability in patients with known coronary artery disease who represent a therapeutic dilemma after they are evaluated with other imaging modalities (Fig. 3-18).

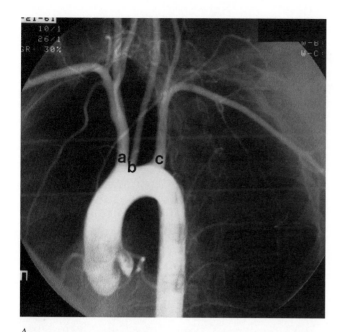

A

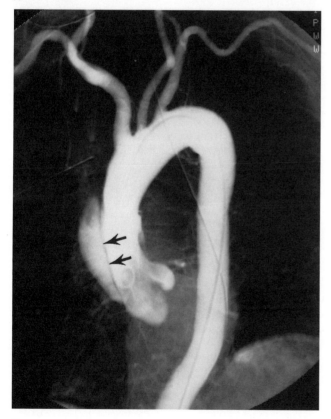

B

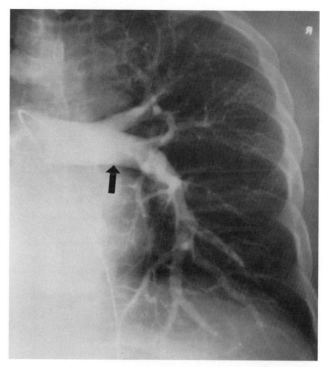

A

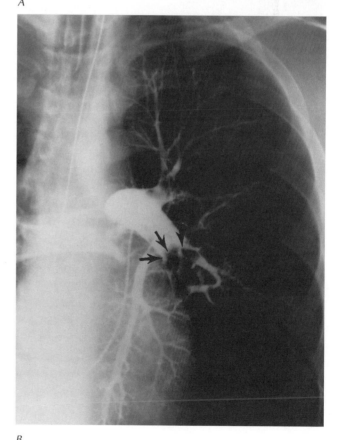

B

FIG. 3-14 (*A*) Normal aortogram in a patient suspected of having traumatic aortic injury. Note the normal origins of the "take-offs" of the right brachiocephalic artery (a), left common carotid artery (b), and left subclavian artery (c) from the arch of the aorta. (*Courtesy of William D. Routh, M.D., Winston-Salem, N.C.*) (*B*) Aortogram in a patient with aortic dissection shows the "flap" as a filling defect in the contrast in the ascending aorta (*arrows*). This entity will be discussed in further detail later in the chapter. (*Courtesy of William D. Routh, M.D., Winston-Salem, N.C.*)

FIG. 3-15 (*A*) Normal left pulmonary angiogram shows the large proximal left pulmonary artery (*arrow*) and the progressive branching of the vascular tree in the left lung. (*B*) Left pulmonary angiogram of a patient clinically suspected of having pulmonary embolus shows the embolus as a filling defect in the contrast in the proximal aspect of the left lower lobe pulmonary artery (*arrows*). (*Courtesy of William D. Routh, M.D., Winston-Salem, N.C.*)

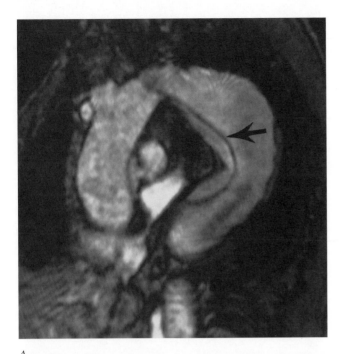

A

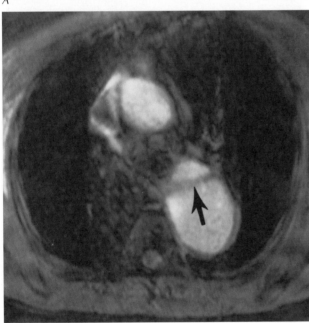

B

FIG. 3-16 Oblique coronal (*A*) and axial (*B*) images of a 75-year-old man with extreme chest pain show an aortic dissection on MR imaging. The flap is identified as the linear low-signal line within the aorta (*arrow*) (note similarity to Fig. 3-14*B*).

TECHNIQUE SELECTION

A potentially bewildering array of imaging tests is used to evaluate the cardiovascular system (see Table 3-1). After a thorough history and physical examination, the initial screening study should always be the plain film, or chest radiograph. Ideally, the PA and lateral views should be ob-

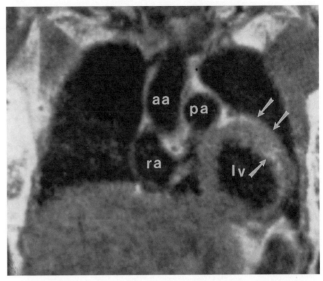

A

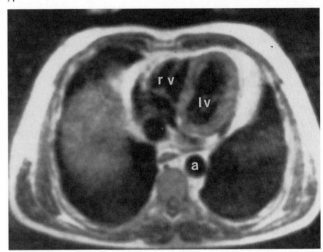

B

FIG. 3-17 (*A*) Normal coronal MR image shows the right atrium (ra), ascending aorta (aa), pulmonary artery (pa), and left ventricle (lv). Note how well the thickness of the myocardium in the left ventricle is depicted with MR imaging (*arrows*). (*B*) Normal MR axial image shows the right ventricle (rv), left ventricle (lv), and descending aorta (a). MR imaging is an excellent way to noninvasively visualize the cardiac and great vessel structures.

tained and with maximum inspiration. This study gives important information about the cardiac contour and the status of the lungs and is a good examination for excluding disorders that would require immediate attention, such as pneumothorax. In the patient requiring cardiovascular monitoring or cardiac pacemaker placement, fluoroscopy is usually employed for correct placement of these devices in the acute setting. Fluoroscopy is also used to monitor imaging tests that require catheter placement and contrast material injection.

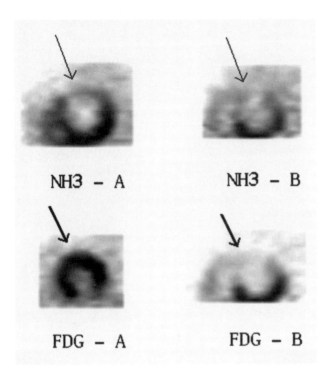

NH3 – A   NH3 – B

FDG – A   FDG – B

FIG. 3-18 The upper images of two patients, *A* and *B*, show NH₃ resting perfusion defects in the left anterior descending artery distribution (*arrows*). The lower images in the same two patients show that the ischemic zone in patient *A* takes up fluorodeoxyglucose (FDG) avidly; this pattern indicates that the ischemic muscle is still viable (*arrow*). Patient *B* has a defect in the FDG images that is identical to the perfusion defect, indicating nonviable muscle or scar tissue (*arrow*).

Depending on the major history and physical examination findings, echocardiography and cardiac angiography are probably the most commonly performed secondary imaging examinations. Echocardiography is a good screening test to assess cardiac and great vessel valvular motion and structural abnormalities, cardiac chamber morphology, and flow. Angiography delineates the structural status of the coronary arterial vessels and can give information on blood flow through the cardiac chambers, valves, and proximal great vessels, mainly in patients with suspected atherosclerosis. Because of its inherent risks, coronary arteriography is usually reserved for patients considered to be at high risk for myocardial ischemic events on the basis of history or results of noninvasive stress testing with electrocardiography, echocardiography, or radionuclide techniques. Which modality is best to use depends on patient characteristics, availability of the imaging technique, and local expertise in interpreting the images.

In patients with suspected pulmonary emboli, the ventilation-perfusion ($\dot{V}/\dot{Q}$) scan can be performed if the chest radiograph is relatively unremarkable (see Chap. 4). This test can confirm the clinically suspected diagnosis of pulmonary embolic disease and often provides a useful "map" of the most suspicious regions of the lung for the angiographer if an angiogram is required for the definitive diagnosis of pulmonary embolism.

Echocardiography, MR imaging, or cardiac angiography may be selected for patients with suspected congenital heart disease. The advantages of MR imaging in this setting are that it is noninvasive, generally needs no contrast material administration, and uses no ionizing radiation—important considerations in pediatric patients. Therefore, MR imaging has the potential to become the preferred pediatric imaging test.

Suspected aortic dissection (either atherosclerotic or traumatic in origin) can be evaluated by TEE, CT, aortography, or MR imaging. TEE has the advantages of being quick and noninvasive, and the examination can be performed expediently at the bedside. MR imaging is advantageous because it is noninvasive, uses no ionizing radiation, is less operator-dependent, and can be performed in multiple planes. Because survival rates often depend on early surgical intervention, availability and timeliness of the examinations are important. The choice of examination should be based on patient characteristics, examination availability, and expertise of the imagers.

In patients whose plain films suggest intrinsic pulmonary or mediastinal processes, contrast-enhanced chest CT is currently the preferred modality. MR imaging may become more important in this situation if it becomes less costly, and PET may play a future role in staging patients with lung cancer and lymphoma.

Finally, regardless of the situation, it is reasonable for the clinician and imager to decide together which imaging tests are most appropriate. In many instances, the next most efficacious and least costly imaging examination is not always clear-cut. In fact, in some circumstances it is not necessary to perform another test because of the limited potential yield from the examination or because there is no adequate therapy for the suspected abnormality.

It is hoped that future recommendations for test selection will be determined by well-designed prospective, unbiased outcomes studies comparing all these modalities in various clinical scenarios. In the meantime, a commonsense approach, taking into consideration the history and physical examination findings, the information gleaned from the plain film, and the potential yield from the array of other available imaging tests, is the most appropriate tack. In all instances, communication between the clinician and imager is critical for the best patient care.

Monitoring Devices

In clinical hospital practice, particularly in the ICU setting, a number of cardiac and great vessel catheters and tubes are used to monitor various parameters in patients. The student should be familiar with the normal routes and positions of these devices, as well as possible malpositions and complications. Table 3-3 lists the most common monitoring devices.

TABLE 3-3   MOST COMMON MONITORING DEVICES

Central venous catheters

Flow-directed arterial catheters

(Swan-Ganz catheter)

Intraaortic counterpulsation balloon pumps

Cardiac pacemakers

Unipolar

Bipolar

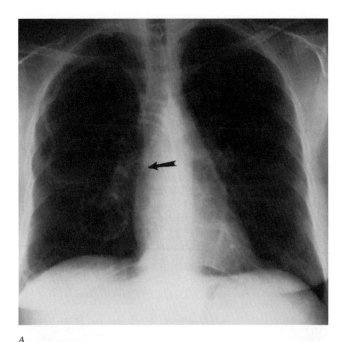

A

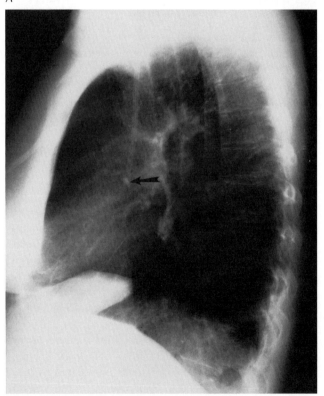

B

FIG. 3-19 PA (*A*) and lateral (*B*) views of a patient whose subclavian catheter placement is normal with its tip in the superior vena cava above the right atrium (*arrows*).

Intrathoracic central venous catheters are used mainly for monitoring central venous pressure (CVP), maintaining proper nutrition, and delivering medication. It is standard practice to request a chest radiograph after catheter placement to verify its location and to check for potential complications. Measurement of CVP is optimally obtained when the tip of the catheter is proximal to the right atrium and distal to the most proximal valves of the large veins. A catheter tip proximal to the veins gives an inaccurate reading of CVP, and a tip too close to the right atrium may cause arrhythmias from right atrial myocardial irritation. Unsatisfactory positioning of the catheter is seen in up to 38 percent of patients, and most of these are not suspected clinically before being discovered on the plain radiographs. Therefore, a postplacement chest film is warranted and appropriate.

The basic venous anatomy of the upper mediastinum should be reviewed and kept in mind when evaluating catheter placement. The most common route of catheter insertion is beneath the clavicle into the subclavian vein. Radiographs obtained after insertion show the catheter following the course of the subclavian vein and curving gently downward to terminate in the superior vena cava (SVC) proximal to the right atrium (Fig. 3-19). A common normal variation of venous anatomy is the persistent left SVC. In this situation, the catheter descends down the left mediastinum before terminating in the left SVC (Fig. 3-20).

The major potential complications from catheter placement are outlined in Table 3-4. For CVP catheters, the major concerns with regard to malpositioning are inaccurate CVP measurement, thrombosis, catheter knotting, and infusion of substances into the mediastinum or pleura.

Flow-directed arterial catheters are also regularly used in cardiac and ICU patients to monitor cardiac output. The most common flow-directed catheter is the Swan-Ganz (SG) catheter. It is usually inserted percutaneously into the left or right subclavian veins and is then "floated" under portable fluoroscopic guidance through the brachiocephalic vein, SVC, right atrium, tricuspid valve, right ventricle, and pulmonic valve and then is directed out into the pulmonary outflow track. It usually terminates in the main pulmonary outflow region or in the proximal right or left pulmonary arteries. The SG catheter tip should be distal to the pulmonary valve and yet be proximal to the

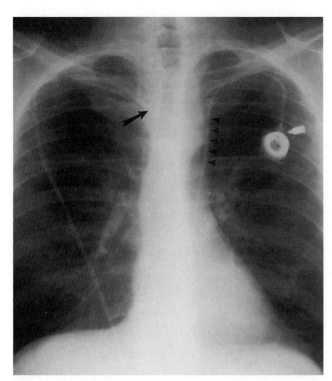

FIG. 3-20 Upright PA chest film in a patient with leukemia shows two central venous catheters. The right subclavian catheter terminates in the superior vena cava (*arrow*). The left subclavian catheter extends into the mediastinum along a persistent left superior vena cava (*arrowheads*).

TABLE 3-4   POTENTIAL COMPLICATIONS OF CATHETERS

Malposition

Catheter knotting/fragmentation

Pneumothorax

Vascular injury

Thrombosis (venous)

Infarction (arterial)

Infection (sepsis)

Air embolism

Endocarditis

Septic emboli

Cardiac arrhythmias

Nerve injury

    Brachial plexus

    Phrenic

    Recurrent laryngeal

Thoracic duct injury

Fistulas

    Arteriovenous

    Venobronchial

    Arteriobronchial

smaller pulmonary arterial vessel lumina so that it will not cause occlusion and, potentially, thrombosis. It may then be intermittently "wedged" into a distal pulmonary artery branch to obtain pulmonary wedge (arterial) pressures (Fig. 3-21).

The most common complication of SG catheter placement is tip malposition. The tip may be positioned in a number of inappropriate vessels or locations, and a chest radiograph should be obtained after catheter insertion to confirm catheter position (Fig. 3-22). Introduction of any catheter into the subclavian vein, because of its close proximity to the lung apex, can cause pneumothorax (Fig. 3-23). Vascular perforation by the catheter and infusion of fluids into the mediastinum or pleura can be diagnosed easily on the plain radiograph (Fig. 3-24). Pulmonary infarction also can result from thrombosis by a flow-directed arterial catheter that is placed too far distally into a small pulmonary artery. This complication can be recognized on the chest film as a wedge-shaped or ill-defined lung opacity distal to the catheter tip (Fig. 3-25).

Another device with which the student should be familiar is the intraaortic counterpulsation balloon pump (IABP). Used in the high-risk cardiac surgery patient with cardiogenic shock, this catheter measures approximately 26 cm in length and is surrounded by a balloon, which inflates with helium or carbon dioxide gas during diastole

and deflates during systole. Deflation during systole decreases afterload and results in diminished left ventricular work and oxygen requirements, whereas inflation of the balloon during diastole increases cardiac pressure to help ensure adequate perfusion of the coronary arteries. The catheter, introduced percutaneously into the thoracic aorta via the common femoral artery or placed into the ascending aorta at the time of surgery, should be positioned so that its tip is distal to the origin of the left subclavian artery. The tip of the catheter has a small radiopaque marker so that this position can be ascertained on the plain radiograph (Fig. 3-26). The major complications of the IAPB result from positioning of its tip proximal to the left subclavian artery, which may cause occlusion of the left subclavian vessel orifice, cerebral artery embolization, or aortic tear.

Cardiac pacemakers are other devices with which the student should be familiar. There are three major types, epicardial, subxiphoid, and transvenous, and there is wide variation in their use in clinical practice today. Unipolar or bipolar pacers may be used, and the most common route of implantation for the transvenous pacers is through the subclavian vein. The unipolar pacer tip normally should be situated near the apex of the right ventricle (Fig. 3-27). The bipolar transvenous pacer has a proximal lead that termi-

nates in the right atrium and a distal lead that should terminate anteriorly within the right ventricle (Fig. 3-28). Transvenous placement of cardiac pacers carries the same potential complications as does placement of any other catheter. The purpose of the chest radiograph after pacemaker insertion is to document the appropriate placement of these leads, to check for complications from placement, and to establish a baseline examination to compare with future chest films.

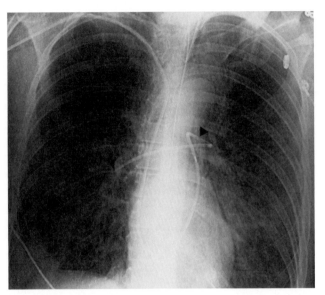

FIG. 3-21 Supine AP chest radiograph of a patient in the ICU shows the tip of the Swan-Ganz catheter positioned normally in the right descending pulmonary artery (*arrow*). Note the curved and coiled path of the catheter in the proximal right pulmonary artery (*arrowhead*).

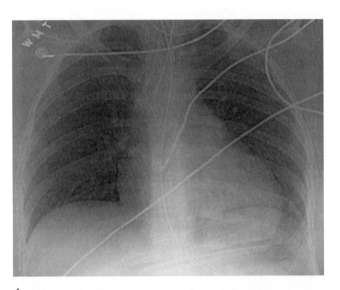

A

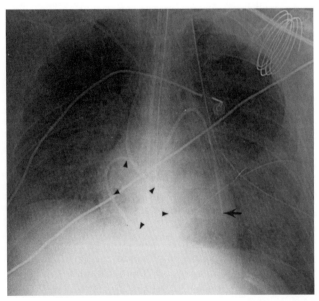

FIG. 3-22 Supine AP chest radiograph of a patient in the ICU in congestive failure shows a Swan-Ganz catheter tip positioned too far distally within the left lower lobe pulmonary artery (*arrow*). Notice the coiled catheter in the right atrium (*arrowheads*).

B

FIG. 3-23 (*A*) Supine AP chest radiograph of a patient in the ICU shows borderline cardiomegaly and clear lung fields. (*B*) Supine AP chest radiograph obtained after placement of left subclavian catheter shows a large left pneumothorax (*arrowheads*). Because the apex of the lung is so close to the entrance of the subclavian catheter, pneumothorax is a rather common complication of subclavian catheter placement.

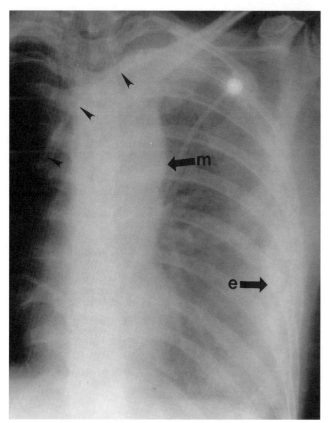

FIG. 3-24 Coned-down view of left side of chest in an ICU patient after placement of the left subclavian catheter (*arrowheads*) shows a large left pleural effusion (e) and widened mediastinum (m). Vascular perforation during the catheter placement resulted in a mediastinal hematoma and left hemothorax. (*Courtesy of Paul Dee, M.D., Charlottesville, Va.*)

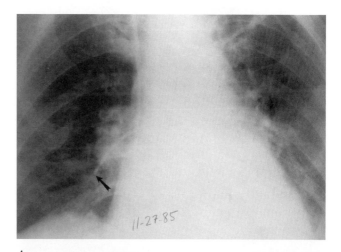

A

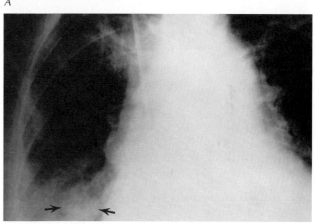

B

FIG. 3-25 (*A*) Supine AP chest radiograph in a patient in the ICU shows the tip of the Swan-Ganz catheter wedged well down into the right lower lobe pulmonary artery (*arrow*). (*B*) Supine AP chest radiograph obtained after removal of the Swan-Ganz catheter in the same patient shows an ill-defined soft-tissue opacity in the right lower lobe, pulmonary infarction from occlusion of the pulmonary artery by the SG catheter (*arrows*).

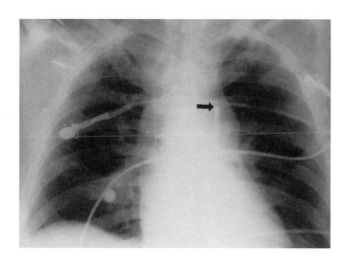

FIG. 3-26 Supine AP film of patient 6 h after coronary artery bypass surgery shows the tip of the IABP in normal position distal to the left subclavian origin (*arrow*).

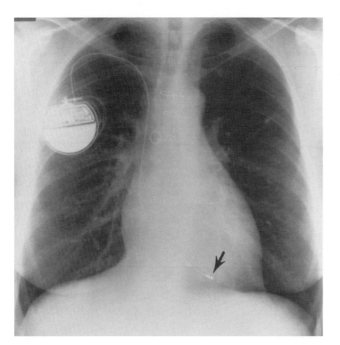

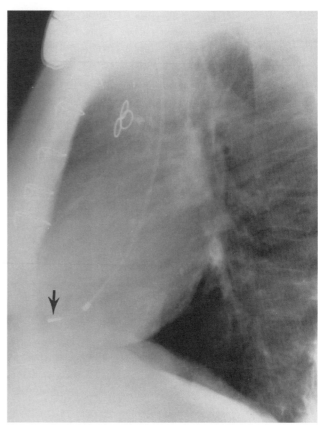

A

FIG. 3-27 Upright PA (*A*) and lateral (*B*) films in a patient with a unipolar pacer. The pacer wire extends through the right atrium and tricuspid valve to terminate in the anterior wall of the right ventricle (*arrows*).

B

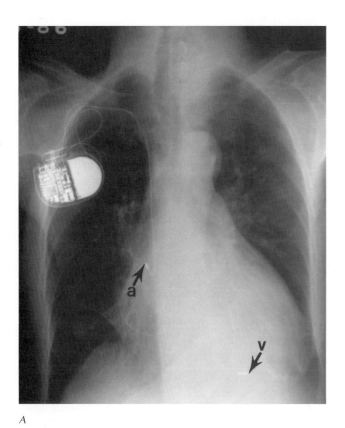

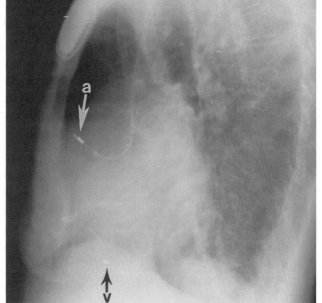

A

B

FIG. 3-28 Upright PA (*A*) and lateral (*B*) views of patient with bipolar pacer show the atrial pacer wire tip (a) in the right atrium and the ventricular wire tip (v) inferiorly in the region of the apex of the right ventricle. These are normal positions for the tips of bipolar pacers.

EXERCISE 3-1: INCREASED HEART SIZE

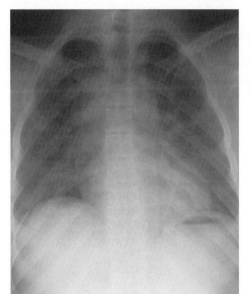

FIG. 3-E-1

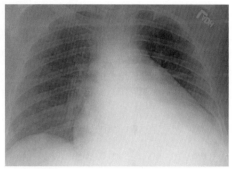

A

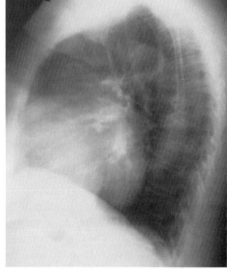

FIG. 3-E-2 *Panels A and B.*

B

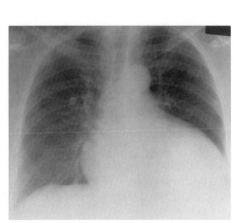

FIG. 3-E-3

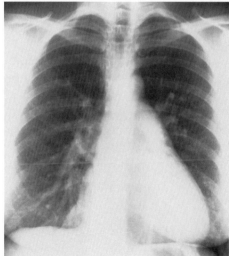

FIG. 3-E-4 *Panel A.*

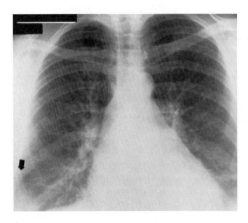

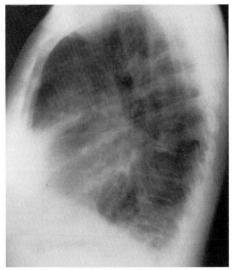

A

FIG. 3-E-5   *Panels A and B.*

B

Clinical Histories:

Case 3-1
A 20-year-old uncooperative man presents with minimal chest pain (Fig. 3-E-1).

CASE 3-2
A 40-year-old woman presents with collagen-vascular disease (Fig. 3-E-2*A*,*B*).

CASE 3-3
A 60-year-old alcoholic man presents with shortness of breath (Fig. 3-E-3).

CASE 3-4
A 28-year-old woman presents with a loud systolic murmur and without cyanosis (Fig. 3-E-4*A*).

CASE 3-5
A 75-year-old man presents with acute shortness of breath and hypotension and a long-standing history of hypertension (Fig. 3-E-5*A*,*B*).

Questions:

3-1.   The most likely diagnosis in Case 3-1 is
   A.   congestive heart failure.
   B.   pericardial effusion.
   C.   intracardiac shunt.
   D.   expiratory phase of respiration film.
   E.   pulmonic stenosis.

3-2.   The most likely diagnoses in Cases 3-2 and 3-3 are
   A.   mediastinal masses.
   B.   intracardiac shunts (atrial septal defect and ventricular septal defect).
   C.   pericardial effusion and cardiomyopathy.
   D.   combined aortic and pulmonary arterial disease.
   E.   technical aberrations.

3-3. The best imaging test to distinguish a mediastinal mass from a cardiac abnormality is
  A. computed tomography.
  B. echocardiography.
  C. thallium scan.
  D. fluoroscopy.
  E. plain film (chest radiographs).

3-4. The most likely diagnosis in Case 3-4 is
  A. Ebstein's anomaly.
  B. mediastinal disease.
  C. intracardiac shunt.
  D. pericardial effusion.
  E. mitral and aortic stenosis.

3-5. The most likely diagnosis in Case 3-5 is
  A. cardiomyopathy.
  B. pulmonary edema.
  C. pericardial effusion.
  D. acute pneumonia.
  E. aortic dissection.

3-6. Is each of the following statements true or false?
  A. The normal cardiothoracic ratio is less than 50 percent.
  B. The major cause of cardiac enlargement is medications.
  C. Kerley's B lines are a prominent plain-film feature of pulmonary edema.
  D. The most common congenital heart lesion is atrial septal defect (ASD).
  E. An intracardiac shunt must be greater than 2 to 1 for pulmonary artery hypertrophy to be visible on the plain film.

3-7. The best imaging test for confirming mediastinal adenopathy suspected on the plain film is
  A. tomography.
  B. MR imaging.
  C. computed tomography.
  D. PET scanning.
  E. echocardiography.

Radiologic Findings:

3-1. This case represents an apparent "enlarged heart" due to an expiratory phase of respiration in this uncooperative patient (*D* is the correct answer to Question 3-1). Note the decreased lung volumes and the elevation of the hemidiaphragms. The resultant crowding of vessels obscures much of the cardiac border. The technique of the PA and lateral plain-film examination should be noted in all cases so as to avoid "diagnosing" diseases that patients do not have.

3-2 and 3-3. Cases 3-2 and 3-3 are examples of a pericardial effusion and cardiomyopathy, respectively (*C* is the correct answer to Question 3-2). Both these patients have similar plain-film findings of the so-called globular or water-bottle configuration of the heart. Figure 3-E-2*C* is an axial CT image from Case 3-2 showing the pericardial effusion (*arrows*).

3-4. This patient has cardiomegaly, increased pulmonary vascularity, and prominent pulmonary arteries, all findings typical of an intracardiac shunt, which in this case

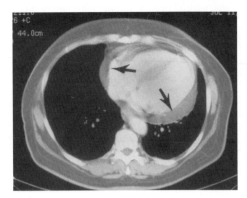

FIG. 3-E-2 (*Panel C*) Axial CT image shows low-density pericardial fluid surrounding the heart (*arrows*).

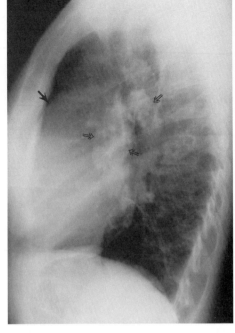

FIG. 3-E-4 (*Panel B*) Lateral view of patient in Case 3-4 shows filling in of the retrosternal space by the enlarged right ventricle (*arrow*) and large right and left pulmonary arteries from the pulmonary arterial hypertension (*open arrows*).

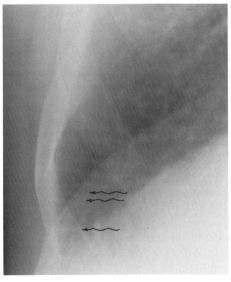

C

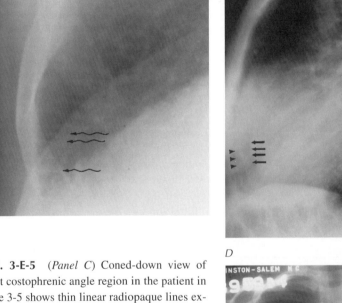

D

FIG. 3-E-5 (*Panel C*) Coned-down view of right costophrenic angle region in the patient in Case 3-5 shows thin linear radiopaque lines extending to the pleural surface. These are Kerley's B lines (thickened interlobular septae) (*arrows*). (*Panel D*) Lateral view of another patient with pericardial effusion showing separation of the epicardial fat (*arrowheads*) from the pericardial fat (*arrows*). Pericardial effusion is sometimes suggested on the lateral chest radiograph if this sign is used. (*Panel E*) Upright PA view of a young child with Ebstein's anomaly shows the globular-shaped heart characteristic of this disorder. (*Courtesy of Thomas E. Sumner, M.D., Winston-Salem, N.C.*)

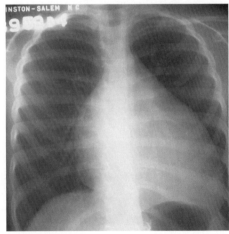

E

was a long-standing ASD (*C* is the correct answer to Question 3-4). The lateral film (Fig. 3-E-4*B*) shows the enlarged pulmonary arteries and ventricular prominence.

3-5. This case (Fig. 3-E-5*A,B*) illustrates cardiomegaly, increased pulmonary vascularity, redistribution of blood flow, and Kerley's B lines (Fig. 3-E-5*A,C, arrows*) typical of pulmonary edema (*B* is the correct answer to Question 3-5).

Discussion:

Pericardial effusion and cardiomyopathy have similar appearances on PA chest films (Cases 3-2 and 3-3). This appearance is often referred to as a globular shape or a water-bottle heart. When this appearance is observed, an echocardiogram is the next best imaging test to differentiate between these two entities. However, this diagnosis may be suggested on the lateral view by a separation of the pericardial and epicardial fat by pericardial fluid, as exhibited in a different patient in Fig. 3-E-5*D* (Fig. 3-9*B*). However, if the clinical question is whether there is a mediastinal mass or a cardiac abnormality, CT is the best test to use (*A* is the correct answer to Question 3-3).

Ebstein's anomaly, mentioned in Question 3-5, is an uncommon type of congenital heart disease that also may result in a globular-shaped appearance of the heart on the chest radiograph. In these patients, the tricuspid valve is downwardly displaced and therefore insufficient, and there is usually an associated ASD. The tricuspid insufficiency results in a massively enlarged right atrium, and the lung vascularity is usually diminished because of decreased flow through the pulmonary vessels. These patients may present with congestive failure early in life, and MRI or cardiac angiography is usually required to make this diagnosis (Fig. 3-E-5*E*).

Increased heart size is a common clinical problem that may be caused by a variety of abnormalities. Cardiac enlargement is diagnosed on the plain film if the cardiothoracic ratio is greater than 50 percent (Statement 3-6*A* is true). The most common cause of enlargement is atherosclerotic cardiovascular disease (Statement 3-6*B* is false), although a large number of other entities may cause an increased cardiac silhouette. If the heart "fails," pulmonary edema from cardiac failure ensues, and Kerley's B lines (interlobular septa dilated with edema fluid) (Fig. 3-E-5*C, arrows*) are generally seen on the radiograph, as Case 3-5 demonstrates (Statement 3-6*C* is true). Intracardiac shunts, especially ASD and ventricular septal defect (VSD), also cause cardiac enlargement because of the increased flow from the internal shunting. VSD is the most common congenital cardiac anomaly (Statement 3-6*D* is false), and the intracardiac shunt must be at least 2 to 1 for the plain film to show recognizable changes (Statement 3-6*E* is true).

Mediastinal masses may occur in a location or a distribution that makes the heart appear enlarged on chest radiographs. At the present time, CT is the next-best test to confirm clinical suspicion of a mass and to evaluate mediastinal adenopathy (*C* is the correct answer to Question 3-7). PET scanning, however, has shown some promise in identifying tumorous nodes that have a normal size and shape on CT scans. PET therefore may be a worthwhile preoperative screening test in the future.

EXERCISE 3-2: ALTERATIONS IN CARDIAC CONTOUR

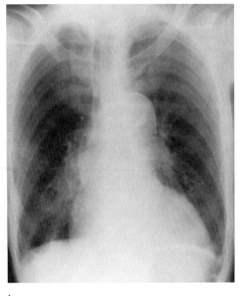
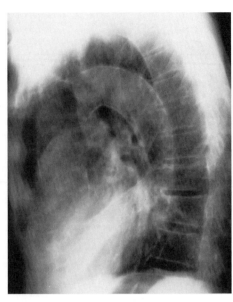

FIG. 3-E-6 *Panels A and B.*

A

B

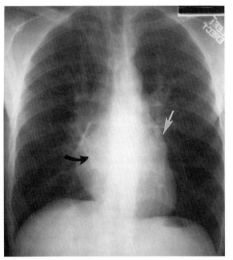
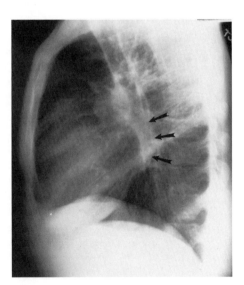

FIG. 3-E-7 *Panels A and B.*

A

B

Clinical Histories:

CASE 3-6
A 65-year-old man presents with a long history of an abnormality seen on his electrocardiogram (Fig. 3-E-6*A,B*).

CASE 3-7
A 30-year-old woman presents with systolic and diastolic murmurs and a history of rheumatic fever as a child (Fig. 3-E-7*A,B*).

CASE 3-8
A 75-year-old man with a history of a myocardial infarction 10 years earlier had this study done as a routine screening examination (Fig. 3-E-8*A,B*).

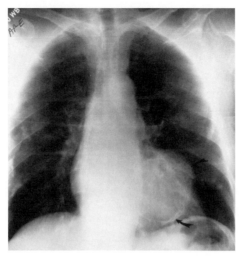

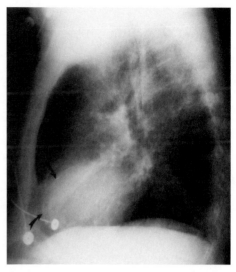

FIG. 3-E-8 *Panels A and B.*

A

B

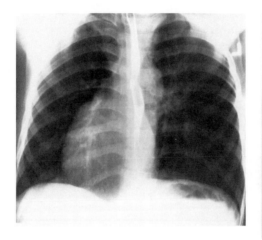

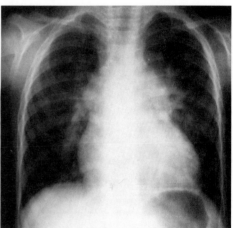

FIG. 3-E-9

FIG. 3-E-10 *Panel A.*

CASE 3-9
A 24-year-old man had this finding on his radiograph immediately after barium swallow (Fig. 3-E-9).

CASE 3-10
A 6-year-old child presents with a history of cardiac complications since birth (Fig. 3-E-10*A*).

Questions:

3-8. In Case 3-6, the most likely cause of the electrocardiographic abnormality is
    A. tetralogy of Fallot.
    B. malingering.
    C. long-standing hypertension.
    D. congenital heart disease.
    E. drug abuse.

3-9. In Case 3-7, the contour abnormality is
    A. left atrial enlargement.
    B. left ventricular hypertrophy.

C. pulmonic stenosis.

D. right atrial enlargement.

E. right ventricular hypertrophy.

3-10. In Case 3-7, the cardiac valve most likely to be involved is the

A. aortic valve.

B. mitral valve.

C. pulmonic valve.

D. tricuspid valve.

E. none of the valves.

3-11. In Case 3-8, what is the cardiac or great vessel contour abnormality?

A. Left atrial enlargement

B. Left ventricular enlargement

C. Right atrial enlargement

D. Left ventricular aneurysm

E. Right ventricular aneurysm

3-12. The diagnosis in Case 3-9 is

A. situs inversus.

B. dextrocardia.

C. technical aberration.

D. tetralogy of Fallot.

E. pulmonary atresia.

3-13. The configuration of the heart in Case 3-10 has been called the

A. the "boot-shaped heart."

B. the "third mogul of the heart."

C. the "snowman appearance."

D. the "double-contour sign."

E. the "water-bottle heart."

Radiologic Findings:

3-6. In this case, the classic findings of enlargement of the left ventricle, characteristic of left ventricular hypertrophy, are seen on both the PA and the lateral films. Extensive aortic calcification and ectasia also are present. The most common cause of left ventricular hypertrophy is long-standing hypertension (*C* is the correct answer to Question 3-8).

3-7. In this case, a double contour to the right side of the heart is seen on the PA film (*black arrow*). There also is an enlarged left atrial appendage (*white arrow*). The lateral film shows enlargement of the left atrial shadow, the superior and posterior region of the cardiac contour (*arrows*) (*A* is the correct answer to Question 3-9). There is increased pulmonary vascularity, and this constellation of findings is characteristic of left atrial enlargement in this patient, who has mitral valvular insufficiency (*B* is the correct answer to Question 3-10).

3-8. The PA and lateral chest films in this case show an enlargement of the left ventricular contour and a focal bulge that has calcification within its margin or wall (*arrows*). The lateral film confirms the calcification (*curved arrows*), and with the patient's history of myocardial infarction 10 years earlier, the most likely diagnosis is a left ventricular aneurysm, which this proved to be (*D* is the correct answer to Question 3-11).

3-9. The asymptomatic patient in this case shows the apex of the heart to be on the right side of the chest and the descending aorta to be in its correct position on the left. These findings are diagnostic of dextrocardia (*B* is the correct answer to Question 3-12).

3-10. In this case, an example of total anomalous pulmonary venous connection or return (TAPVR), a prominent mediastinal shadow, cardiomegaly, and increased vascularity are seen. These findings are sometimes referred to as the "snowman appearance" of the heart. The snowman is caused by the dilated vertical vein connecting the confluence of veins to the innominate vein on the left and the dilated superior vena caval shadow on the right (*C* is the correct answer to Question 3-13).

Discussion:

Alterations of the normal cardiac contour are common clinical scenarios. The most common contour abnormality is probably dilatation or hypertrophy of the left ventricle from long-standing hypertension, as exhibited by the 65-year-old man in Case 3-6. Left ventricular enlargement is first suggested on the PA view by an increase in the CT ratio to over 50 percent and by a prominence of the apex of the cardiac contour. Size of the left ventricle also can be estimated from the lateral projection. The junction at which the inferior vena cava (IVC) contacts the left ventricle on the lateral film is an important landmark for this measurement (see Fig. 3-7). Two centimeters above this IVC-cardiac junction, the left ventricular shadow should not project more than 1.8 cm directly posteriorly. If the left ventricle projects more than 2 cm behind this junction, left ventricular hypertrophy or left ventricular enlargement should be suspected (Fig. 3-E-6*C,D*).

Left atrial enlargement (LAE), as shown in Case 3-7, occurs mainly with left-sided obstructive lesions such as mitral stenosis or mitral regurgitation, usually as a result of rheumatic fever or collagen-vascular disease. The major sign of LAE on the PA view is the so-called double contour of the right heart border. This double soft-tissue shadow is caused by the protrusion of the dilated left atrium to the right of the spine and its projection behind the dilated right atrial border (Fig. 3-E-7*A, black arrow*). Another sign of LAE is dilatation of the left atrial appendage. The left atrial appendage region is the area immediately adjacent to and below the left main bronchus, which, when enlarged, causes an extra soft-tissue density to the left heart border. This has been called the "third mogul" of the left cardiac border (Fig. 3-E-7*A, white arrow*). LAE also causes a separation or splaying of the left and right mainstem bronchi that can be seen on the PA chest radiograph. This measurement is referred to as the *carinal angle* and normally measures between 60 and 120 degrees. With LAE, the angle may be increased. Widening of this an-

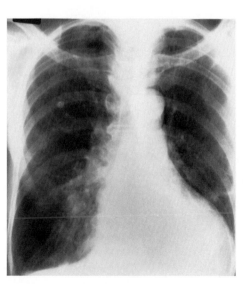
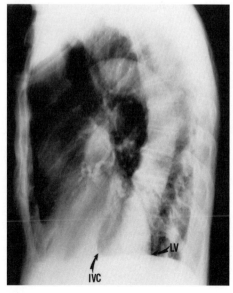

C   *D*

FIG. 3-E-6   PA (*Panel C*) and lateral (*Panel D*) views of patient with long-standing aortic stenosis show left ventricular prominence with displacement of the cardiac apex on the PA view and marked displacement of the left ventricular shadow (LV) in relation to the inferior vena cava (IVC) on the lateral view. (*Courtesy of Caroline Chiles, M.D., Winston-Salem, N.C.*)

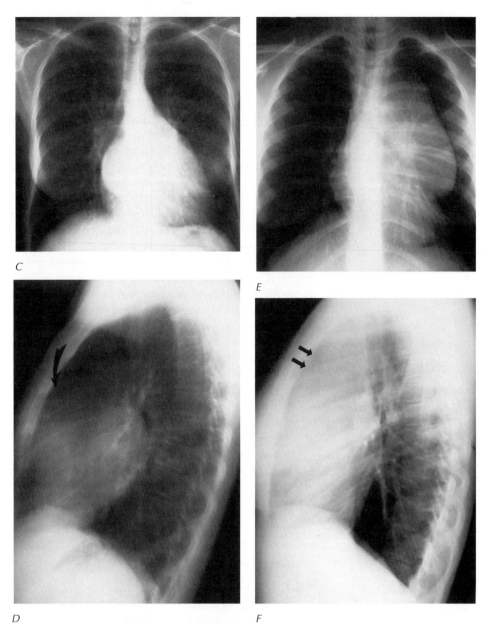

C

D   *F*

FIG. 3-E-7 PA (*Panel C*) and lateral (*Panel D*) views of patient with long-standing mitral stenosis show the double contour on the PA view and filling in of the retrosternal space on the lateral
view (*curved arrow*). Right ventricular hypertrophy or dilatation will be manifested as soft-tissue
density in the retrosternal space on the lateral view. PA (*Panel E*) and lateral (*Panel F*) views of patient with night sweats show an anterior mediastinal mass that fills in the retrosternal space on the
lateral view (*arrows*). A CT scan (*Panel G*) in the same patient shows the location of the anterior
mediastinal mass (*arrows*) adjacent to the aortic arch. Biopsy of the mass was interpreted as
Hodgkin's disease.

gle also can be caused by subcarinal adenopathy, and in patients thought to have this abnormality, CT is recommended, as outlined in the preceding exercise.

The left atrium makes up the posterior cardiac shadow just above the left ventricle
(*LA* in Fig. 3-7). Left atrial enlargement is recognized on the lateral film by enlargement
and posterior displacement of the left atrial shadow (Fig. 3-E-7*B, arrows*). If the LAE is
caused by mitral stenosis, a diligent search should be made for calcification in the mitral
valve annulus.

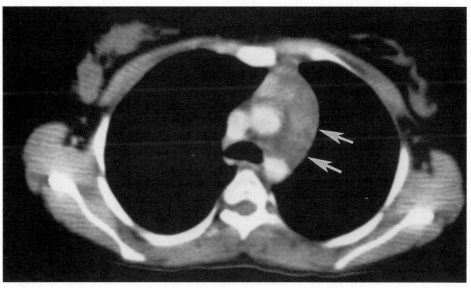

FIG. 3-E-7   (*Continued*)

G

Right ventricular enlargement (RVE) or hypertrophy (RVH) results most commonly from pulmonic stenosis or right-sided heart failure from a variety of disorders. In this cardiac contour abnormality there is an increase in the soft-tissue density within the retrosternal clear space that is best seen on the lateral film (Fig. 3-E-7*C,D*). On the PA film, an occasional uplifting of the apex of the heart also may be seen. However, anterior mediastinal masses also may cause retrosternal fullness and should be included in the differential diagnosis. When the cause is not clear from the plain film, CT and MRI are the next most appropriate tests to differentiate between these two diagnostic considerations (Fig. 3-7-*E–G*).

In the United States aneurysms (localized areas of dilatation of the heart), as shown in the patient in Case 3-8, are almost always caused by the sequelae of myocardial infarction. Aneurysms are usually diagnosed on the PA chest radiograph as localized soft-tissue outpouchings or irregularities at the apical or anterolateral segments of the left ventricular cardiac contour. The diagnosis often can be confirmed on the lateral view, as was true in this patient. A linear rim of dystrophic calcification may develop within the nonviable myocardium in the aneurysm after the infarction. With fluoroscopy, aneurysms show paradoxical enlargement during systole while the remainder of the heart is contracting. Since there is stasis of blood in the aneurysm, blood clots develop within the aneurysm and may be a source of distal emboli. The next most appropriate tests to evaluate suspected left ventricular aneurysms are echocardiography and MRI. The advantage of MRI is that it is less technique-dependent than echocardiography. Other causes of left ventricular aneurysm include Chagas' disease, cardiomyopathy, trauma, myocarditis, and myocardial abscess.

Dextrocardia, as shown in Case 3-9, is usually recognized easily on the PA chest radiograph. However, this finding may be overlooked if the left and right designations on the film are marked incorrectly or are misinterpreted. In most cases of dextrocardia, the aorta descends on the left side, and the patient is asymptomatic. If the aorta descends on the right side, a number of other abnormalities should be considered (Table 3-5). The works listed in the Bibliography provide more in-depth discussion of this topic.

The snowman appearance of the cardiac shadow, shown in Case 3-10, is caused by the congenital anomaly of TAPVR. In this disorder, the right atrium receives both the systemic and the pulmonary venous blood flow. Obviously, therefore, some form of intracardiac communication (usually a large ASD) is essential for these patients' survival. The right side of the snowman's head is formed by the dilated SVC, and the left side of the head is caused by a large remnant of the left anterior cardinal vein (the so-called ver-

TABLE 3-5   SOME CONGENITAL CARDIAC LESIONS ASSOCIATED WITH RIGHT AORTIC ARCH

Lesion	Approximate Incidence (%)
Corrected great vessel malposition	50
Asplenia syndrome	30–40
Truncus arteriosus	35
Tetralogy of Fallot	
With pulmonary atresia	50
Classic	25
Complete transposition of the great vessels with VSD and pulmonic stenosis	5–10
Tricuspid valve atresia	5
Large VSD	2

tical vein) draining all the pulmonary veins from behind the left atrium up to the left brachiocephalic or innominate vein. The body of the snowman is represented by the dilated right atrium and ventricle; the atrium bulges to the right, and the ventricle expands to the left and superiorly, producing a convex cardiac border comprising the displaced left atrium and ventricle (Fig. 3-E-10*B*).

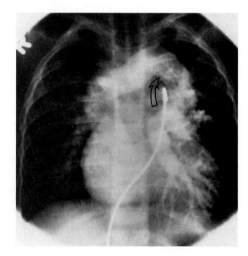

FIG. 3-E-10   (*Panel B*) Angiogram of the patient in Case 3-10 shows that the left side of the snowman's head is formed by the left anterior cardinal vein (vertical vein) draining all the pulmonary veins from behind the left atrium up to the left brachiocephalic vein (*open arrow*). (*Courtesy of Laurence B. Leinbach, M.D., Winston-Salem, N.C.*)

EXERCISE 3-3: PULMONARY VASCULARITY

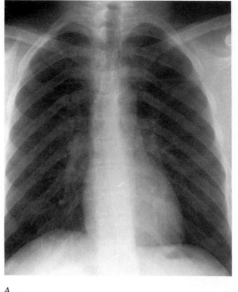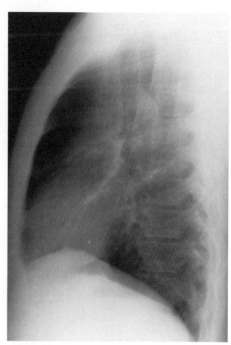

FIG. 3-E-11 *Panels A and B.*

A

B

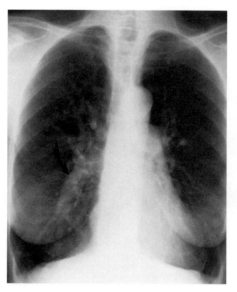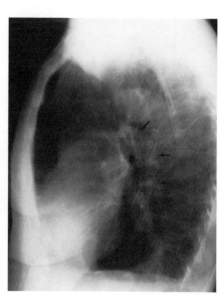

FIG. 3-E-12 *Panels A and B.*

A   *B*

Clinical Histories:

CASE 3-11
A 28-year-old man is examined in the Emergency Department for chest pain and shortness of breath (Fig. 3-E-11).

CASE 3-12
A 65-year-old woman presents with a 100-pack-year history of smoking (Fig. 3-E-12).

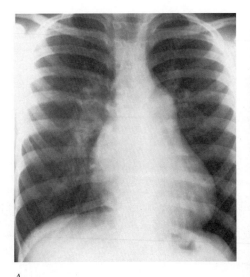 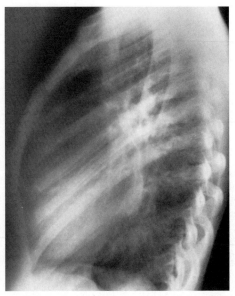

A

FIG. 3-E-13   *Panels A and B.*

B

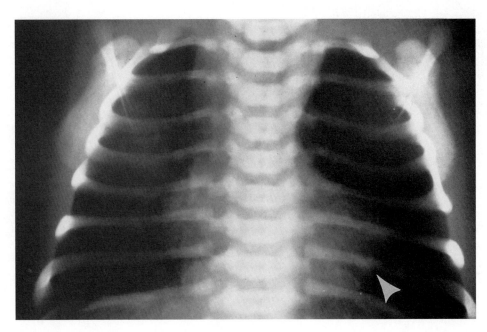

FIG. 3-E-14   *Panel A.*

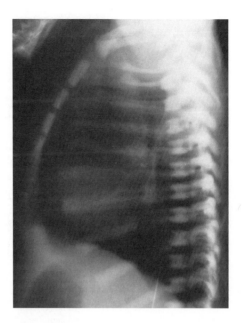

FIG. 3-E-14 *(Continued) Panel B.*

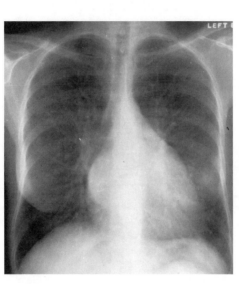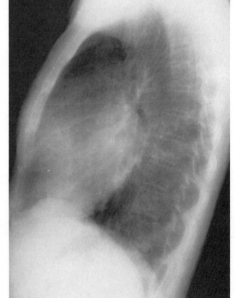

FIG. 3-E-15 *Panels A and B.*

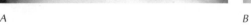

A   *B*

CASE 3-13
An acyanotic 22-year-old man presents with a systolic murmur (Fig. 3-E-13).

CASE 3-14
A 6-year-old child presents with intermittent cyanosis (Fig. 3-E-14).

CASE 3-15
A 50-year-old woman presents with acute shortness of breath (Fig. 3-E-15).

Questions:

3-14. The most likely cause of the patient's symptoms in Case 3-11 is
    A. pneumonia.
    B. pulmonary edema.
    C. interstitial lung disease.
    D. hysterical anxiety reaction.
    E. pneumothorax.

3-15. The curved arrow in Case 3-12 (Fig. 3-E-12*A*) is directed to the
    A. right atrium.
    B. ascending aorta.
    C. right descending pulmonary artery.
    D. main pulmonary artery.
    E. pneumonia.

3-16. The arrows in Case 3-12 (Fig. 3-E-12*B*) are outlining which structure?
    A. Left pulmonary artery
    B. Descending aorta
    C. Right pulmonary artery
    D. Atelectasis
    E. Pneumonia

3-17. The most likely diagnosis in Case 3-13 is
    A. aortic stenosis.
    B. pulmonic stenosis.
    C. VSD.
    D. pulmonary edema.
    E. normal chest radiograph.

3-18. The characteristic shape of the cardiac silhouette in Case 3-14 is the
    A. third mogul.
    B. snowman appearance.
    C. boot-shaped heart.
    D. double-contour sign.
    E. water-bottle heart.

3-19. The characteristic cardiac appearance in Case 3-14 is associated with which of the following diagnoses?
    A. Ebstein's anomaly
    B. Tetralogy of Fallot
    C. Mitral stenosis
    D. Aortic stenosis
    E. Aortic aneurysm

3-20. The most likely etiology of the radiographic findings in Case 3-15 is
    A. cardiac failure with pulmonary edema.
    B. pulmonic stenosis with pneumonia.
    C. pulmonary embolism.
    D. pneumomediastinum.
    E. pneumothorax.

Radiologic Findings:

3-11. In this case, the chest radiograph was normal in a 28-year-old man seen in the Emergency Department for left-sided chest pain. The electrocardiogram also was normal, and there was no obvious cause for the patient's pain. He had just stopped medication for a psychiatric illness and was hysterical (*D* is the correct answer to Question 3-14). Note the well-demarcated pulmonary vessels in the perihilar regions and the branching or arborization of these vessels into the lung fields. There are more pulmonary vascular markings in the bases of the lung on this upright film because of gravitational effects.

3-12. This case is an example of chronic obstructive pulmonary disease (COPD). The large central pulmonary arteries indicate pulmonary arterial hypertension. The curved arrow in Fig. 3-E-12*A* identifies the enlarged right descending pulmonary artery (*C* is the correct answer to Question 3-15). The generalized proximal pulmonary artery enlargement is confirmed on the lateral film (Fig. 3-E-12*B*) by the extremely prominent left pulmonary artery (*arrows*) (*A* is the correct answer to Question 3-16). Note the attenuation of vessels in the periphery of the lungs. This constellation of findings is typical of emphysema and COPD. There is also extreme bullous disease, which results in an overall appearance of hyperlucency of the lungs.

3-13. This case shows increased pulmonary vascularity in a 22-year-old patient with VSD (*C* is the correct answer to Question 3-17). Notice the large central pulmonary arteries, the increased linear opacities radiating out into the lung fields, and the relatively uniform distribution of the pulmonary vascular shadows. In patients with long-standing intracardiac shunts and pulmonary hypertension, the pulmonary arterial resistance may get so high that there is actually a reversal of the intracardiac shunt from right to left. This situation is called the *Eisenmenger complex*. In these patients the central pulmonary arteries are quite large, but the peripheral pulmonary vascularity is decreased, or attenuated, because of their extensive atherosclerotic changes caused by long-standing hypertension.

3-14. This case shows the characteristic boot-shaped heart of tetralogy of Fallot (T of F) (*C* is the correct answer to Question 3-18 and *B* is the correct answer to Question 3-19). Note the uplifted cardiac apex caused by the enlarged right ventricle (*white arrowhead*). These patients typically have decreased pulmonary vascularity, as exhibited in this child.

3-15. This case is an example of a long-standing hypertension in a patient with shortness of breath and pulmonary edema from cardiac failure (*A* is the correct answer to Question 3-20). Note the increased cardiac silhouette size, the increased perihilar opacities, and the altered distribution of blood flow to the upper lung zones. In this woman, the cause of the pulmonary edema was cardiac failure from myocardial infarction.

Discussion:

The reader will remember from cadaveric dissections that the appearance of the pulmonary vascularity is very similar to the branching of a tree. The main pulmonary arteries are large, the lobar arteries are smaller, and each branching segment becomes progressively smaller with arborization. On the chest radiograph, this pattern is manifested by linear opacities or shadows that are much more prominent in the central portion of the chest and gradually get less prominent as they arborize toward the periphery of the lung, as in the normal person in Case 3-11. The right descending pulmonary artery (RDPA) is one important landmark on the PA chest film on which we should concentrate (see Fig. 3-6). In the normal chest, the lateral border of the RDPA is usually very well demarcated, and the artery usually measures less than 15 mm in its widest diameter.

Hypertrophy or dilatation of this vessel is caused by a variety of abnormalities (Table 3-6). COPD, because of the resultant pulmonary hypertension, is the most common cause of pulmonary arterial hypertension and is shown in the patient in Case 3-12.

Intracardiac shunts that result in increased pulmonary arterial flow also can enlarge the pulmonary vascular tree and increase vascularity. The most common lesions showing increased vascularity without cyanosis are ASD, VSD, and patent ductus arteriosus (PDA). The main cardiac lesions with cyanosis and increased pulmonary vascularity are transposition of the great vessels, truncus arteriosus, and TAPVR; these signs are also seen in about 15 percent of patients with tricuspid atresia. The standard texts listed in the Bibliography at the end of the chapter provide in-depth discussions of these entities.

Case 3-13 is an example of a VSD with resultant increased vascularity. The other common cause of pulmonary artery prominence is mitral disease (either stenosis or regurgitation), which is usually accompanied by prominent vascular markings seen diffusely throughout the lung fields (see Case 3-7).

Tetralogy of Fallot, as shown in Case 3-14 in a cyanotic child, results in decreased pulmonary vascularity because of the associated pulmonic stenosis. The differential diagnosis for decreased vascularity in a cyanotic person includes trilogy of Fallot (pulmonic stenosis with an ASD) and tricuspid atresia.

Pulmonary edema, as exhibited in Case 3-15, regardless of the cause, is another process that causes the increase in the pulmonary vascularity seen on chest radiographs (further discussion in the next chapter). Perihilar indistinctness, caused by perivascular and interstitial edema, may obliterate the borders of the pulmonary vascular tree. Associated findings are redistribution of blood flow to the apices, Kerley's B lines, and pleural effusions (Fig. 3-E-5C). This woman was hypoxemic, and her condition was evolving into a myocardial infarction as this film was obtained.

TABLE 3-6   CAUSES OF PULMONARY ARTERIAL HYPERTENSION

Chronic obstructive pulmonary disease (COPD)

Left-sided obstructive lesions

    Mitral stenosis

    Intracardiac shunts

Recurrent pulmonary emboli

Idiopathic (by exclusion)

EXERCISE 3-4: VASCULAR ABNORMALITIES

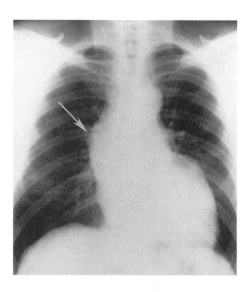

FIG. 3-E-16

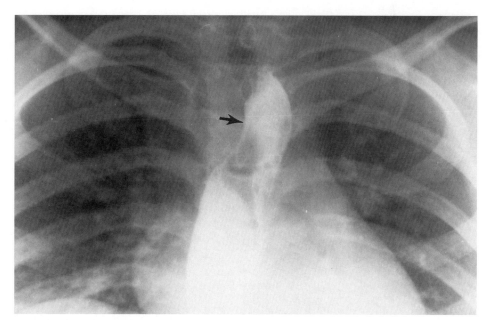

FIG. 3-E-17 *Panel A.*

Clinical Histories:

CASE 3-16
A 67-year-old man presents with a long history of hypertension (Fig. 3-E-16).

CASE 3-17
A 25-year-old man presents with chest fullness; film from barium swallow (Fig. 3-E-17*A*).

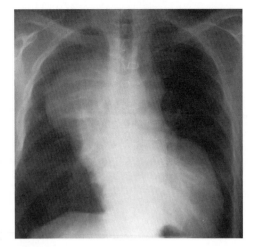

FIG. 3-E-18   *Panel A.*

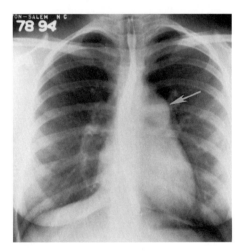

FIG. 3-E-19   *Panel A.*

FIG. 3-E-20

CASE 3-18
A 76-year-old man presents with substernal chest pain (Fig. 3-E-18*A*).

CASE 3-19
A 22-year-old man presents with differential pulses in the legs and arms (Fig. 3-E-19*A*).

CASE 3-20
A 38-year-old man presents with a systolic murmur (Fig. 3-E-20).

Questions: **3-21.** Match each case with the appropriate diagnosis:

Diagnosis	**Case**
(1) Right aortic arch	_____
(2) Aortic aneurysm	_____
(3) Aortic ectasia in elderly person	_____
(4) Coarctation of the aorta	_____
(5) Pulmonary artery dilatation	_____

3-22. The arrowhead in Fig. 3-E-19 refers to

    A. metastatic disease.

    B. fibrous dysplasia.

    C. fractures.

    D. rib notching.

    E. normal irregularities.

3-23. The arrow in Fig. 3-E-19 is showing

    A. aortic ectasia.

    B. aortic constriction.

    C. pulmonary artery dilatation.

    D. adenopathy.

    E. embolic changes.

Radiologic Findings:

3-16. In this case, aortic ectasia (*arrow*) is seen in a patient who has had coronary artery bypass surgery and has a history of long-standing hypertension (Diagnosis 3).

3-17 and 3-18. Case 3-17 is an example of a right-sided aortic arch in a patient without cardiac symptoms (Diagnosis 1), and Case 3-18 shows a localized dilatation in the region of the ascending aorta characteristic of an aortic aneurysm (Diagnosis 2). In fact, this is a film of the patient in Case 3-16, 9 years later. The CT image (Fig. 3-E-18*B*) and the angiogram (not shown) confirmed the large ascending aneurysm.

3-19. This case shows rib notching (*arrowhead*) (*D* is the correct answer to Question 3-22) and a localized constriction of the proximal descending aorta (*arrow*) (*B* is the correct answer to Question 3-23). These findings are diagnostic of coarctation of the aorta (Diagnosis 4).

3-20. This case is an example of pulmonary artery dilatation (*arrow*) in a patient with pulmonic stenosis (Diagnosis 5).

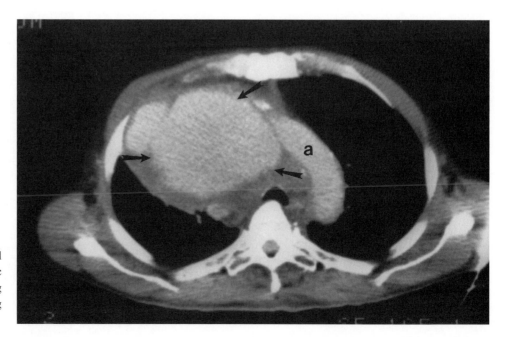

FIG. 3-E-18 (*Panel B*) Axial CT image shows large aortic aneurysm (*arrows*) originating from the proximal ascending portion of the aortic arch (a).

Discussion:

Anomalies of the major vessels are commonly encountered on the chest film. The aortic arch is an easily recognized shadow. On the PA projection, the aorta originates in the middle of the chest in the substernal region and then arches superiorly and slightly to the left (hence "the aortic arch"); then it curves, crosses the mediastinum at an oblique angle, and continues as the descending thoracic aorta (see Fig. 3-6). The configuration of the aorta changes during life. In the young person, the aortic arch is narrow and smooth, and the descending thoracic segment is very straight. In the older patient with atherosclerotic disease, as shown in Case 3-16, the aorta becomes ectatic or "uncoiled," creating a larger, more distinct shadow in the mediastinum and showing an undulating pattern in the descending thoracic portion.

Other abnormalities of the aortic arch are uncommon. Congenital aortic anomalies include left aortic arch with aberrant branching, right aortic arch, complete double aortic arch, and incomplete double aortic arch. The most prominent of these aberrations is the right aortic arch, which occurs in 1 in 2500 people. It can be diagnosed on the plain film by noting an indentation to and slight deviation of the right side of the trachea and displacement of the SVC shadow, as shown in Case 3-17 (Fig. 3-E-17A,B, *arrows*). The barium swallow also can demonstrate esophageal compression by the aorta as it crosses from right to left in the lower chest (Fig. 3-E-17B, *arrowheads*). Great vessel branching from this anomaly is variable and may be delineated by MRI or angiography. The congenital cardiac lesions associated with a right aortic arch have already been listed in Table 3-5.

Aneurysms or dilatations of the aorta, shown in Case 3-18, are other aortic anomalies most often caused by atherosclerosis. They may be saccular or fusiform in shape, and symptoms include chest pain, hoarseness from compression of the recurrent laryngeal nerve, postobstructive atelectasis from compression of a bronchus, and dysphasia from esophageal compression. However, aneurysms are discovered most commonly as an incidental finding on an imaging study done for other reasons. An aneurysm of the ascending or transverse aortic segments shows a focal soft-tissue bulge adjacent to the aortic shadow, usually with curvilinear calcification in its wall. A saccular aneurysm of the descending aorta may be misdiagnosed as a mediastinal mass, especially if it does not contain linear calcification. In these cases, as mentioned previously, CT or MR imaging

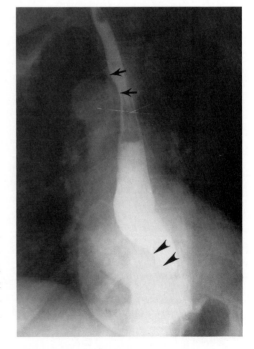

FIG. 3-E-17 (*Panel B*) AP view of a barium swallow in a patient with right aortic arch shows extrinsic compression of the esophagus by the right-sided arch (*arrows*). As the aorta crosses to the left, it causes compression of the distal esophagus (*arrowheads*). (*Courtesy of Thomas E. Sumner, M.D., Winston-Salem, N.C.*)

is the next best imaging modality to perform. Other causes of aneurysms are infection, especially fungal in origin (mycotic aneurysm), syphilis, trauma, and cystic medial necrosis associated with Marfan's syndrome.

A special type of aneurysm is the dissecting aneurysm, which is usually caused by atherosclerosis with medial layer necrosis. This is a disorder in which blood dissects, or extrudes, into the aortic wall between a separation or tear of the intima, and diffuse widening of the aortic shadow results. This process may begin anywhere along the course of the thoracic aorta, and the exact location is very important because it has therapeutic implications. Aortic dissections that are proximal to the origin of the left subclavian artery (type A dissections) are traditionally treated medically, whereas those which begin distal to the left subclavian artery (type B dissections) can be treated surgically. The definitive diagnosis of aortic dissection is best made by aortography, but CT with contrast enhancement, MR imaging, and ultrasonography also are useful in diagnosing this disorder, and MR imaging may eventually replace aortography in this clinical setting (see Fig. 3-17).

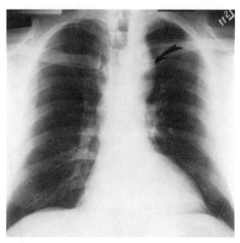

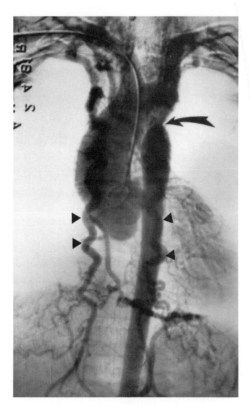

B

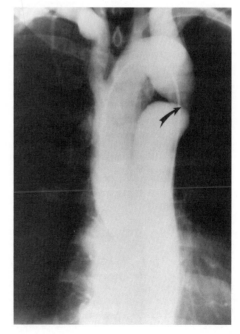

C

D

FIG. 3-E-19   (*Panel B*) Aortogram of the patient in Case 3-19 shows the characteristic constriction in the descending aorta (*curved arrow*) and the dilated intercostal veins (*arrowheads*). (*Panel C*) Upright PA view of a patient with pseudocoarctation shows the high ascending aorta (*arrow*). (*Panel D*) Aortogram of the same patient shows the characteristic kink of the aorta (*arrow*). Note the lack of dilated intercostal arteries.

The abnormality in Case 3-19 is coarctation of the aorta. This disorder is a localized partial obstruction of the aorta at the junction of the aortic arch and descending aorta near the ductus arteriosus (the in utero connection between the aorta and pulmonary arteries) or ligamentum arteriosum (the fibrous remnant of the ductus arteriosus in the adult). Coarctation is caused by a fibrous ridge and results in partial obstruction to aortic flow. About one-half of these patents also have bicuspid aortic valves. Patients with coarctation have elevated upper extremity blood pressure and decreased lower extremity blood pressure. A systolic ejection murmur also may be heard. Because of the partial aortic obstruction, collateral systemic channels form mainly through the intercostal arteries and result in the characteristic rib notching seen in this disorder (Fig. 3-E-19*B*).

Pseudocoarctation of the aorta is widely believed to be a part of the spectrum of coarctation. However, patients with this abnormality have no significant aortic obstruction and do not have differential upper and lower extremity pulses. The aorta is instead kinked at the site of the ligamentum arteriosum, and the position of the ascending aorta is more vertical and rises unusually higher, making the curve of the aorta tighter (Fig. 3-E-19*C,D*).

EXERCISE 3-5: HEART AND GREAT VESSEL CALCIFICATIONS

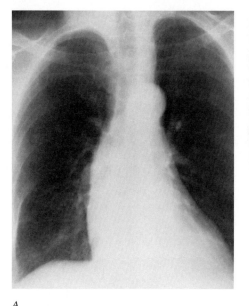
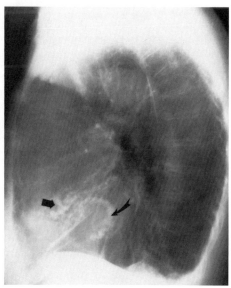

A

B

FIG. 3-E-21 *Panels A and B.*

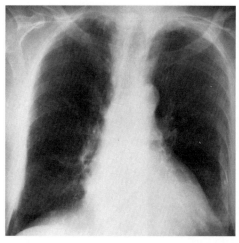
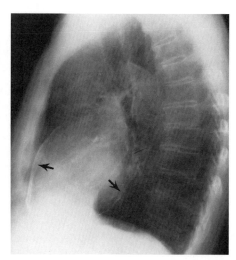

FIG. 3-E-22 *Panels A and B.*

A

B

Clinical Histories:

CASE 3-21

A 75-year-old patient presents with "lots of murmurs" when examined by a medical student who was on the first day of clinical rotations (Fig. 3-E-21*A,B*).

CASE 3-22

A 70-year-old patient is seen and tells the medical student that she had been very sick as a younger woman but did not know her diagnosis at that time (Fig. 3-E-22).

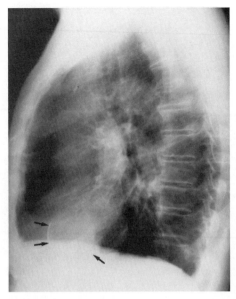

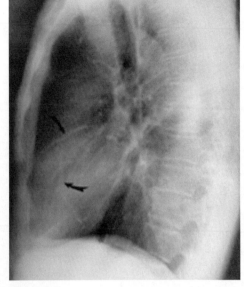

FIG. 3-E-23   **FIG. 3-E-24**

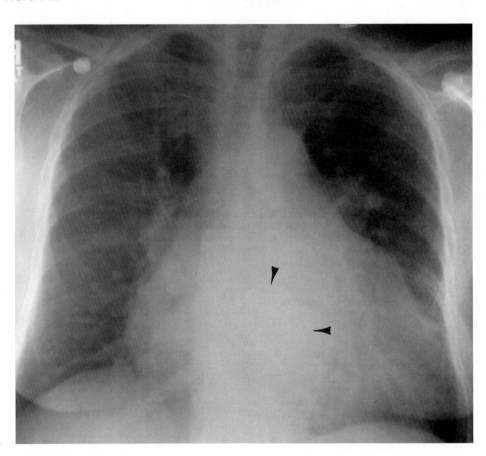

FIG. 3-E-25   *Panel A.*

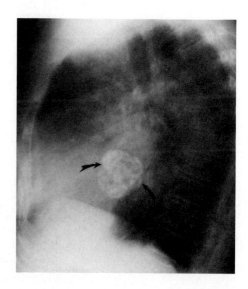

FIG. 3-E-25   *(Continued) Panel B.*

CASE 3-23

A 65-year-old man with a long history of hypertension was hospitalized 6 years ago with an acute illness. This is a current lateral chest radiograph (Fig. 3-E-23).

CASE 3-24

A 66-year-old man presents with long-standing diabetes mellitus. This is a current lateral chest radiograph (Fig. 3-E-24).

CASE 3-25

A woman presents with shortness of breath and decreased exercise tolerance. These are current PA and lateral chest radiographs (Fig. 3-E-25A,B).

Questions:

3-24. In Case 3-21 (Fig. 3-E-21B), the straight arrow refers to
   A.   the mitral valve.
   B.   the tricuspid valve.
   C.   the aortic valve.
   D.   a pulmonary embolus.
   E.   a pericardial calcification.

3-25. In Case 3-21 (Fig. 3-E-21B), the curved arrow on the lateral chest radiograph is pointing to the region of the
   A.   mitral valve.
   B.   aortic valve.
   C.   tricuspid valve.
   D.   pericardial calcification.
   E.   pulmonary embolus.

3-26. In Case 3-22 (Fig. 3-E-22B), the arrows are pointing to
   A.   a pulmonary infiltrate.
   B.   a pericardial effusion.
   C.   a pericardial calcification.
   D.   an ascending aortic aneurysm.
   E.   a descending thoracic aortic aneurysm.

3-27. In Case 3-23 (Fig. 3-E-23), the arrows on the lateral chest radiograph point to calcifications within which cardiac structure?
   A.   Pericardium
   B.   Mitral valve
   C.   Aortic valve
   D.   Tricuspid valve
   E.   Left ventricle

3-28. In Case 3-24 (Fig. 3-E-24), the curved arrows point to calcification within the region of which cardiac structure?
   A.   Aortic valve
   B.   Mitral valve
   C.   Pericardium
   D.   Coronary artery
   E.   Aortic aneurysm

3-29. In Case 3-25 (Fig. 3-E-25*A,B*), the arrows and arrowheads point to
   A.   a calcified mediastinal mass.
   B.   a calcified left atrial myxoma.
   C.   pulmonary embolus calcification.
   D.   aortic valve calcification.
   E.   mitral valve calcification.

Radiologic Findings:

3-21. The PA and lateral chest films in this case show irregular linear calcifications in two areas, best seen on the lateral projection. Anteriorly, the curved linear calcifications denoted by the straight arrow reside in the aortic valve (*C* is the correct answer to Question 3-24). The curved arrows posteriorly point to calcification within the mitral valve annulus (*A* is the correct answer to Question 3-25). This patient had rheumatic fever as a young adult, and the calcifications in the aortic valve and mitral annulus resulted from this infection.

3-22. This case shows pericardial calcification in a patient who had viral pericarditis as a young child (*C* is the correct answer to Question 3-26). Note that the calcification is seen much better on the lateral view.

3-23. The lateral chest radiograph in this case shows linear calcification in a focal area overlying the left ventricular shadow. This calcification resides in a left ventricular aneurysm that this man developed after a myocardial infarction 6 years earlier (*E* is the correct answer to Question 3-27).

3-24. The lateral chest radiograph in this case shows small linear tram track calcifications overlying the exact course of the coronary arteries. These calcifications represent coronary artery calcification in a patient with long-standing diabetes (*D* is the correct answer to Question 3-28).

3-25. This case is difficult. A circular, heavily calcified area overlying the left atrium is seen in both the PA (*arrowheads*) and lateral (*curved arrows*) projections. These calcifications resided within a left atrial tumor, a myxoma that was causing the patient's symptoms of shortness of breath and decreased exercise tolerance (*B* is the correct answer to Question 3-29).

Discussion:

Calcifications, present in almost any area of the cardiovascular system, may be either metastatic or dystrophic in origin. Metastatic calcifications are usually caused by soft-tissue precipitation in patients with hypercalcemia. Dystrophic soft-tissue calcifications are responses to tissue injury or degeneration and have no metabolic cause. They can be seen in practically any of the soft-tissue components of the cardiovascular system. We will concentrate on calcifications that can be seen on the plain film, although CT in general is a more sensitive test for delineating subtle calcifications. The most common site of calcification seen on the plain chest radiograph is within the aorta, usually in elderly patients with long-standing atherosclerotic cardiovascular disease or diabetes. In this instance, the calcification is linear and is associated with the aortic wall (Fig. 3-E-6*A,B*). These calcific deposits also may be present in aneurysms (Fig. 3-E-8*A,B*).

The aortic valve and mitral valve annulus are the most common intracardiac regions to demonstrate dystrophic calcification, usually secondary to long-standing stenosis or insufficiency from rheumatic fever. Bicuspid valves also may show this type of calcification. The lateral film (Fig. 3-E-21*C*) is best for deciding which valve is calcified. A line drawn from the hilum (*C*) obliquely and downward to intersect the anterior cardiophrenic angle (*N*) will project behind aortic calcifications (*A*). Calcifications that lie in back of this line are usually mitral annulus calcifications (*M*).

Pericardial calcification as in Case 3-22 is seen in approximately 50 percent of patients with constrictive pericarditis. It has a characteristic curvilinear appearance outlining the location of the pericardium and is most often appreciated on the less pulsatile right heart border (Fig. 3-E-22*A,B*).

Myocardial calcification, as is seen in left ventricular aneurysms, was discussed in the exercise on altered cardiac contour and is shown in a slightly different form in Case 3-23 (Fig. 3-E-23). Thin, focal, linear calcifications overlying the left ventricle should be considered as aneurysms, and echocardiography or MR imaging should be performed to exclude this diagnosis.

Calcifications within the wall of the coronary arteries, as exhibited in Case 3-24, are recognized on the plain film as thin, linear, calcific deposits corresponding to the course of the coronary arteries. Usually caused by long-standing hypertension or diabetes, this finding is significant because these patients have a high incidence of obstructive coronary artery disease.

Case 3-25 is an example of the rare primary cardiac neoplasm that may calcify and be detected initially on the plain film. The cardiac tumor that most commonly calcifies is the left atrial myxoma, and calcification occurs in about 10 percent of these extremely rare lesions (Fig. 3-E-25*A,B*). Rarely, myocardial metastatic disease (such as osteosarcoma) or other primary cardiac tumors may calcify. Finally, primary mediastinal neoplasms such as teratomas may rarely show calcification. In these patients, CT should be performed expeditiously to diagnose these lesions and to provide a "map" for biopsy or surgery.

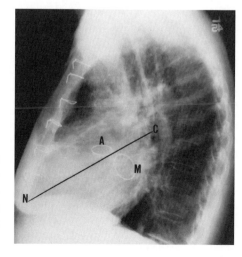

FIG. 3-E-21 (*Panel C*) Lateral view of a patient who had undergone replacement of the aortic (A) and mitral (M) valves. The line CN connects the carina and the anterior cardiophrenic angle. Aortic valves usually lie above this line and mitral valves below it.

EXERCISE 3-6: MONITORING DEVICES

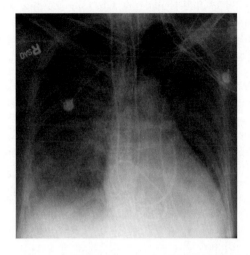

FIG. 3-E-26

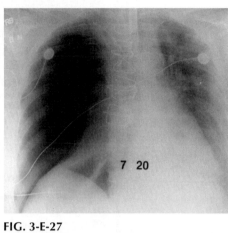

FIG. 3-E-27

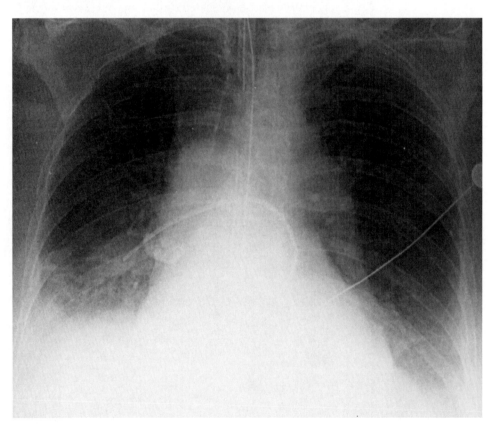

FIG. 3-E-28

Clinical Histories:

CASE 3-26
A routine supine portable chest radiograph is obtained after SG catheter placement (Fig. 3-E-26).

CASE 3-27
A supine chest radiograph is obtained after a difficult CVP placement (Fig. 3-E-27).

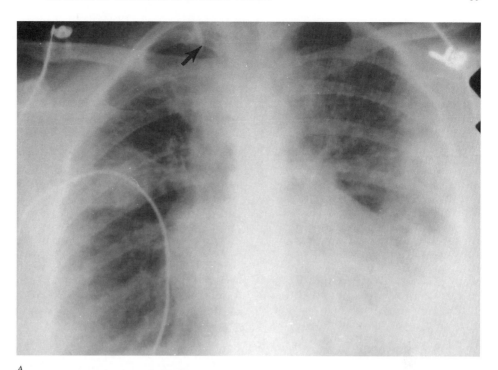

A

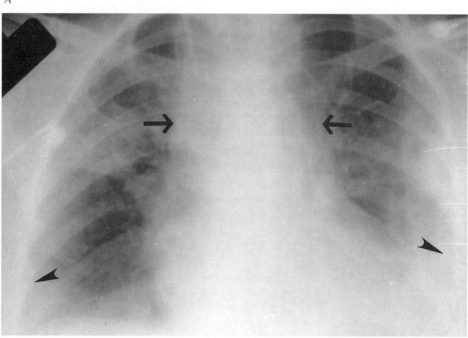

FIG. 3-E-29 *Panels A and B.*

B

CASE 3-28
A routine supine chest radiograph is obtained in an ICU patient after manipulation of the SG catheter (Fig. 3-E-28).

CASE 3-29
A supine chest radiograph is done at 8 A.M. after placement of a right internal jugular catheter (Fig. 3-E-29A), and a supine film is done 1.5 h later after the patient experienced extreme substernal chest pain (Fig. 5-E-29B).

Questions:

3-30. The complication of SG catheter placement in Case 3-26 is
  A. malposition of the tip.
  B. pneumothorax.
  C. perforation.
  D. catheter coiling.
  E. catheter thrombosis.

3-31. The complication of CVP catheter placement in Case 3-27 (Fig. 3-E-27) is
  A. malposition of the tip.
  B. pneumothorax.
  C. perforation.
  D. catheter coiling.
  E. catheter thrombosis.

3-32. The major potential risk of the SG catheter position in Case 3-28 (Fig. 3-E-28) is
  A. inaccurate pulmonary pressures.
  B. perforation.
  C. bleeding.
  D. infarction.
  E. arteriovenous malformation.

3-33. The complication of catheter placement in Case 3-29 (Fig. 3-E-29*A,B*) is
  A. mediastinal hemorrhage.
  B. pneumothorax.
  C. pneumomediastinum.
  D. pulmonary infarction.
  E. myocardial infarction.

Radiologic Findings:

3-26. The supine portable chest radiograph obtained after SG catheter placement in this case (Fig. 3-E-26) shows the catheter coiled within the right ventricle before it terminates in the proximal main pulmonary artery (*D* is the correct answer to Question 3-30). This coiling of the catheter in the right ventricle may cause thrombosis or arrhythmia, and it was necessary to reposition this catheter after this film was obtained.

3-27. The supine chest radiograph in this case (Fig. 3-E-27) shows a right pneumothorax after a difficult CVP placement (*B* is the correct answer to Question 3-31). Pneumothorax is one of the potential complications of subclavian venous catheterization because the apex of the lung is only approximately 0.5 cm below the subclavian vein. Therefore, a needle approach under the clavicle may puncture the apex of the lung and produce a pneumothorax. Fortunately, this is not a very common complication of CVP catheterization.

3-28. In this case, the chest radiograph obtained after manipulation of the SG catheter (Fig. 3-E-28) shows the tip of the catheter to be wedged out the right descending pulmonary artery. This catheter extends beyond the larger proximal artery and does have the potential to cause pulmonary infarction (*D* is the correct answer to Question 3-32). Routine chest radiographs are obtained after SG catheter placement to document the tip of the catheter and to make sure that there are no other complications from the catheter placement.

3-29. In this case, there are two supine chest films. Figure 3-E-29A shows cardiomegaly and was obtained after a right internal jugular catheter was inserted (*arrow*). The tip of the catheter can be seen superimposed over the right apex of the lung. At this time there is no complication from the catheter placement, despite the cardiomegaly and ill-defined opacity, which proved to be pneumonia, in the right upper lobe. The next supine film was done 2 h later (Fig. 3-E-29B) and shows widening of the mediastinum and increasing cardial/pericardial silhouette (*arrows*). Associated pleural effusions are also seen (*arrowheads*). The patient was experiencing substernal chest pain, and a CT scan obtained later showed that this catheter tip had perforated the internal jugular vein and was in the mediastinum. These findings represent a mediasternal and pleural hemorrhage after vessel perforation by the catheter (*A* is the correct answer to Question 3-33).

Discussion:

As mentioned in the subsection on monitoring devices within the chapter, a number of catheters can be inserted into the heart and great vessels to monitor various hemodynamic parameters, particularly in the ICU setting. Table 3-3 lists the most common monitoring devices, and Table 3-4 shows the most common complications from placement of these devices. We have reviewed the normal placement of catheters and some of the more common related complications. The student should be familiar with this aspect of radiography in the ICU setting, and the Bibliography at the end of the chapter provides further in-depth learning.

The heart and great vessels present an interesting and demanding diagnostic challenge to the physician. A thorough history and physical examination are the initial steps to generate a differential diagnosis and to decide which imaging tests are necessary to limit these possibilities. The choice of imaging tests ideally should be made in consultation with the imager, taking into consideration potential morbidity, cost, and availability of the technology and the interest and expertise of the imager. Students should be aware that careful decision making has the potential to decrease the cost of medical care in the United States.

BIBLIOGRAPHY

Elliott LP (ed): *Cardiac Imaging in Infants, Children, and Adults.* Philadelphia, Lippincott, 1991.

Gedgaudas E et al: *Cardiovascular Radiology.* Philadelphia, Saunders, 1985.

Higgins CB: *Essentials of Cardiac Radiology and Imaging.* Philadelphia, Lippincott, 1992.

Swischuk LE, Sapire DW: *Basic Imaging in Congenital Heart Disease,* 3d ed. Baltimore, Williams & Wilkins, 1986.

Swischuk LE: *Plain Film Interpretation in Congenital Heart Disease,* 2d ed. Baltimore, Williams & Wilkins, 1979.

4

RADIOLOGY OF THE CHEST

Caroline Chiles
Robert H. Choplin

The chest radiograph is the most frequently performed radiographic study in the United States. It should almost always be the first radiologic study ordered for evaluation of diseases of the thorax. The natural contrast of the aerated lungs provides a window into the body to evaluate the patient for diseases involving the heart, lungs, pleurae, tracheobronchial tree, esophagus, thoracic lymph nodes, thoracic skeleton, chest wall, and upper abdomen. In both acute and chronic illnesses, the chest radiograph allows one to detect a disease and monitor its response to therapy. For many disease processes (e.g., pneumonia and congestive heart failure), the diagnosis can be established and the disease followed to resolution with no further imaging studies. There are limitations to the chest radiograph, and diseases may not be sufficiently advanced to be detected or may not result in detectable abnormalities. Other imaging methods are needed to complement the conventional chest radiograph. These imaging methods include computed tomography (CT), magnetic resonance imaging (MRI), ultrasound (US), and radionuclide studies. These techniques, their clinical uses, and case studies are included in this chapter.

TECHNIQUES

Conventional Radiography

THE POSTEROANTERIOR AND LATERAL CHEST RADIOGRAPHS

The simplest conventional studies of the chest are posteroanterior and lateral chest radiographs taken in a radiographic unit specially designed for these studies. The x-rays travel through the patient and expose a receptor from which the image is recorded. Most commonly, the receptor is an intensifying screen and radiographic film, but there are several types of digital radiographic receptors in use as well. Computed radiography and large field-of-view image intensifiers are two types of these receptors. The digital images may be printed on film by laser printers or viewed on monitors. The two views of a chest radiograph are taken in projections at 90 degrees to each other with the patient's breath held at the end of a maximum inspiration. The first view is obtained as the patient faces the film cassette with the x-ray beam source positioned 6 ft behind him or her. Since the x-ray beam travels in a posterior-to-anterior direction, this view is called a *posteroanterior* (PA) chest radiograph. Another view is then obtained with the patient turned 90 degrees with the left side against the film cassette and the arms overhead. The x-ray beam travels from right to left through the patient, and this is called a *left lateral view.* Anatomic features of the chest that are readily identifiable on plain radiographs are shown in Figs. 4-1 and 4-2.

OTHER RADIOGRAPHIC PROJECTIONS

In some clinical situations, patients may not be able to stand or sit upright for the conventional PA and lateral radiographs, and a film must be taken with the patient's back turned to the film cassette and the x-ray beam traversing the patient in an anterior-to-posterior direction. These radiographs are called *anteroposterior* (AP) radiographs. They may be taken in the x-ray department but are more commonly obtained as portable studies at the patient's bedside.

Films also may be obtained with the patient lying on one side in a decubitus position with the x-ray beam traversing the patient either PA or AP along a horizontal plane. These films are designated as *lateral decubitus films.* A left lateral decubitus radiograph indicates that the left side of the patient is dependent against the table. A

right lateral decubitus radiograph indicates that the right side of the patient is dependent against the table. Films may be taken with the patient lying on the back with the x-ray beam traversing from side to side in a horizontal direction. These films are designated *cross-table lateral films.* Finally, films may be taken with the patient lying on one side with the x-ray beam traversing from side to side in a vertical direction. In our department, these films are designated *lateral recumbent films.*

THE PORTABLE CHEST RADIOGRAPH

If the clinical situation prevents the patient from coming to the radiology department, a chest radiograph may be obtained at the patient's beside, and these are almost always AP radiographs. The AP portable radiograph does not provide as much information as PA and lateral chest radiographs for a number of reasons. Because it is a single view, lesions are not as easily or accurately localized along the AP axis of the thorax. The patients for whom these films are obtained are usually quite ill and cannot be positioned as well as patients traveling to the x-ray department. Such

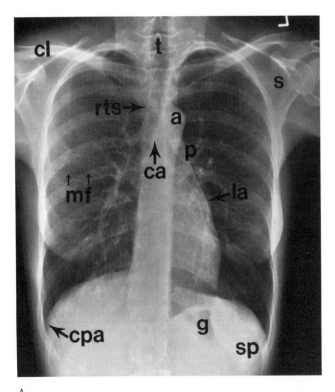

A

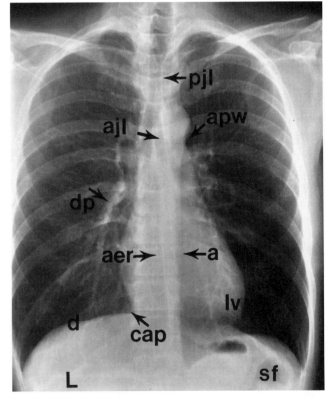

B

FIG. 4-1 Normal radiographic anatomy. Posteroanterior chest radiographs. [Key to Figs. 4-1 and 4-2: a = aorta; aer = azygoesophageal recess; ajl = anterior junction line; apw = aortopulmonary window; bi = bronchus intermedius; ca = carina; cap = cardiophrenic angle; cpa = costophrenic angle; cl = clavicle; d = diaphragm; dp = descending (or interlobar) pulmonary artery; g = gastric air bubble; ivc = inferior vena cava; L = liver; la = left atrium; lpa = left pulmonary artery; lul = left upper lobe bronchus; lv = left ventricle; m = manubrium; mf = minor fissure; MF = major fissure; p = main pulmonary artery; pjl = posterior junction line; rpa = right pulmonary artery; rts = right tracheal (or paratracheal) stripe; rul = right upper lobe bronchus; rv = right ventricle; s = scapula; sf = splenic flexure of colon; sp = spleen; svc = superior vena cava; t = trachea; v = vertebral body.]

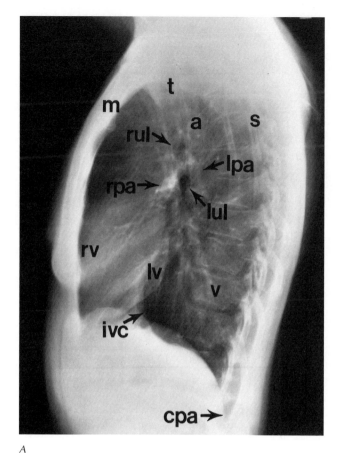

A

FIG. 4-2 Normal radiographic anatomy. Lateral chest radiographs. (See Fig. 4-1 for key.)

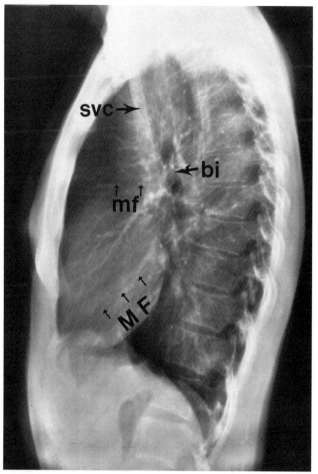

B

patients frequently cannot cooperate by holding their breath at total lung capacity. A mobile x-ray generator is typically not as powerful as a fixed x-ray generator, and longer exposure times are therefore necessary to obtain sufficient film exposure. The quality of portable chest radiographs, therefore, is often inferior to that of PA and lateral radiographs as a result of both respiratory and cardiac motion. X-ray grids are used to reduce scatter radiation and improve image quality. Grids are used for most conventional chest films done in radiology departments where fixed equipment is present. Grids are not usually used for portable radiographs, and the result is a high proportion of scattered x-rays that degrade the image. Paradoxically, the portable radiograph may be more expensive than conventional PA and lateral chest radiographs owing to extra labor and equipment costs in obtaining a bedside radiograph.

FLUOROSCOPY OF THE CHEST

Fluoroscopy is performed by placing the patient in a radiation beam and capturing the image on an image intensifier. While the radiation beam is on, the images provide a real-time evaluation of the patient. The images may be permanently recorded on film, magnetic or optical media, or intermittently as spot films. The equipment is not dedicated to chest evaluation. Depending on the task to be accom-

plished, the fluoroscopy equipment ranges from relatively simple to the complex biplane units designed for angiography.

Computed Tomography of the Chest

Computed tomography (CT) produces axial slices of the chest, virtually eliminating superimposition of structures. The patient lies on a table within the circular gantry of the CT scanner. Several types of scanners are available, but all project x-rays at multiple angles through a single plane of the patient. The table may be advanced in increments while the radiographic beam is off or smoothly at precise speeds while the x-ray beam is on. The information about the attenuation of the multiple x-ray beams is processed by a computer, which reconstructs the data to produce images of the patient. The scan may take several minutes to an hour, depending on the type of CT scanner used and the number of axial images obtained. Intravenous contrast material is frequently administered for opacification of arteries and veins within the mediastinum and hila to facilitate recognition of abnormal masses or lymph nodes. Anatomic features of the chest that are readily identifiable on CT scans are shown in Figs. 4-3 and 4-4.

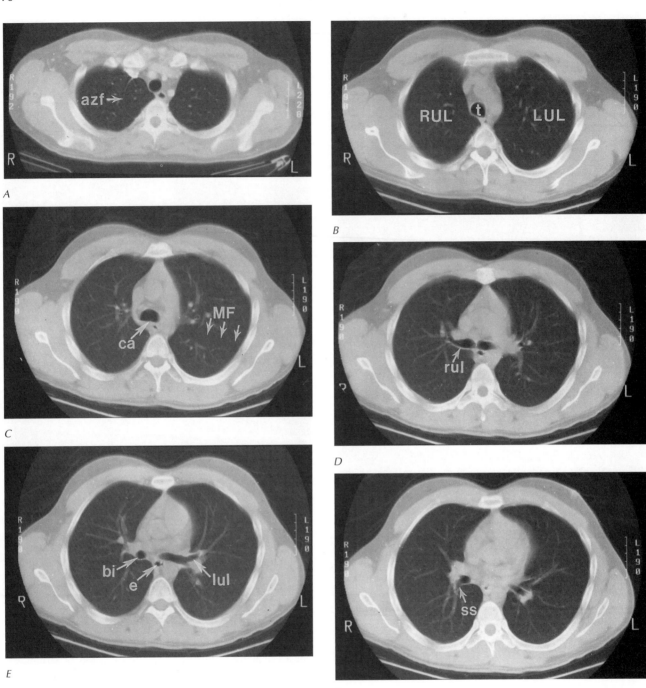

FIG. 4-3 Normal CT anatomy. Axial scans of the chest, contiguous slices at 1 cm collimation, lung window settings. [Key to Figs. 4-3 and 4-4: a = aorta; aa = ascending aorta; arch = transverse section of the aortic arch; azf = azygos fissure (normal variant); azv = azygos vein; bb = basilar segmental bronchi of lower lobes; bi = bronchus intermedius; ca = carina; cc = common carotid artery; cl = clavicle; da = descending aorta; dp = descending (or interlobar) pulmonary artery; e = esophagus; hazv = hemiazygos vein; h = humerus; im = internal mammary artery and vein; ipv = inferior pulmonary vein; ivc = inferior vena cava; ivs = interventricular septum; l = liver; la = left atrium; lbv = left brachiocephalic vein; lcc = left common carotid artery; Li = lingula segment of the left upper lobe; lij = left internal jugular vein; LLL = left lower lobe; lpa = left pulmonary artery; lsa = left subclavian artery; lul = left upper lobe bronchus; LUL = left upper lobe; lv = left ventricle; m = manubrium; MF = major fissure; r = rib; ra = right atrium; rba = right brachiocephalic artery; rbv = right bronchiocephalic vein; rij = right internal jugular vein; RLL = right lower lobe; RML = right middle lobe; rml = right middle lobe bronchus; rpa = right pulmonary artery; rsa = right subclavian artery; rsv = right subclavian vein; RUL = right upper lobe; rul = right upper lobe bronchus; rv = right ventricle; rvot = right ventricular outflow tract; s = scapula; ss = bronchus to superior segment of lower lobe; st = sternum; svc = superior vena cava; t = trachea; th = thyroid; v = vertebral body.]

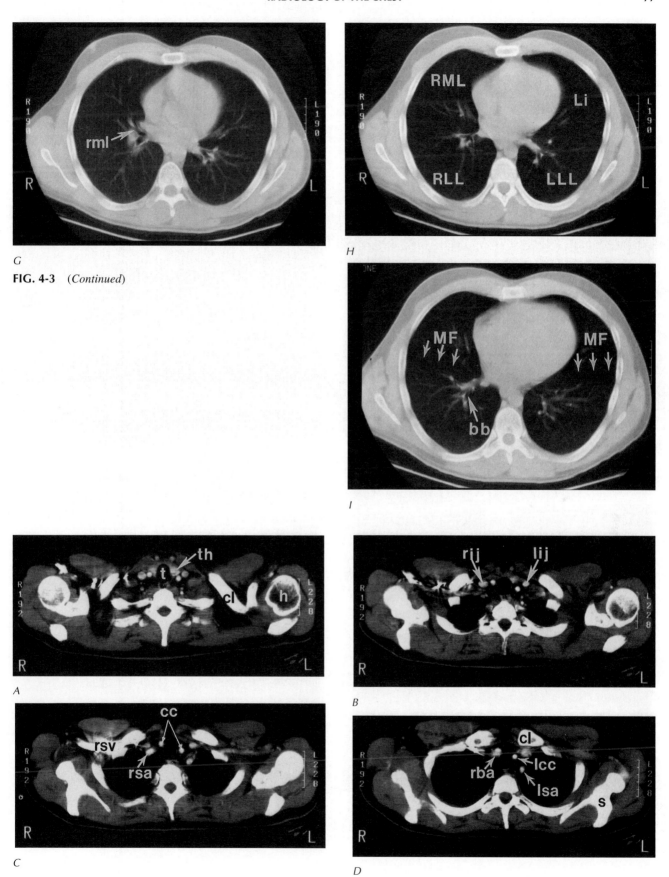

G

FIG. 4-3   (*Continued*)

H

I

A

B

C

D

FIG. 4-4   Normal CT anatomy. Axial scans of the chest, contiguous slices at 1 cm collimation, soft-tissue (mediastinal) window settings. (See Fig. 4-3 for key.)

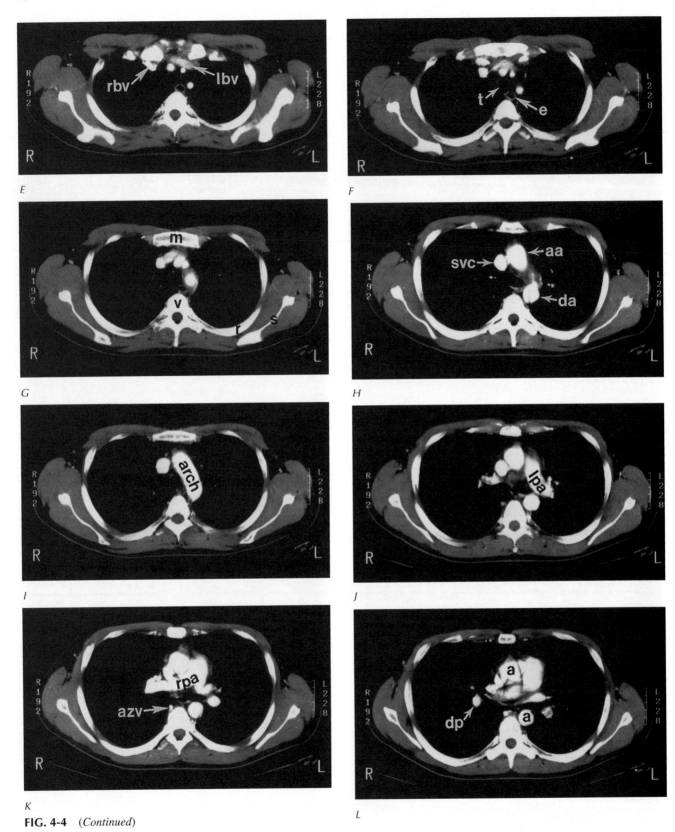

FIG. 4-4 *(Continued)*

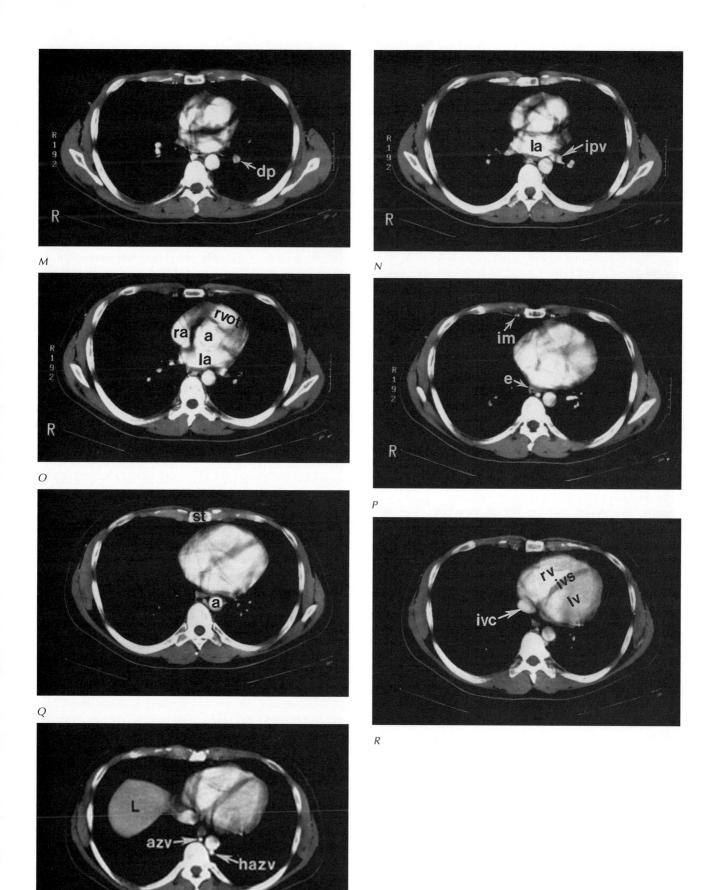

FIG. 4-4 (*Continued*)

Ultrasonography of the Chest

Sonographic images depict the transmission of sound waves into the body and their reflection. When a sound wave encounters air, it is almost completely reflected. The air within the lungs precludes sonographic imaging of them unless they are consolidated. On the other hand, fluid and soft tissues are often well depicted by this technique. Ultrasound equipment consists of the transducer, which emits the ultrasound waves and records their reflections, a computer to control the emissions and process the reflections, and a recording device. Ultrasound units come in a variety of sizes and offer a range of functions. The larger ones are usually placed in the x-ray department, whereas the smaller ones are portable and may be used throughout a hospital or imaging center. The images are sectional ones and are freely oriented by changing the position of the hand-held transducer.

Magnetic Resonance Imaging of the Chest

For magnetic resonance (MR) imaging the patient is placed in a strong magnetic field that is altered locally with radio-frequency waves. The changes in the patient's tissues are recorded as they return to the steady state. An MR imaging machine consists of the magnet, the coils that apply magnetic gradients, the radiofrequency coils, and computers to control the imaging and process the raw data. The MR imaging gantry is a tubular or C-shaped device in which the patient is usually placed in a supine position. A major advantage of MR imaging is that the patient is not exposed to ionizing radiation. A second advantage is that MR imaging offers a wider range of soft-tissue contrast than does CT. MR images may be acquired in any plane, and coronal and sagittal as well as axial images are commonly used. MR imaging does not require administration of intravenous contrast material to identify vessels, since no signal is recovered from flowing blood with spin-echo techniques. Any vascular structure containing flowing blood appears black (signal void) on spin-echo sequences, making the distinction between vessels and lymph nodes readily apparent even without intravenous contrast administration. In patients with allergy to x-ray contrast media, MR imaging may be the preferred examination. A major disadvantage of MR imaging in the thorax is its inability to provide adequate images of aerated or partially aerated lungs. Other disadvantages include decreased spatial resolution relative to CT and degradation of the image by cardiac and respiratory motion. In addition, patients with pacemakers, intraorbital metal fragments, retinal tacks, and some ferromagnetic prostheses cannot safely be placed within the magnetic field generated by the MR imaging scanner. The entire examination may take as little as 30 min or as long as several hours depending on the number of MR imaging sequences obtained. Anatomic features of the chest that are readily identifiable on MR images are shown in Figs. 4-5 and 4-6.

Nuclear Medicine

Nuclear medicine techniques used in evaluating diseases of the thorax include ventilation-perfusion ($\dot{V}/\dot{Q}$) scanning, scanning for sites of inflammation with white cells labeled with gallium-67 or indium-111, and scanning with tumor-seeking radiopharmaceuticals for tumor staging. The $\dot{V}/\dot{Q}$ scan is the imaging study of choice for a patient with suspected pulmonary thromboembolism. The $\dot{V}/\dot{Q}$ scan is non-invasive, and when results are negative, fewer than 10 percent of patients have pulmonary thromboembolism. The ventilation study is typically performed with the patient inhaling 10 to 30 mCi of xenon-133 while images are obtained with a scintillation camera (Fig. 4-7A). Wash-in images are obtained for two consecutive 120-s periods, an equilibrium image is obtained, and then wash-out images are obtained over 30- to 60-s periods in posterior and left and right posterior oblique projections. This portion of the study takes about 15 min. The perfusion scan is obtained by intravenously injecting 2 to 4 mCi of technetium-99m–labeled macroaggregated albumin containing 200,000 to 700,000 particles. The particles range in size from 10 to 100 μm, and they lodge in capillaries and capillary arterioles, accurately reflecting pulmonary blood flow (Fig. 4-7B). The scintillation camera is set so that it obtains anterior, posterior, both posterior oblique, and both anterior oblique projections for 750,000 counts per image. The perfusion study takes about 30 min to perform.

Other radionuclide scans used for the evaluation of suspected pulmonary disease include gallium-67 citrate scans, in which gallium accumulates in leukocytes and in some tumors. After 5 mCi of gallium-67 citrate is injected intravenously, scans are obtained at 24 to 72 h, allowing time for blood background and colon activity to clear. Abnormal increase in activity in the lungs may be focal or diffuse and may correspond to disease activity in inflammatory diseases, including sarcoidosis, radiation pneumonitis, and idiopathic pulmonary fibrosis, as well as in pneumonia and lung abscess. Gallium activity within the lung is usually reported as a gallium index, which is the product of an intensity of 0 to 4 (4 = area of greatest activity, usually the liver) multiplied by the percentage of total lung area involved. The maximum gallium index is 400 (intensity of 4×100 percent involvement). Gallium has affinity for some tumors, including lymphomas, and can be used to detect occult sites of tumor either at presentation or during recurrence.

Another test that can be used to detect occult sites of infection is the indium-111–labeled white blood cell (WBC), or leukocyte, scan. The serous layer of an 80-mL blood sample taken from the patient is centrifuged to produce a white blood cell button. The 1 to 2 mCi of indium-111 is added to the resuspended white blood cells. The labeled white blood cells are reinjected into a peripheral vein, and scanning is performed 24 to 48 h after injection. The activity accumulates in sites of infection, and this test could be used to distinguish between pneumonia or lung

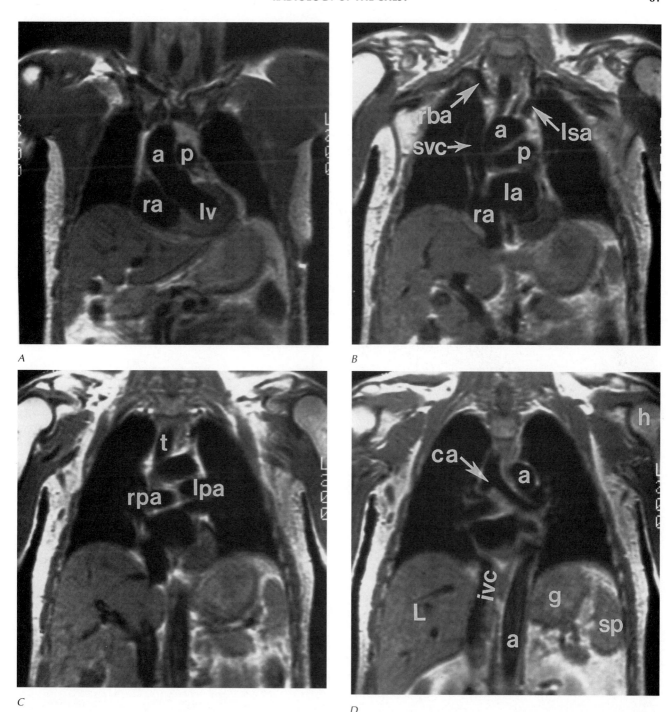

A

B

C

D

FIG. 4-5 Normal MR imaging anatomy. Coronal spin-echo images of the thorax. [Key to Figs. 4-5 and 4-6: a = aorta; aa = ascending aorta; arch = transverse section of the aortic arch; azv = azygos vein; bi = bronchus intermedius; ca = carina; da = descending aorta; dp = descending (or interlobar) pulmonary artery; e = esophagus; g = gastric fundus; h = humerus; im = internal mammary artery and vein; ipv = inferior pulmonary vein; ivc = inferior vena cava; ivs = interventricular septum; k = kidney; L = liver; la = left atrium; lcc = left common carotid artery; lpa = left pulmonary artery; lsa = left subclavian artery; lv = left ventricle; m = manubrium; p = pulmonary artery; pc = pericardium; ra = right atrium; rba = right brachiocephalic artery; rca = right coronary artery; rpa = right pulmonary artery; rv = right ventricle; rvot = right ventricular outflow tract; sp = spleen; spv = superior pulmonary vein; st = sternum; svc = superior vena cava; t = trachea; v = vertebral body.].

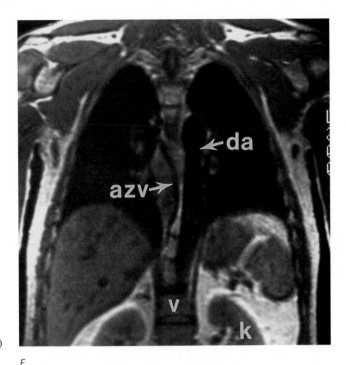

FIG. 4-5 *(Continued)*

E

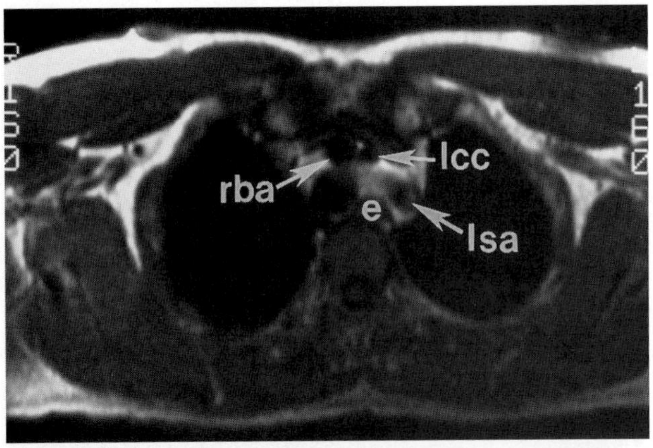

A

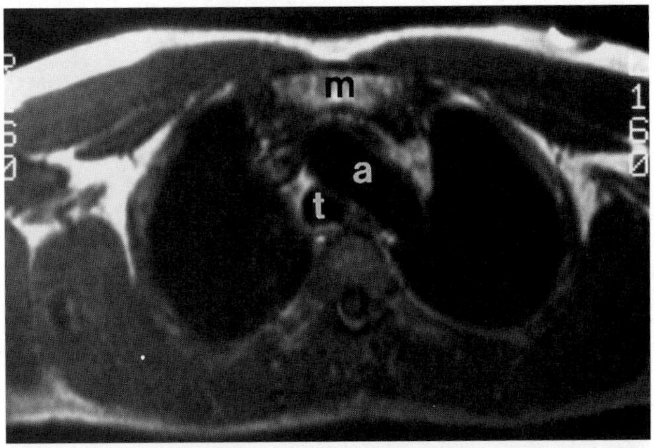

B

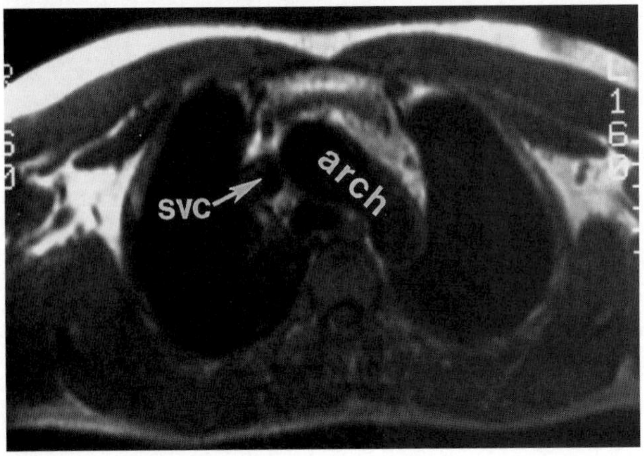

C

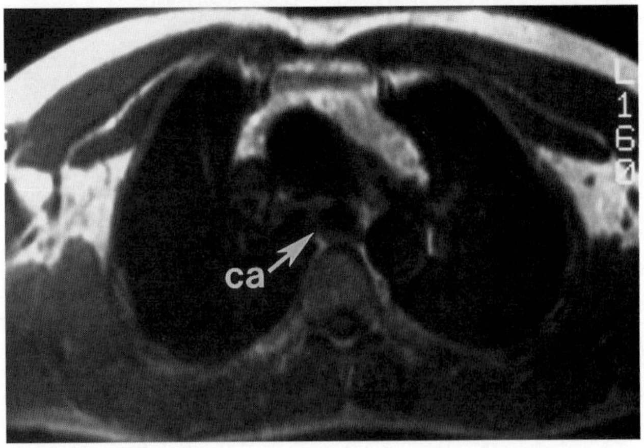

D

FIG. 4-6 Normal MR imaging anatomy. Axial spin-echo images of the thorax. (See Fig. 4-5 for key.)

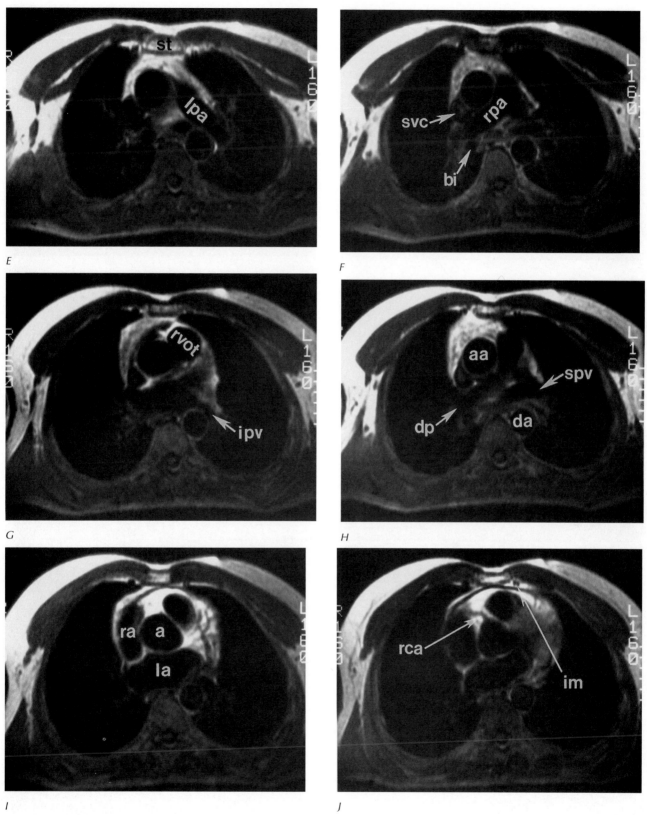

FIG. 4-6 (*Continued*)

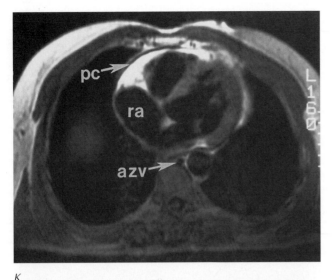

K

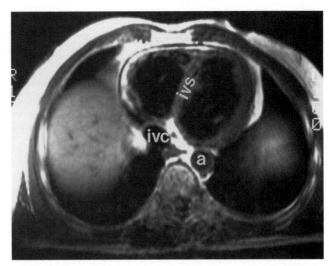

L

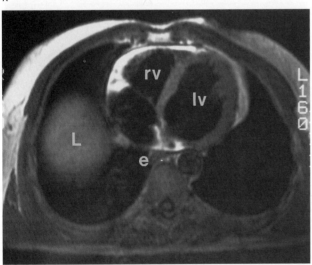

M

FIG. 4-6 (*Continued*)

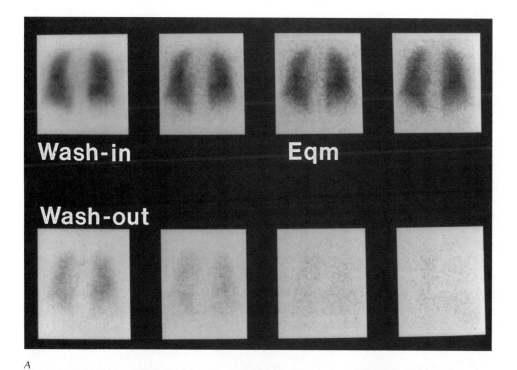

A

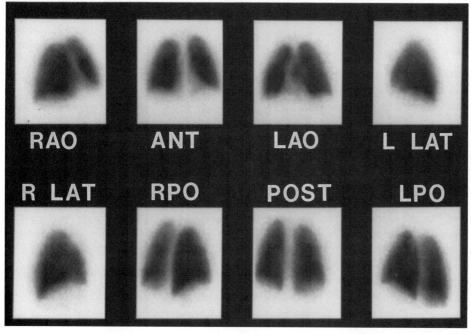

B

FIG. 4-7 (*A*) Ventilation scan performed in the posterior projection shows normal wash-out of the xenon-133 gas and no retention of gas in any regions on the wash-out views (Eqm = equilibrium). (*B*) Normal perfusion scans are performed in eight projections of equal profusion of radionuclide throughout all segments of the lungs (RAO = right anterior oblique; ANT = anterior; LAO = left anterior oblique; LLAT = left lateral; RLAT = right lateral; RPO = right posterior oblique; POST = posterior; LPO = left posterior oblique).

abscess and noninfectious lung diseases. In practice, this test is infrequently obtained for pulmonary disease, since CT almost always localizes abnormalities precisely and fiberoptic bronchoscopy is very effective for diagnosis of pulmonary abnormalities.

Tomography is also available for radionuclide imaging as two other techniques. Single photon emission computed tomography (SPECT) is used for photon emitters (technetium-99m, indium-111, iodine-123). The primary advantage of SPECT is the ability to depict anatomy in three dimensions. SPECT may be used to improve the spatial resolution of radionuclide imaging, including perfusion scans, and gallium-67– and indium-111–labeled WBC scans. A positron-emission tomography (PET) scanner resembles a CT scanner and uses positron emitters (fluorine-18, carbon-11). Today, the most widely used positron emitter is fluorine-18 deoxyglucose (FDG), which is used as a metabolic tracer. The raised metabolic rate can be used to distinguish neoplasm and inflammation from normal tissue. Although PET provides tomographic images, the spatial resolution (0.7 to 1.0 cm) is somewhat inferior to that of CT.

TECHNIQUE SELECTION

The number of diseases and clinical situations for which a chest radiograph may be indicated is so large that an exhaustive listing of individual indications is prohibitive. As a general rule, however, conventional radiographs should be obtained for any patient with symptoms suggesting disease of the heart, lungs, mediastinum, or chest wall. In addition, a chest radiograph is indicated for patients with systemic disease that have a high likelihood of secondary involvement of those structures. Examples of the former are pneumonia and congestive heart failure and of the latter are a primary extrathoracic neoplasm and connective-tissue disease.

In an acutely ill patient, the portable chest radiograph is an invaluable tool for monitoring the patient's cardiopulmonary status. These radiographs are also used for monitoring of life-support hardware, such as central venous access catheters, nasogastric tubes, and endotracheal tubes.

Fluoroscopy provides real-time imaging of the chest. Fluoroscopy may be used to evaluate the motion of the diaphragm in a patient with suspected diaphragmatic paralysis. A paralyzed hemidiaphragm has sluggish motion as the patient breathes, and as the patient takes in a quick breath of air, it moves paradoxically upward as the normal hemidiaphragm moves downward ("sniff test"). Fluoroscopy and fluoroscopically positioned spot films are also useful for identification of calcification within a pulmonary nodule, within coronary arteries, and within cardiac valves. Fluoroscopic guidance is commonly used for percutaneous transthoracic needle biopsy of lung masses.

Since the three dimensions of the thorax are captured on a single two-dimensional chest radiograph, superimposition of structures within the thorax may result in confusing shadows. Because CT provides images without this overlap, it is used frequently to clarify confusing shadows identified on conventional radiographs (Table 4-1). These examinations are also used to detect disease that is occult because of small size or a hidden position. Because of its wider range of density discrimination, CT can demonstrate mediastinal and chest wall abnormalities earlier than is possible with conventional chest radiography. Abnormalities of hilar structures can be identified on CT scans because of the decreased overlap of the complex structures of the hilum. CT scans of the chest are ordered routinely for oncology patients both for evaluation of the extent of disease at presentation and for monitoring response to therapy or progression of disease. CT is useful for evaluation of the lung parenchyma, since thin sections (1 to 2 mm thick) reveal great anatomic detail. Thin-section CT [or high-resolution CT (HRCT)] may enable detection of occult pulmonary parenchymal disease and may be used for following the course of known pulmonary disease. Because intravenous contrast material may be administered, vascular structures may be evaluated, and the technique may be useful in patients with aortic dissection, aortic aneurysm, and superior vena caval obstruction. Because the cost of CT is approximately 10 to 20 times that of PA and lateral chest radiographs, CT is not practical for monitoring the course of disease on a daily basis.

Ultrasonography is useful for imaging the soft tissues of the chest wall, heart, and pericardium, as well as fluid collections within the pleural space. Large, mobile pleural effusions are usually aspirated without sonographic guidance, since these collect predictably within dependent

TABLE 4-1   INDICATIONS FOR CT OF THE CHEST

Clarification of abnormal chest radiograph findings

Staging of lung cancer and esophageal cancer

Detecting metastatic disease from extrathoracic malignancy

Evaluation of a solitary pulmonary nodule

Suspected mediastinal or hilar mass

Evaluation of chronic pulmonary disease (thin-section or high-resolution CT)

Suspected pleural tumor or empyema

Determining source of hemoptysis (e.g., bronchiectasis)

CT-guided percutaneous needle aspiration of lung and mediastinal masses

CT-guided pleural drainage

areas of the thorax. On the other hand, loculated pleural fluid collections may be difficult to aspirate without guidance, and the most appropriate entrance site may be marked with sonography for easier access. Ultrasonography has been used for guidance for biopsy of peripheral lung lesions as well.

MR imaging of the thorax is used most commonly for cardiovascular imaging, but there are indications for MR imaging in mediastinal and pulmonary parenchymal imaging as well (Table 4-2). MR imaging is helpful when bronchogenic carcinoma is suspected of invading vascular structures, including the cardiac chambers, pulmonary arteries and veins, and superior vena cava. In a patient with suspected Pancoast's (superior sulcus) tumor, MR imaging is preferred to CT because of the ability to obtain images in coronal and sagittal planes. The apex of the lung can be difficult to evaluate on axial images alone because of partial-volume effects.

The diseases and situations for which nuclear medicine techniques are helpful are determined for the most part by the radioactive tracer, and these have been outlined in the Technique section (Table 4-3).

TABLE 4-2   INDICATIONS FOR MR IMAGING OF THE CHEST

Evaluation of a mediastinal mass

Suspected Pancoast (superior sulcus) tumor

Superior vena cava syndrome

Staging of lung cancer, when CT suggests invasion of the heart, great vessels, chest wall, diaphragm

Suspected aortic dissection

Evaluation of the mediastinum and hilum in patients with allergy to iodinated contrast media

Congenital and acquired heart disease

TABLE 4-3   INDICATIONS FOR NUCLEAR MEDICINE IMAGING OF THE CHEST

Suspected pulmonary thromboembolism ($\dot{V}/\dot{Q}$ scan)

Staging of inflammatory disease (e.g., sarcoidosis) (gallium scan)

Detecting recurrence of lymphoma (gallium scan)

Detecting infection (indium-111–labeled WBC scan)

Differentiation of benign and malignant pulmonary nodule (PET)

Detecting recurrent or metastatic tumor (PET)

EXERCISE 4-1: THE OPAQUE HEMITHORAX

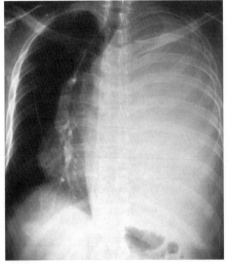

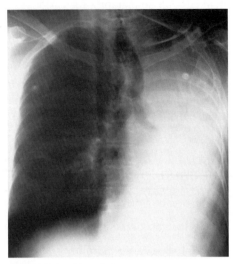

FIG. 4-E-2   *(Panel A)*

FIG. 4-E-1   *(Panel A)*

Clinical Histories: **CASE 4-1**
A 40-year-old man presents with fever and dyspnea (Fig. 4-E-1*A*).

CASE 4-2
A 62-year-old man presents with dyspnea that has increased over 2 days (Fig. 4-E-2*A*).

Questions: **4-1.**   The most likely diagnosis for Case 4-1 is
          A.   massive left pleural effusion.
          B.   total atelectasis of the left lung.
          C.   right pneumothorax.
          D.   aplasia of the left lung.
          E.   mediastinal hematoma.

4-2.   The most likely diagnosis for Case 4-2 is
          A.   left pleural effusion.
          B.   collapse of the left lung.
          C.   right pneumothorax.
          D.   collapse of the right lung.
          E.   mediastinal hematoma.

Radiologic Findings: 4-1. In this case, a frontal chest radiograph (Fig. 4-E-1*A*) shows that the left hemithorax is opaque. Signs of mass effect are present and suggest a space-occupying lesion in the left hemithorax. There is shift of the mediastinum toward the *contralateral* hemithorax, as evidenced by shift of the trachea and right heart border to the right. If a nasogastric tube were in place, esophageal shift could be inferred from the shift of the nasogastric tube. Space-occupying lesions also cause inferior displacement of the hemidiaphragm. Although the diaphragm itself is not visible, when the process is on the left, one can infer that the diaphragm is depressed by the inferior displacement of the gastric air bubble. Mass effect also may widen the distance between ribs. In this patient, the space-occupying lesion was a large left pleural effusion resulting from tubercu-

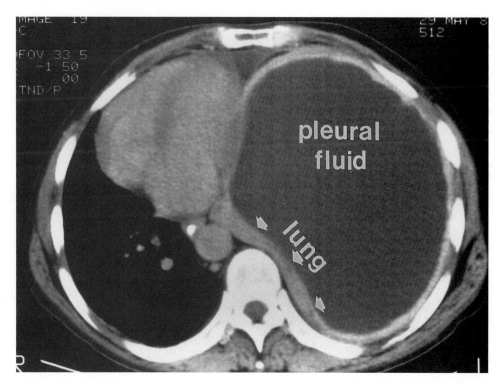

FIG. 4-E-1 (*Panel B*) Axial CT scan of the chest shows filling of the left pleural space by fluid, with compression of the left lung and displacement of the mediastinal contents in the right hemithorax. The pleural fluid in this case represented tuberculous empyema.

lous empyema. A chest CT scan (Fig. 4-E-1*B*) in this patient shows the large pleural effusion and complete collapse of the underlying left lung against the medial aspect of the left hemithorax (*A* is the correct answer to Question 4-1).

4-2. A frontal chest radiograph in this case (Fig. 4-E-2*A*) shows that the left hemithorax is also opaque. In contrast to the patient in Fig. 4-E-1*A*, the patient in Fig. 4-E-2*A* has signs of volume loss within the left hemithorax. There is mediastinal shift toward the *ipsilateral* hemithorax, as evidenced by shift of the trachea and the right heart border into the left hemithorax. If more air were visible within the stomach, one would expect that it would be higher in the left upper quadrant of the abdomen than is normally seen because of elevation of the left hemidiaphragm. The mediastinal window of the chest CT examination (Fig. 4-E-2*B*) shows the mediastinal shift to the left and total consolidation of the left lung (*arrows*). There is a small left pleural effusion (*arrowheads*). The lung window of the chest CT examination (Fig. 4-E-2*C*) shows that the right lung is aerated. In this patient the left lung collapse is due to a bronchogenic carcinoma in the left main bronchus. This case exhibits the signs of volume loss, as opposed to mass effect (*B* is the correct answer to Question 4-2).

Discussion:

This exercise reviews the principal signs that allow one to distinguish mass effect from volume loss. The mass effect caused by a tumor or by a large pleural effusion expands the hemithorax and displaces the trachea, mediastinum, and diaphragm away from the mass. There may be a subtle increase in the distance between ribs. Volume loss, on the other hand, decreases the size of the hemithorax, and the trachea, mediastinum, and diaphragm move toward the involved hemithorax. The distance between the ribs on the abnormal side will be slightly decreased. In both chest radiographs shown above, the left lung is collapsed. In Fig. 4-E-1*A*, the opacification of the left hemithorax occurs as a result of massive left pleural effusion, and the left lung is collapsed as a result of both compression by the fluid present within the left pleural space and a loss of the negative intrapleural pressure that keeps the lung in close juxtaposition to the chest wall. In Fig. 4-E-2*A*, the collapse is due to obstruction of the left main bronchus, resulting in atelectasis (airlessness) of the left lung.

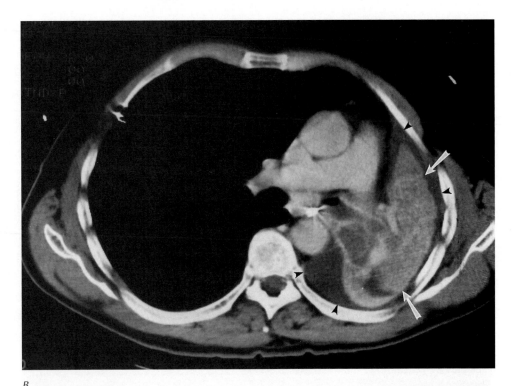

B

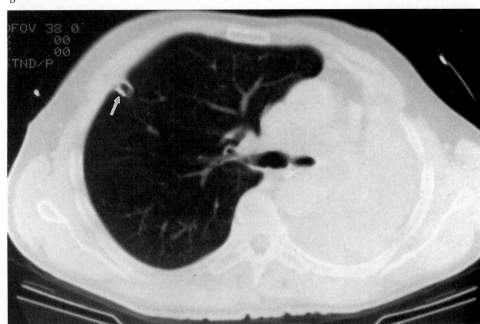

FIG. 4-E-2 (*Panel B*) CT scan shows mediastinal shift to the left, consolidation of the entire left lung (*arrows*), and small pleural effusion surrounding the left lung (*arrowheads*). (*Panel C*) Lung window shows that the right lung is overexpanded to compensate for the left lung atelectasis. A right-sided chest tube (*arrow*) is noted incidentally.

C

EXERCISE 4-2: LOBAR ATELECTASIS

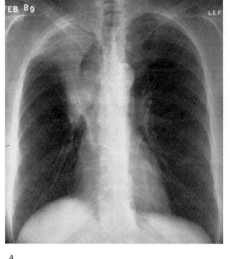

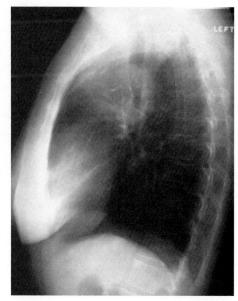

FIG. 4-E-3 (*Panels A and B*)

A

B

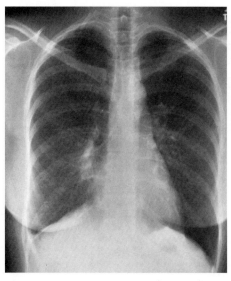

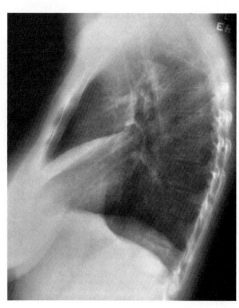

FIG. 4-E-4 (*Panels A and B*)

A

B

Clinical Histories:

CASE 4-3
A 61-year-old woman presents with dyspnea (Fig. 4-E-3).

CASE 4-4
A 45-year-old woman presents with chronic cough (Fig. 4-E-4).

FIG. 4-E-5 (*Panels A and B*)

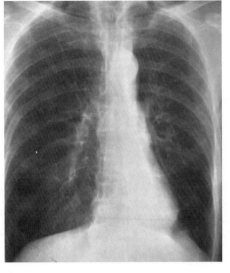

A

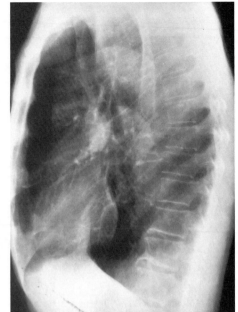

B

FIG. 4-E-6 (*Panels A and B*)

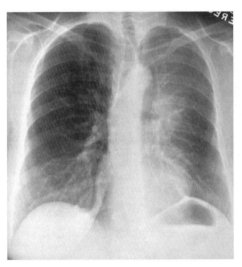

A

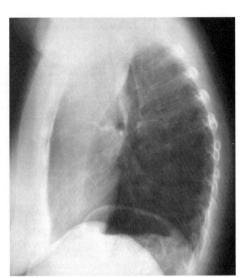

B

CASE 4-5
A 62-year-old man presents with a cough productive of blood-tinged sputum (Fig. 4-E-5A,B).

CASE 4-6
A 49-year-old woman presents with cough (Fig. 4-E-6).

Questions:

4-3. In Fig. 4-E-3, the inferior margin of the opacity in the right upper thorax is due to
A. the major fissure in right upper lobe (RUL) collapse without a hilar mass.
B. the minor fissure in RUL collapse with a hilar mass.
C. the minor fissure in RUL collapse without a hilar mass.
D. the major fissure in RUL collapse with a hilar mass.

4-4. In Fig. 4-E-4, all the following are true with regard to right middle lobe collapse except
A. a triangular opacity is superimposed on the heart on the lateral radiograph.
B. the right heart border is obscured.
C. the minor fissure is inferiorly displaced.
D. the right heart border is shifted to the left.

4-5. In Fig. 4-E-5A,B, signs of left lower lobe collapse include all the following except
A. obscuration of the lateral wall of the descending thoracic aorta.
B. inferior displacement of the left hilum.
C. obliteration of the posterior aspect of the left hemidiaphragm on the lateral view.
D. triangular opacity in the left retrocardiac area on the frontal view.
E. shift of the major fissure toward the anterior chest wall on the lateral view.

4-6. In Fig. 4-E-6, signs of left upper lobe collapse include all the following except
A. A crescent of air around the transverse section of the aortic arch resulting from hyperexpansion of the superior segment of the left lower lobe.
B. anterior displacement of the left major fissure on the lateral view.
C. obscuration of the left heart border.
D. tracheal deviation to the left.
E. inferior displacement of the left hilum.

Radiologic Findings:

4-3. In Fig. 4-E-3, there is opacity in the right upper lobe that is sharply marginated on its inferior border. Volume loss is evidenced by the slight displacement of the trachea into the right hemithorax, the position of the right heart border further to the right of the thoracic spine than normal, and the slight elevation of the right hemidiaphragm, which is normally 1 to 1.5 cm higher than the left hemithorax. The pulmonary vessels of the right hilum are obscured by opacity in the right upper thorax. The configuration of the inferior margin of the opacity is that of a reverse S or S on its side. The S sign of Golden describes the appearance of the minor fissure in right upper lobe collapse, which is due to bronchogenic carcinoma. In this case, bulky right hilar lymph node enlargement has caused extrinsic compression of the right upper lobe bronchus and has resulted in right upper lobe collapse. The right hilar mass tethers the medial aspect of the minor fissure to its normal midthoracic position, whereas the lateral aspect of the minor fissure moves freely and collapses superiorly. In patients in whom the minor fissure is incomplete, collateral air drift across the canals of Lambert and the pores of Kohn may allow a lobe to remain aerated despite complete obstruction of its bronchus. In Fig. 4-E-3A, hyperexpansion of the superior segment of the right lower lobe produces the ovoid lucency on the medial aspect of the collapsed right upper lobe. On the lateral radiograph, a V-shaped opacity is seen at the lung apex. A masslike opacity is superimposed on the suprahilar area, corresponding to a combination of tumor and atelectatic lung (*B* is the correct answer to Question 4-3). In patients with right upper lobe collapse without a hilar mass, the fissure is able to rotate in a more straight line and does not result in the reverse S sign. The major fissure is oriented in a coronal plane and is not normally visualized on the frontal chest radiograph. Therefore, the major fissure would not account for the opacity seen on the frontal chest radiograph, either with or without a hilar mass.

4-4. In Fig. 4-E-4, the right heart border is obscured by adjacent opacity on the PA radiograph. The heart is in the midthorax in approximately its normal position. The heart border has not been displaced to the left. On the lateral radiograph, a narrow triangular opacity is superimposed on the heart. The apex of the triangle points toward the hilum, and the base of the triangle is against the anterior chest wall. This is a collapsed right middle lobe. The right hemidiaphragm is slightly elevated, but there are no other signs of volume loss. Right middle lobe collapse may have minimal impact on the overall volume in the right hemithorax because it is the smallest of the pulmonary lobes, and the upper and lower lobes can expand to compensate for its volume loss. Right middle lobe collapse, unlike other lobar collapse, is often due to benign causes and results from extrinsic pressure because of enlarged lymph nodes, which totally surround the bronchus. This enlargement is most frequently due to granulomatous disease of an infectious or noninfectious nature (*D* is correct answer to Question 4-4).

4-5. When the left lower lobe collapses, the result is a triangular opacity, which can be quite subtle, behind the heart. Secondary signs of volume loss, however, should prompt one to look closely for the collapse. These signs include a shift of the trachea and heart to the left (note that the right heart border is now superimposed on the thoracic spine), inferior displacement of the left hilum, and elevation of the left hemidiaphragm. On the lateral radiograph, the right hemidiaphragm is visible along its entire contour. However, the left hemidiaphragm is obscured posteriorly because it is in contact with the collapsed left lower lobe. Since it is tethered medially by the inferior pulmonary ligament, the left lower lobe collapses posteriorly and medially (Fig. 4-E-5*C*). The major fissure is displaced *posteriorly,* as well as rotated into a more sagittal orientation than the normal coronal orientation. All the statements in Question 4-5 are correct except shift of the major fissure toward the *anterior* chest wall on the lateral view (*E* is the correct answer to Question 4-5). You may have noted the large lung volumes in this patient, which are due to centrilobular emphysema. In this patient, who has a long history of cigarette smoking, a squamous cell carcinoma in the left lower lobe bronchus was responsible for the collapsed left lower lobe.

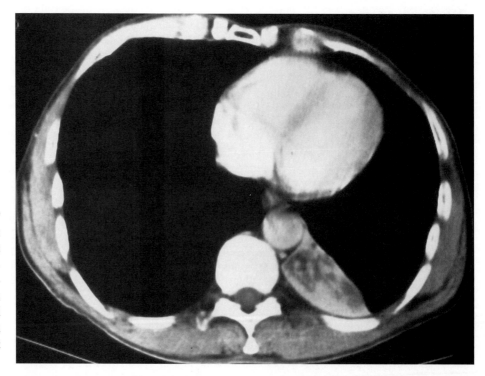

FIG. 4-E-5 (*Panel C*) Axial CT scan shows a triangular mass within the posteromedial aspect of the left hemithorax. This represents the collapsed left lower lobe. The branching areas of decreased attenuation within the mass represent mucoid impaction within the obstructed bronchi. Note the shift of the heart toward the left hemithorax.

4-6. The primary sign of volume loss in Fig. 4-E-6*B* is anterior displacement of the left major fissure on the lateral radiograph. The collapsed left upper lobe is opaque as a result of both airlessness and postobstructive pneumonitis. When there is little pneumonitis within the obstructed lobe, the left upper lobe can collapse completely behind the anterior chest wall so that only a narrow band of opacity is visible behind the sternum. In this situation, the diagnosis may be suggested by the secondary signs of volume loss. Note the shift of the trachea to the left and the slight elevation of the left hemidiaphragm. The left lower lobe is hyperexpanded. The hyperexpanded superior segment of the left lower lobe produces a crescent of air around the transverse section of the aortic arch on the PA radiograph. A thin opaque line is visible at the apex of the left hemidiaphragm on the PA radiograph. Presence of this line, called a *juxtaphrenic peak,* should prompt one to look for upper lobe collapse. The hilum may be displaced anteriorly in left upper lobe collapse, but it is never displaced inferiorly. Option *E* inferior displacement of the left hilum, is therefore false (*E* is the correct answer to Question 4-6). Since the lingular bronchus arises from the left upper lobe bronchus, the lingular segment of the left upper lobe is collapsed as well in this patient. The lingula is adjacent to the left heart border and is responsible for the obscuration of the left heart border in left upper lobe collapse.

Discussion:

The term *atelectasis* refers to volume loss, or airlessness, within the lung. The term *collapse* is often used to describe complete atelectasis of an entire lobe or an entire lung. Atelectasis can occur as a result of several pathophysiologic processes. Obstruction of a bronchus by bronchogenic carcinoma should always be considered in an adult with lobar atelectasis. The tumor may be within the bronchus (endobronchial), as occurs with squamous cell carcinoma or small cell undifferentiated carcinoma. The tumor may be outside the bronchus, and enlarged lymph nodes may cause extrinsic compression of the bronchus. In a child, aspiration of a foreign body is a more likely cause of obstruction of a bronchus. Complete obstruction of a lobar bronchus may not always result in lobar collapse because pathways of collateral ventilation are present within the lung. The pores of Kohn and the canals of Lambert allow collateral air drift between adjacent areas of lung but do not extend across pleural surfaces. The visceral pleural surface that covers the lung creates the interlobar fissures (minor fissure, major fissure) that separate lobes of the lungs. These fissures are not always complete, however, and may not extend entirely across the lung. When the right upper lobe bronchus is occluded, for example, the right upper lobe may remain partially aerated as a result of collateral air drift from the right middle lobe around an incomplete minor fissure. Obstruction of smaller airways can occur as a result of mucous plugs, which are often present in intubated patients and in patients with chronic small airways disease.

Passive atelectasis occurs as a result of a space-occupying process within the pleural space. This is also called *relaxation atelectasis,* since the lung is no longer exposed to the negative intrapleural pressure that normally keeps the lung apposed to the chest wall. Any space-occupying pleural process, including a large pneumothorax (air in the pleural space), pleural effusion, hemothorax (blood in the pleural space), or pleural tumor, can cause atelectasis within the underlying lung. *Cicatrization atelectasis* describes the volume loss that occurs as a result of pulmonary scarring. *Adhesive atelectasis* occurs when there is a loss of the pulmonary surfactant that maintains the surface tension that keeps alveoli open. Adhesive atelectasis occurs with pulmonary embolism and with respiratory distress syndrome of the newborn. Atelectasis of small areas of lung is often referred to as *subsegmental atelectasis* and may be recognized as linear bands of opacity, often at the lung bases.

It is helpful to remember the normal positions of the hemidiaphragms, trachea, mediastinum, and hila so that displacement of these structures can be readily noted. In most patients, the left hilum appears slightly higher than the right, since the left hilar opacity is predominantly due to the left pulmonary artery arching over the left main bronchus. The right hemidiaphragm is usually 1.0 to 1.5 cm higher than the left hemidiaphragm.

The trachea should be in the midline, and the spinous processes of the upper thoracic vertebrae should be superimposed on the center of the tracheal air column. The right heart border normally lies just to the right of the thoracic spine. Subtle signs of volume loss may be more readily appreciated by comparison of the patient's radiograph with baseline radiographs taken previously.

EXERCISE 4-3: AIRSPACE DISEASES

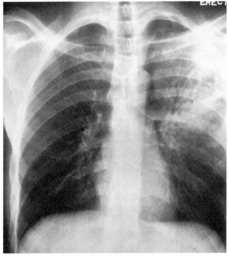

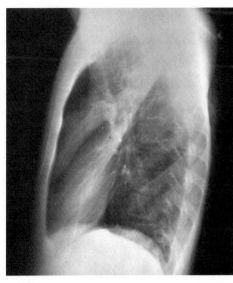

FIG. 4-E-7 (*Panels A and B*)

A

B

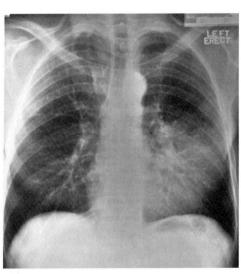

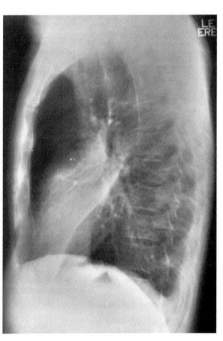

FIG. 4-E-8 (*Panels A and B*)

A   *B*

Clinical Histories:

CASE 4-7
A 32-year-old man presents with fever, cough, and hemoptysis (Fig. 4-E-7*A,B*).

CASE 4-8
A 57-year-old man presents with fever and a cough productive of purulent sputum (Fig. 4-E-8).

Questions:

4-7. Which of the following is not an accurate description of the opacity in the left upper lobe in Fig. 4-E-7*A,B*?
   A. Lobar distribution
   B. Ill-defined margins
   C. Reticular pattern
   D. Air bronchograms
   E. Airspace disease

4-8. For Fig. 4-E-8, which one of the following best explains the opacity in the left hemithorax?
   A. Collapse of the left upper lobe due to bronchial obstruction
   B. Airspace consolidation of the lingula
   C. Empyema loculated within the left major fissure
   D. Carcinoma in the left upper lobe

Radiologic Findings:

4-7 and 4-8. Both these patients have opacity in the left upper lobe. In the patient in Fig. 4-E-7, the opacity is in the upper lung and obscures the margin of the aortic arch. The opacity extends down to the hilum but does not obscure the left heart border. In the patient in Fig. 4-E-8, the opacity is lower in the hemithorax and obscures the lateral margin of the heart. On the lateral view of each patient, the posterior margin is sharply demarcated by the major fissure, indicating the lobar nature of the process. Radiolucent structures that exhibit a branching pattern are noted to arborize through both opacities.

Discussion:

The patient in Fig. 4-E-7 has primary tuberculosis (*Mycobacterium tuberculosis*), manifested as pneumonia in the anterior and apicoposterior segments of the left upper lobe. The patient in Fig. 4-E-8 has pneumococcal pneumonia (*Streptococcus pneumoniae*) in the superior and inferior lingula segments of the left upper lobe. The opacity seen on both radiographs is best described as airspace disease. The alveoli, or airspaces, that are normally filled with air have become filled with exudate. The exudate-filled alveoli surround the bronchi so that the air-filled bronchi are visible as radiolucent branching structures within the more radiopaque background (Fig. 4-E-7*C*). Airspace disease is often either lobar, multilobar, or diffuse in distribution. The process may appear initially as

FIG. 4-E-7 (*Panel C*) Close-up view of the left upper lobe shows an ill-defined infiltrate, that is radiopaque. Arborizing through this opacity are radiolucent branching structures representing the air-filled bronchi (air bronchograms) (*arrows*).

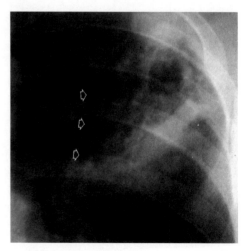

C

multiple ill-defined nodules that rapidly coalesce. These nodules are the shadows of fluid-filled acini. They are 6 to 10 mm in diameter and always have ill-defined margins. The margins of these coalescing opacities are difficult to outline. Although there can be associated volume loss as the surfactant within the alveoli is lost, the signs of volume loss are often subtle and do not account for the opacity seen within the lung. Once air-space disease is identified, an attempt should be made to determine its cause. Airspace disease that appears suddenly or exhibits change over hours to days is due either to pulmonary hemorrhage or to contusion, pneumonia, or pulmonary edema (blood, pus, or water). The patient's clinical history, physical examination, and laboratory data help to determine the most likely diagnosis.

In these two patients with fever and productive cough, pneumonia is likely (*B* is the correct answer to Question 4-8). On the other hand, a patient with rib or sternal fractures as a result of blunt chest trauma is more likely to have pulmonary contusion. Pulmonary edema, which may occur as a result of either cardiogenic or noncardiogenic disease, is discussed later in this chapter.

A reticular pattern is one in which the opacities are linear in nature and the lines range from quite thin to several millimeters thick. The opacities are oriented in multiple directions and may appear to overlap so as to create the appearance of a net. This pattern is not present (*C* is the correct answer to Question 4-7).

EXERCISE 4-4: DIFFUSE LUNG INFILTRATES

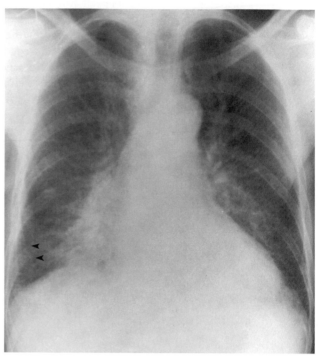

FIG. 4-E-9

Clinical History: **CASE 4-9**
A 69-year-old man presents with progressive dyspnea, orthopnea, and pedal edema and a history of hypertension (Fig. 4-E-9).

Question: 4-9. Which of the following best describes the chest radiograph in Fig. 4-E-9?
  A. Normal heart size and alveolar pulmonary edema
  B. Cardiomegaly, interstitial pulmonary edema, and small bilateral pleural effusions
  C. Unilateral interstitial disease
  D. Cardiomegaly and oligemia in the right lung

Radiologic Findings: 4-9. Frontal chest radiograph (Fig. 4-E-9) shows mild enlargement of the heart and indistinct vascularity, particularly at the lower lungs. Interlobular septal lines (*arrowheads*) are visible adjacent to both lower costophrenic angles.

Discussion: Pulmonary edema can be divided into two major categories: *cardiogenic edema* and *noncardiogenic edema*. Cardiogenic edema occurs as a result of elevation of pulmonary capillary pressure, which is usually due to pulmonary venous hypertension. Noncardiogenic edema occurs as a result of disorders that increase pulmonary capillary permeability. With both types of edema, there is a net movement of fluid out of the microvasculature and into the pulmonary interstitium and alveoli. The most common cause of pulmonary edema is left ventricular failure, which may be due to atherosclerotic coronary artery disease, mitral or aortic valvular disease, myocarditis, or cardiomyopathy. Cardiogenic edema is preceded by pulmonary venous hypertension, which is associated with redistribution of pulmonary blood flow from dependent regions of the lung to nondependent regions. In the erect patient, the radiographic sign of this redistribution is an increase in size of vessels in the upper lungs and a decrease in the caliber of pulmonary vessels in the lung bases. Radiographically, it is often difficult to distinguish pulmonary arteries from pulmonary veins, but for purposes of determination of flow redistribution, the distinction is ignored, and multiple vessels are measured at equal distances from the hilum or chest wall.

When seen end-on, normal bronchoarterial bundles may appear as adjacent circles of equal diameter, with the artery opaque and the bronchus lucent. The pulmonary arteries and bronchi are located together in the same interstitial space and arborize adjacent to each other. The pulmonary veins return blood to the heart in a separate interstitial space and have a slightly different arborization pattern. As the pulmonary venous pressure increases, fluid leaks from the pulmonary capillaries into the adjacent interstitium. This interstitial pulmonary edema may be identified by peribronchial cuffing, indistinctness of the perivascular margins, perihilar haziness, and thickening of the interlobular septa and interlobar fissures. As the pulmonary capillary pressure increases further, fluid spills into the alveoli, producing a symmetrical appearance of airspace filling that is predominantly perihilar (central) and basilar in distribution. Cardiogenic edema is greatest in dependent regions of the lungs. In supine patients, the dependent regions are the posterior segments of the upper lobes and the superior and posterior basilar segments of the lower lobes. The central pattern of pulmonary edema has been called "bat-wing" edema. As the pulmonary edema worsens, the pulmonary and pleural lymphatics clear fluid from the lungs, and pleural effusions will develop. In congestive heart failure, the pleural effusions are generally small to moderate in size, and there is typically more fluid within the right pleural space than the left. Isolated left pleural effusion is unlikely to be due to congestive heart failure. In cardiogenic edema, the heart size with be increased. The cardiothoracic (*CT*) ratio is a guide to determining cardiac enlargement. The transverse dimension of the heart is divided by the transverse diameter of the thorax at the same level. When the cardiothoracic ratio is greater than 0.5, cardiomegaly is often (but not always) present. When possible, both the PA and lateral projections should be used to determine cardiac volume. Cardiomegaly may be more readily recognized when comparison is made with prior radiographs. Comparison requires a similar depth of inspiration and similar positioning of the patient (AP versus PA, supine versus erect).

Noncardiogenic edema, or "capillary leak" edema, may be due to a number of conditions, including adult respiratory distress syndrome (ARDS), fat embolism, amniotic fluid embolism, drug overdose, near drowning, and acute airway obstruction. The cause of pulmonary edema in patients with intracranial injury or tumor (neurogenic pulmonary edema) is uncertain. Similarly, the cause of high-altitude pulmonary edema is incompletely understood. The common radiographic findings in noncardiogenic edema are symmetrical, diffuse areas of airspace filling that is often patchier in appearance and more peripheral in distribution. The heart size is usually normal; pleural effusions and septal lines are typically absent.

Renal failure and volume overload may result in pulmonary edema, which may be chronic. When the amount of edema is small to moderate, patients are often reasonably well compensated and are able to carry out many activities of daily living.

EXERCISE 4-5: AIRWAY DISEASE

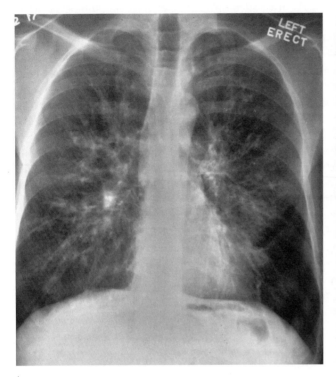

A

FIG. 4-E-10   (*Panels A and B*)

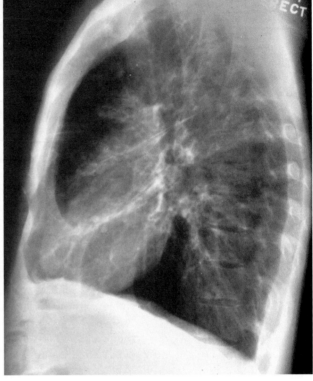

B

Clinical History:	**CASE 4-10** A 22-year-old man is seen who has had chronic cough and copious mucus production since childhood (Fig. 4-E-10*A,B*).

Question:	**4-10.** All the following are accurate descriptors of this patient's chest radiographs except
	    A. increased lung volume.
	    B. thickened bronchovascular bundles.
	    C. enlargement of the hila.
	    D. right paratracheal lymphadenopathy.
	    E. tram track lines.

Radiologic Findings:	4-10. The most prominent radiographic finding in Fig. 4-E-10*A* is coarse thickening of the bronchovascular bundles as they radiate from the hila. Thickened bronchial walls may be identified as tram track lines in the left lower lobe behind the heart and just medial and caudal to the interlobar pulmonary artery on the right. *Tram track lines* refer to the appearance of the nearly parallel walls of bronchi oriented longitudinally. Careful inspection shows that these are present throughout both lungs and are located near the hila. Bronchial walls also project as ring-shaped opacities near the hila (note that one projects into the middle of the left interlobar pulmonary artery). Both these structures represent the thick walls of dilated bronchi (bronchiectasis). The hila themselves are

slightly enlarged as a result of a combination of enlarged hilar lymph nodes and mild pulmonary arterial hypertension. The lung volume is significantly increased. The diaphragms are flatter than normal, especially on the lateral radiograph. The anterior clear space (retrosternal area) is larger and more radiolucent than normal. The right tracheal stripe, on the other hand, is normal, and there is no evidence of right paratracheal lymphadenopathy (*D* is the correct answer to Question 4-10).

Discussion:

The cause of this patient's bronchiectasis is cystic fibrosis. The mucus in patients with cystic fibrosis is thickened, and these patients do not have normal tracheobronchial clearance. This abnormal clearance may cause mucoid impaction, and atelectasis and pneumonia are frequent complications. Bronchiectasis also can occur as a result of pneumonia in patients without cystic fibrosis. In these patients, the bronchiectasis is more likely to be confined to a single lobe, often a lower lobe. Bronchiectasis is divided into three groups: cylindrical, fusiform (or varicose), and saccular (or cystic). These three groups not only describe the appearance of the abnormal bronchi but also give an indication as to its severity. Cylindrical bronchiectasis, the mildest form, is reversible and appears as thick-walled bronchi that fail to taper normally. The more severe forms, fusiform and saccular, are irreversible. Fusiform bronchiectasis has a beaded appearance, whereas the bronchi in saccular bronchiectasis end with clubbed, cystic areas. If the severe forms are localized, surgical resection may be curative. Medical therapy with bronchodilators and, when necessary, antibiotics is used when surgery is not indicated.

Bronchography was formerly the standard method of diagnosing bronchiectasis (Fig. 4-E-10*C,D*). Currently, CT is the method of choice for determining the presence and extent of bronchiectasis. It has the advantages of being less invasive and more readily tolerated by the patient. When the bronchus is perpendicular to the CT plane of section, bronchiectasis is identified as ring shadows adjacent to an opaque circle. The ring represents the thickened, dilated bronchial walls. The opaque circles represent the pulmonary artery adjacent to the dilated bronchus. Images from this patient show a combination of varicose and cystic bronchiectasis (Fig. 4-E-10*E,F*). When the bronchus lies within the plane of section of the CT scan, the dilated bronchial walls project as roughly parallel lines near a vessel (Fig. 4-E-10*G*).

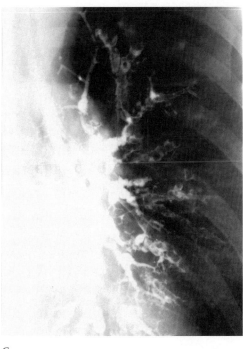

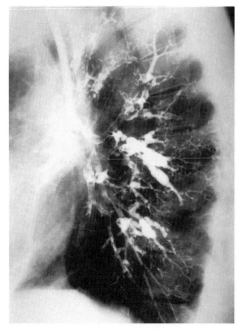

FIG. 4-E-10 Frontal (*Panel C*) and lateral (*Panel D*) views of a bronchogram in another patient shows bronchi in the left lung that are beaded and dilated rather than smoothly tapering.

C

D

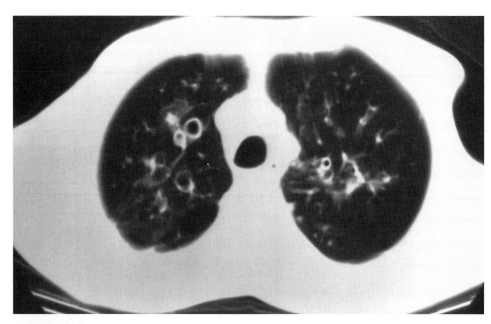

E

F

FIG. 4-E-10 (*Panels E–G*) Axial CT images (lung window settings) show multiple, dilated, thick-walled bronchi. Air-fluid levels (*arrow*) are present within areas of cystic bronchiectasis in this patient with cystic fibrosis. At the lung bases (*G*), thick-walled bronchi are seen longitudinally (*arrowhead*) as they remain within the imaging plane.

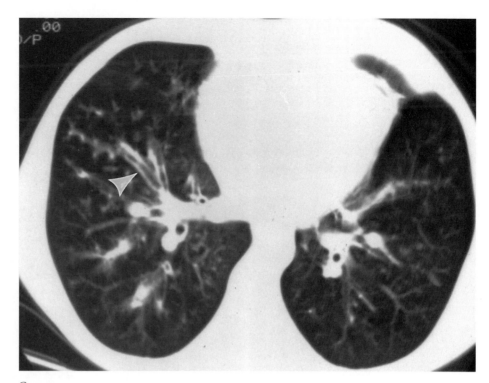

G

FIG. 4-E-10   (*Continued*)

EXERCISE 4-6: SOLITARY PULMONARY NODULE

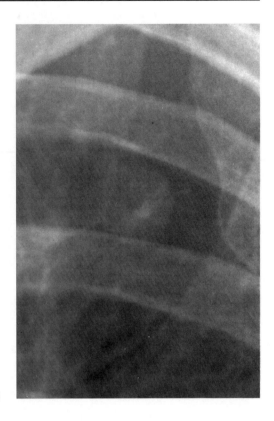

FIG. 4-E-11   *(Panel A)*

Clinical History:

CASE 4-11
A 53-year-old man is scheduled for coronary artery bypass grafting. A close-up view of the left upper lobe from a preoperative chest radiograph is shown (Fig. 4-E-11*A*).

Question:

4-11. Characteristics suggesting that a nodule is benign are
    A.   size of the nodule does not change over 2 years.
    B.   it contains central calcification.
    C.   CT attenuation values within the nodule are over 200 Hounsfield units (HU).
    D.   all of the above.

Radiologic Findings:

    4-11. The close-up view of the left upper lobe shows a nodule that is smoothly marginated and has a region of central opacity indicating a calcified central nidus.

Discussion:

Bronchogenic carcinoma, particularly adenocarcinoma, frequently presents as a solitary pulmonary nodule in the periphery of the lung. A new solitary pulmonary nodule or nodule of indeterminate age, therefore, should be considered a possible malignancy. The most common cause of a solitary pulmonary nodule is a granuloma, typically the result of prior granulomatous infection, such as tuberculosis or histoplasmosis. These can be identified frequently as granulomas because of characteristic patterns of calcification.

    In attempting to determine whether or not a nodule is benign, the characteristics to consider are the age of the patient, any history of previous malignancy, and the nodule's growth rate, density, shape, and edge characteristics. The most important of these are the growth rate and density. If a nodule has had *no* growth over a 2-year period and has calcification of the types associated with benign causes, then the nodule is almost certainly benign. Because of the importance of time in assessing growth, comparison with old films is the most important test and the least expensive method of determining whether a nodule is benign. A 2-year interval is approximately four volume-doubling times for an average lung carcinoma; therefore, an increase in diameter of one-third to one-half of the nodule would be expected. The absence of growth over a 2-year period is evidence that the nodule is stable in size and must therefore be benign. If radiographs demonstrate growth over this 2-year interval, then the nodule should be assumed to be malignant.

If the nodule is diffusely and completely calcified (Fig. 4-E-11*B*), if it is calcified centrally (Fig. 4-E-11*C*), or if it has a laminated pattern (Fig. 4-E-11*D*), then it may be assumed to be benign. Calcification may not be apparent on the initial radiograph because the most commonly used technique for chest radiography obscures subtle calcification. Demonstration of calcification may require fluoroscopy or repeated chest radiography with low-kilovoltage technique to enhance its depiction. When it is not clear from these studies whether calcification is present, CT should be used to identify it. CT has an extended range of tissue discrimination in comparison with plain films. The presence of calcification within a pulmonary nodule can be determined by evaluating the attenuation values within a region of interest (ROI) centered over the nodule (Fig. 4-E-11*E–G*). Air within the lung measures −800 HU, noncalcified nodules measure 30 to 100 HU, and calcified nodules measure over 200 HU. Nodules with somewhat dense calcification can

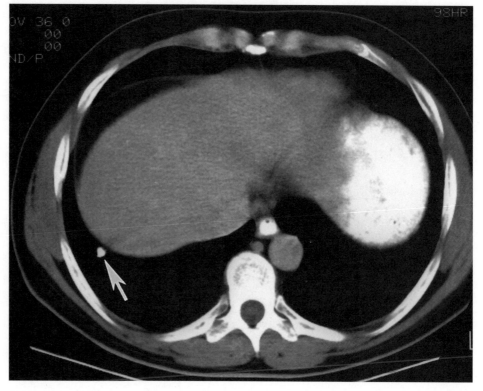

B

FIG. 4-E-11   (*Panel B*) CT scan at a level through the lower lungs shows a nodule (*arrow*) that is completely calcified. Note that the density of the nodule is equal to that of bone. (*Panel C*) Close-up view of the right lower lung shows a nodule with soft-tissue density and a central nidus of increased density representing a calcified central nidus (*arrow*). (*Panel D*) CT scan at the level of the aortic arch shows a nodule in the left lung that has laminar calcification and central and peripheral soft-tissue den-sity (*arrow*). (*Panel E*) CT scan just above the aortic arch shows a nodule in the right upper lobe (*arrow*) with at least two eccentric regions of calcification. (*Panel F*) A region of interest has been drawn on the nodule (*arrow*). (*Panel G*) The Hounsfield units in each pixel in the region of interest are demonstrated. Note the very high numbers in the central portion of the lesion, indicating calcification within those pixels.

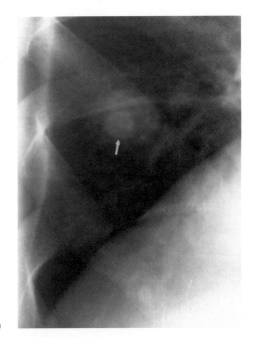

FIG. 4-E-11 (*Continued*)

C

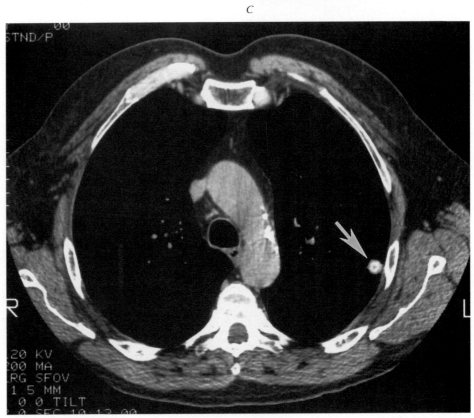

D

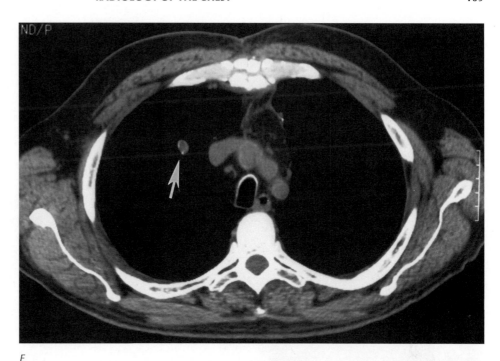

E

FIG. 4-E-11 (*Continued*)

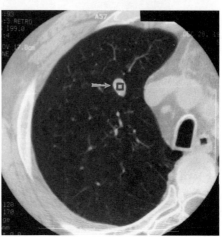

F

Pat. ID: 1004657   Series: 3
Report #1   Image: 17

	306	307	308	309	310	311	312	313	314	315	316
164	-10	14	85	87	53	61	54	22	16	26	-3
165	-7	19	75	78	69	113	112	37	-1	11	12
166	9	3	17	45	113	205	220	114	17	-9	-2
167	23	0	12	89	232	374	370	225	77	-23	-40
168	4	-7	61	207	410	529	437	248	68	-56	-63
169	-21	22	130	301	504	557	363	131	9	-57	-46
170	13	41	187	331	440	424	219	31	-18	-17	-41
171	39	42	164	289	312	239	80	-34	-22	5	-48
172	38	25	122	235	227	102	-17	-74	-33	-6	-68
173	53	47	78	150	139	54	-34	-26	5	-10	-121
174	26	26	29	76	79	28	14	49	26	-68	-228

G

FIG. 4-E-11 (*Continued*)

be identified easily, but subtle amounts of calcification may require a special phantom for accurate determination. Nodules with attenuation values between 0 and 200 HU are not necessarily malignant; they just do not have enough calcification to be categorized unequivocally as benign.

If a nodule is not calcified, or if it has shown growth over a 2-year period, it should be considered as a possible malignancy, and further assessment should be dictated by the clinical circumstances. Most patients will need evaluation for possible surgical resection and tissue biopsy to determine the cause.

Note that the margins of the lesion, whether smooth or spiculated, are of no value in determining the benignity or malignant potential of a lesion. Only uniform or central calcification, absence of growth over a 2-year period, or CT attenuation values over 200 HU throughout the nodule are reliable noninvasive indicators of benignity (*D* is the correct answer to Question 4-11).

EXERCISE 4-7: PULMONARY NEOPLASM

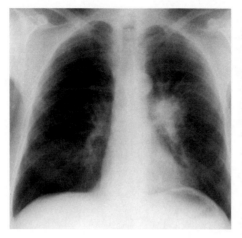

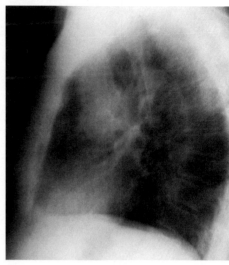

FIG. 4-E-12 (*Panels A and B*)

A

B

| Clinical History: | **CASE 4-12**
A 64-year-old man presents with cough and weight loss and a 50-pack-year history of tobacco use (Fig. 4-E-12*A,B*). |

Question:

4-12. The best description of the chest radiographs in Fig. 4-E-12*A,B* is
   A. mass in the left upper lobe.
   B. left upper lobe collapse.
   C. mediastinal mass.
   D. consolidation of the left upper lobe.
   E. enlargement of the left pulmonary artery.

Radiologic Findings:

4-12. The chest radiographs show a round opacity projecting just laterally and cephalad to the left hilum. Because the medial margin of the opacity can be seen, a mediastinal mass is excluded. The left pulmonary artery can be seen through the opacity and is normal in size. On the lateral view, the opacity maintains a round shape and projects over the anterior portion of the chest. The opacity is smaller than the volume of the left upper lobe, and no air bronchograms are present; this excludes consolidation of the left upper lobe as an answer. The posterior margin of the opacity is not a long straight or gently curving line, as is the major fissure, and therefore, left upper lobe atelectasis is not the correct answer. The one best description of the radiographic findings is mass in the left upper lobe (*A* is the correct answer to Question 4-12). In a patient with cough, weight loss, and a history of tobacco use, bronchogenic carcinoma should be the primary consideration. A CT examination in this patient (Fig. 4-E-12*C*) shows the mass in the anterior segment of the left upper lobe, which is contiguous with the superior left hilum. A CT-guided percutaneous biopsy of this mass was positive for squamous cell carcinoma.

Discussion:

There are more than 150,000 new cases of lung cancer, or bronchogenic carcinoma, in the United States each year. *Bronchogenic carcinoma* is the more appropriate term, since most of them arise from the epithelium of the airways and not the lung per se. Since early recognition and surgical resection offer the patient the best chance for cure, it is impor-

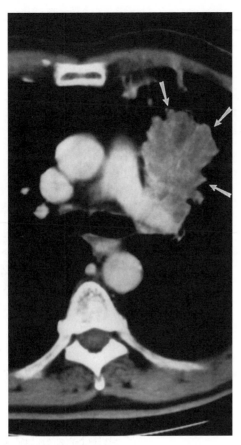

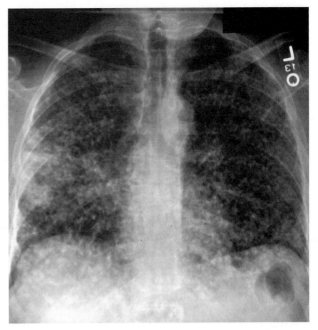

D

C

FIG. 4-E-12 (*Panel C*) Axial CT scan (mediastinal window setting) shows a lobulated mass (*arrows*) within the left upper lobe. The fact that the mass is adjacent to the left pulmonary artery explains why the left hilum is somewhat obscured on the chest radiograph. (*Panel D*) Diffuse pulmonary nodules represent bronchioalveolar cell carcinoma in this patient. (*Panel E*) An air-fluid level is present within a thick-walled cavitary mass at the right lung apex. This represented squamous cell carcinoma.

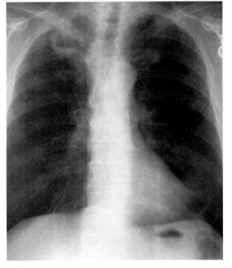

E

tant to be familiar with the variety of radiographic appearances of lung cancer. Four major cell types account for almost 90 percent of all lung cancers. The major cell types are squamous cell, adenocarcinoma, large cell, and small cell. For therapeutic purposes, lung cancer is divided into small cell and non-small cell carcinoma. This distinction is necessary because small cell bronchogenic carcinoma is almost always widespread at the time of diagnosis and is best treated by chemotherapy and radiation therapy. Non-small cell bronchogenic carcinoma, on the other hand, is best treated by surgical resection when the tumor is confined to one lung and regional lymph nodes. The typical radiographic appearance of small cell carcinoma is bulky hilar or mediastinal lymph nodes or both, and the primary tumor sometimes is visible as a nodule within the lung.

Non-small cell bronchogenic carcinoma includes adenocarcinoma, squamous cell carcinoma, and large cell carcinoma. Adenocarcinoma, the most common cell type, typically appears as a solitary pulmonary nodule in the periphery of the lung. Bronchioalveolar cell carcinoma is a subtype of adenocarcinoma that may present as either lobar airspace disease or as diffuse ill-defined pulmonary nodules (Fig. 4-E-12*D*). Bronchioalveolar cell carcinoma rarely may present as a solitary pulmonary nodule. The sec-

TABLE 4-4   TNM STAGING SYSTEM

Tumor		Node		Metastasis	
T_1	A tumor 3 cm or less in greatest diameter limited to the lung, and without invasion proximal to a lobar bronchus	N_0	No lymph node metastases	M_0	No distant metastases
T_2	A tumor larger than 3 cm; a tumor that invades the visceral pleura or produces collapse or consolidation of less than an entire lung; the tumor must be more than 2 cm distal to the carina	N_1	Metastases to ipsilateral hilar lymph nodes	M_1	Distant metastases present
T_3	A tumor invading parietal pleura, chest wall, diaphragm, or mediastinal pleura or pericardium; a tumor less than 2 cm from the carina or producing collapse or consolidation of an entire lung	N_2	Metastases to ipsilateral mediastinal or subcarinal lymph nodes		
T_4	A tumor of any size with invasion of the mediastinum or involving heart, great vessels, trachea, esophagus, vertebral body, or carina or producing malignant pleural effusion	N_3	Metastases to contralateral hilar or mediastinal lymph nodes, or scalene or supraclavicular lymph nodes		

ond most common cell type, squamous cell carcinoma, is associated with cigarette smoking and most often is found as an endobronchial tumor resulting in lobar collapse (see Fig. 4-E-2A). The endobronchial tumor is visible bronchoscopically, and sputum cytology is frequently diagnostic in this tumor. Squamous cell carcinoma also can appear radiographically as a solitary cavitary mass (Fig. 4-E-12E) or noncavitary mass. Large cell carcinoma is the least frequent cell type. Its appearance is that of a bulky lesion within the lung.

When non-small cell lung cancer is diagnosed, the patient undergoes a series of clinical and radiologic studies to determine the stage of the tumor. In the TNM staging system (Table 4-4), the categories of disease are stage I, II, IIIa, IIIb, or IV (Table 4-5). Stages I, II, and IIIa are surgically resectable. Patients with either stage IIIb or stage IV disease are not surgical candidates but are treated with chemotherapy, radiation therapy, or both. In addition to helping define which treatment the patient should receive, the stage of the tumor helps provide prognosis. Patients with stage I disease have a 60 percent 5-year survival rate. Patients with stage IV disease have a 10 percent 5-year survival rate.

TABLE 4-5   STAGING CLASSIFICATIONS

Stage I	Stage II	Stage IIIa	Stage IIIb	Stage IV
$T_1 N_0 M_0$	$T_1 N_1 M_0$	$T_{1-3} N_2 M_0$	T_4 any N M_0	any T any N M_1
$T_2 N_0 M_0$	$T_2 N_1 M_0$	$T_3 N_0 M_0$	any T $N_3 M_0$	
		$T_3 N_1 M_0$		

EXERCISE 4-8: MULTIPLE PULMONARY NODULES

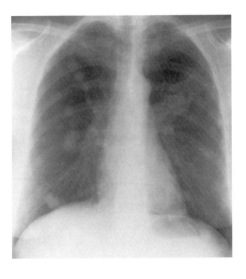

FIG. 4-E-13   *(Panel A)*

Clinical History:

CASE 4-13
A 70-year-old woman is seen with uterine carcinoma treated with surgical resection 3 years previously. A chest radiograph obtained as part of a routine follow-up examination is shown (Fig. 4-E-13*A*).

Question:

4-13. The most likely cause of the multiple pulmonary nodules is
   A.   metastasis.
   B.   herpes simplex pneumonia.
   C.   histoplasmosis.
   D.   Wegener's granulomatosis.
   E.   arteriovenous malformations.

Radiologic Findings:

   4-13. The chest radiograph shows multiple, smoothly marginated, solid nodules in both lungs. These are water-density nodules that are distributed diffusely and have varying sizes. The heart is normal in size and shape.

Discussion:

The radiographic pattern of multiple pulmonary nodules is frequently encountered. The clinical setting has considerable influence on the differential diagnosis in such cases and should always be taken into account when assessing patients with this pattern. However, the differential diagnosis may be narrowed by assessing the absolute size of the nodules, the uniformity of their size, their marginal characteristics, whether or not they are calcified, and whether or not they are cavitary. In adults, the most common causes of multiple nodules are metastatic neoplasm and infectious disease. Metastatic neoplasm may result from carcinoma, sarcoma, or lymphoma. Pulmonary metastases may be of any size and number. In contrast to inflammatory nodules, nodular pulmonary metastases are often of variable diameters. Metastases are usually of soft-tissue density similar to muscle or blood. Metastases may be calcified if the patient has a sarcoma that makes bone or cartilage (e.g., osteosarcoma). Calcified pulmonary nodules are encountered more frequently in patients with healed fungal or mycobacterial disease. Differentiation is often made by the clinical setting or review of old films, but determination of the correct diagnosis may require tissue confirmation.

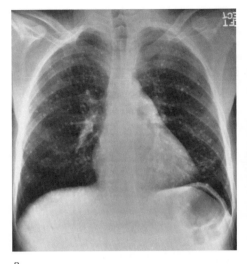

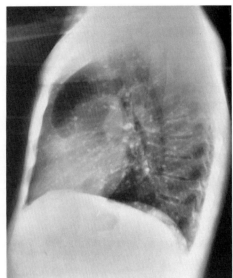

FIG. 4-E-13 Frontal (*Panel B*) and lateral (*Panel C*) chest radiographs show multiple, small, rather dense nodules scattered throughout both lungs; these calcified nodules are the residua of prior *Histoplasmosa* infection. Tuberculosis also can produce calcified granulomata.

B

C

Multiple pulmonary nodules also may be due to infectious disease, particularly fungal or mycobacterial infections. In the United States, the most common fungal infection is histoplasmosis (Fig. 4-E-13*B,C*), although there are regional variations. Infectious nodules are often not as sharply defined as metastases. This is especially true if the nodules represent acinar shadows. In these instances, the nodule is approximately 5 to 10 mm in diameter and is ill-defined or fuzzy on its margin. Acinar nodules develop in patients with viral pneumonias such as herpes pneumonia or chicken pox pneumonia.

Multiple pulmonary nodules also may develop in a wide variety of other disorders, including Wegener's granulomatosis and arteriovenous malformations. Option *A* is the correct answer.

EXERCISE 4-9: CAVITARY DISEASE

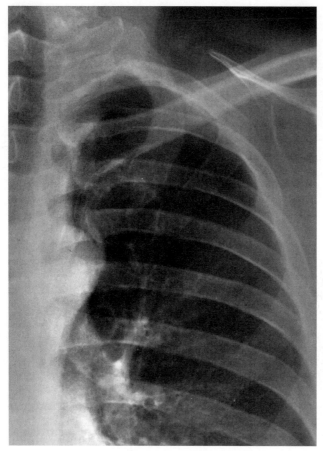

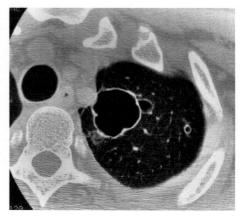

B

FIG. 4-E-14   *(Panels A and B)*

A

Clinical History:

CASE 4-14

A 27-year-old man presents with a history of intravenous drug use and a 2-week history of fever and malaise (Fig. 4-E-14*A,B*).

Question:

4-14. The chest radiographic findings could be explained by any of the following except
A. multiple abscesses due to *Staphylococcus aureus.*
B. pneumatoceles due to *Pneumocystis carinii.*
C. Wegener's granulomatosis.
D. multiple cavities due to *Mycobacterium avium*-intracellulare.
E. metastases from Kaposi's sarcoma.

Radiologic Findings:

4-14. A close-up view of the chest radiograph (Fig. 4-E-14*A*) and CT image (Fig. 4-E-14*B*) of the left upper lobe show multiple thin-walled cavitary lesions. A left pneumothorax is also present. There is no hilar or mediastinal lymph node enlargement. The heart and skeleton are normal.

Discussion:

Inflammatory lesions are the most common cause of lung cavities. The number of cavities may range from one to many. A wide variety of infecting organisms may result in

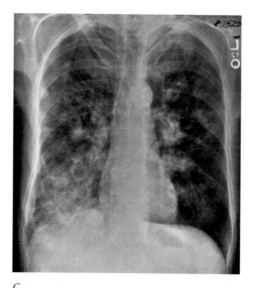

FIG. 4-E-14 Frontal chest radiograph (*Panel C*) and CT scan (*Panel D*) of a 60-year-old man with a previous squamous cell carcinoma of the pharynx. Chest radiograph shows multiple pulmonary nodules, many of which have cavitated, in both lungs.

C

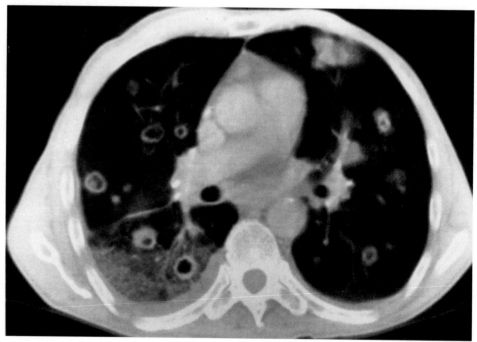

D

cavitation, and the radiograph is nonspecific as to etiology. There is considerable overlap in appearances from the various organisms, so culture or histologic evaluation is the only satisfactory means of identifying the cause. If the lesion is single, a cavitating pneumonia should be the first consideration, especially if the patient is febrile. If multiple cavities are present, the infection is likely due to hematogenous dissemination (septic emboli), and a source for this dissemination should be sought. The source could be right-sided endocarditis or infected venous thrombi. *Staphylococcus aureus* pneumonias are frequently seen in intravenous drug users and usually appear as multiple cavities. These usually have thin walls (2 to 4 mm) that are slightly indistinct on their outer borders.

As the AIDS epidemic has progressed, it has been recognized that patients with *Pneumocystis carinii* pneumonia may develop cavitary lesions in the lungs. These cavities may be reversible and result from pneumatoceles, or they may be due to a slowly progressive granulomatous reaction. The cavities are usually in the upper lobes and are thin-walled. Pneumothorax can result when a peripheral cavity ruptures through the visceral pleura into the pleural space.

Cavities may result from pulmonary vasculitis, of which Wegener's granulomatosis is the prototype. Neoplasia, either primary or secondarily involving the lung, also may cavitate (Fig. 4-E-14*C,D*). This patient is rather young to have neoplasia. If he did have AIDS and Kaposi's sarcoma, it is unusual for that to cavitate (*E* is the correct answer to Question 4-14).

EXERCISE 4-10: OCCUPATIONAL DISORDERS

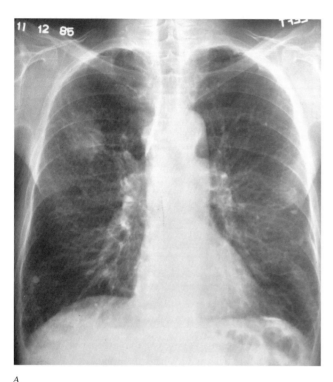

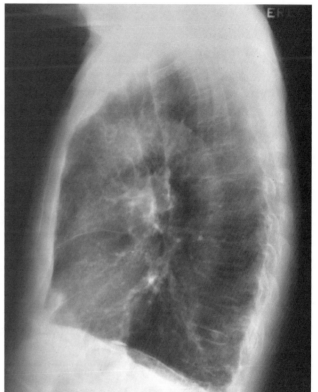

A

FIG. 4-E-15   *(Panels A and B)*

B

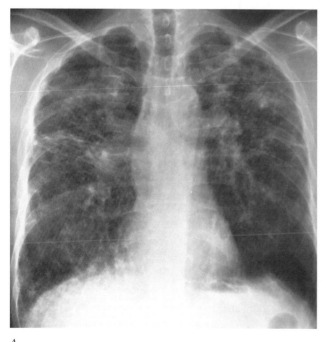

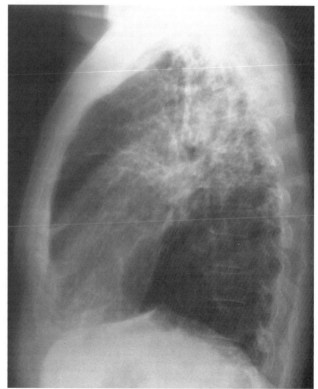

A

FIG. 4-E-16   *(Panels A and B)*

B

Clinical Histories:

CASE 4-15

A 64-year-old man, who previously worked in a naval shipyard, presents with a cough productive of blood-tinged sputum (Fig. 4-E-15A,B).

CASE 4-16

A 55-year-old man presents who worked as a coal miner for 30 years (Fig. 4-E-16A,B).

Questions:

4-15. The most likely diagnosis in Fig. 4-E-15A,B is
A. progressive massive fibrosis due to silicosis.
B. pneumonia in a patient with chronic interstitial lung disease.
C. lung cancer in a patient with asbestosis.
D. rounded atelectasis in a patient with asbestosis.
E. berylliosis.

4-16. The most likely diagnosis in Fig. 4-E-16A,B is
A. progressive massive fibrosis due to silicosis.
B. pneumonia in a patient with chronic interstitial lung disease.
C. lung cancer in a patient with asbestosis.
D. rounded atelectasis in a patient with asbestosis.
E. berylliosis.

Radiologic Findings:

4-15. The dense radiopaque lines projecting adjacent to the left diaphragmatic surface on the PA radiograph and over both diaphragmatic surfaces on the lateral radiograph represent calcified pleural plaques. These are better seen on the oblique radiograph (Fig. 4-E-15C) and on the CT (Fig. 4-E-15D). When the pleural plaques are seen en face on the PA radiograph, they produce irregular opacities over the left midlung. These opacities have been described as having a "holly leaf" appearance. At the lung bases, a network of fine lines is superimposed over the normal vascular shadows. These reticular markings represent interstitial pulmonary fibrosis, which almost certainly represents asbestosis. Also present is a 3.5-cm mass in the anterior segment of the right upper lobe. This is a primary bronchogenic carcinoma (C is the correct answer to Question 4-15). The oval convexity in the lower right paratracheal region represents regional metastasis to the lower right paratracheal lymph node.

4-16. The patient in Fig. 4-E-16A,B has a myriad of small, rounded pulmonary opacities (nodules) that in some areas have coalesced to form larger pulmonary masses. The nodules are predominantly located in the upper lobes. There is also bilateral hilar lymph node enlargement, which is more evident on the lateral radiograph. Bilateral upper lobe volume loss is indicated by upward displacement of the hila. The superolateral margin of the large opacity is relatively straight, and there is emphysema lateral to it. Nodular diseases that have an upper lobe preponderance include silicosis, sarcoidosis, and eosinophilic granuloma. In this patient with a history of working in coal mines, the most likely of these is silicosis, or coal worker's pneumoconiosis (A is the correct answer to Question 4-16).

Discussion:

The two most commonly encountered occupational lung diseases in the United States are asbestosis and silicosis. Development of these diseases is dose-dependent, and there is a latent period of many years between exposure and disease. Asbestos-related diseases occur after exposure to asbestos particles, which are found in many types of insulation, fireproofing materials, concrete, and brake linings. The patient with asbestos exposure is at an increased risk of developing lung cancer. If the patient also smokes, there is an additive risk, and these patients may be as much as 100 times more likely to develop lung cancer than the nonsmoking individual with no asbestos exposure.

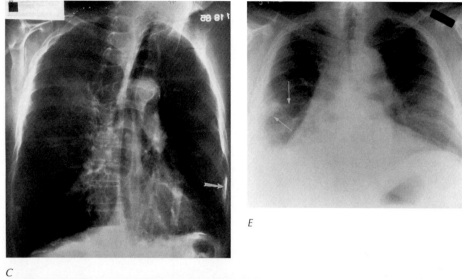

E

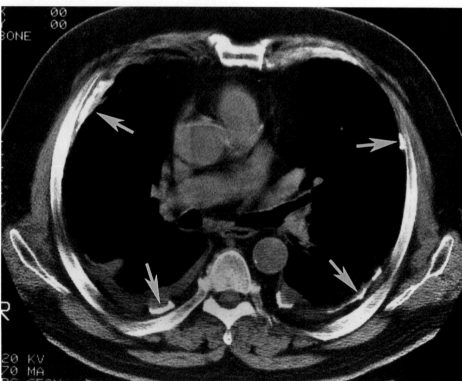

C

D

FIG. 4-E-15 (*Panel C*) Left anterior oblique radiograph shows calcified pleural plaques over the left anterior lung (*arrow*) and over both hemidiaphragms. These are typical of the parietal pleural plaques seen in asbestos exposure. (*Panel D*) Axial CT image (mediastinal window setting) shows bilateral calcified pleural plaques (*arrows*), as well as pleural thickening posteriorly. (*Panel E*) Frontal chest radiograph of a 56-year-old man with right-sided chest pain shows pleural opacity on the right with extension into the minor fissure (*arrows*). The patient was exposed to asbestos 20 years earlier. (*Panels F,G*) CT scans through the upper thorax and midthorax show loss of volume in the right hemithorax, with pleural thickening encircling the lung (*arrows*), representing malignant mesothelioma.

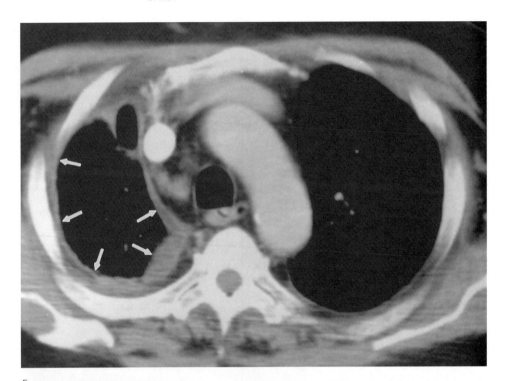

F

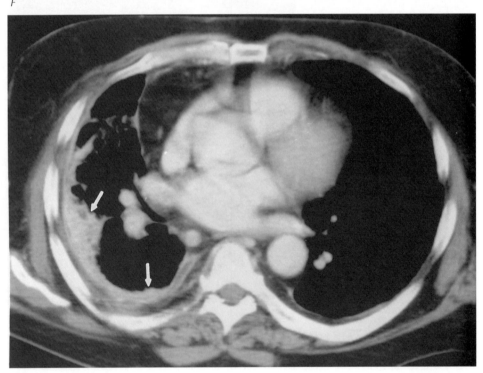

FIG. 4-E-15 *(Continued)*

G

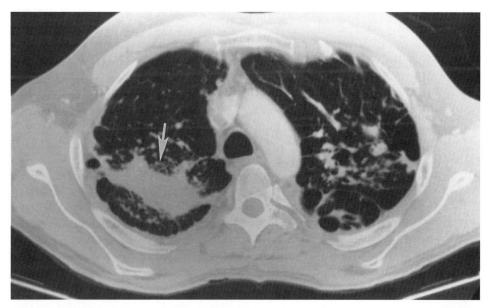

C

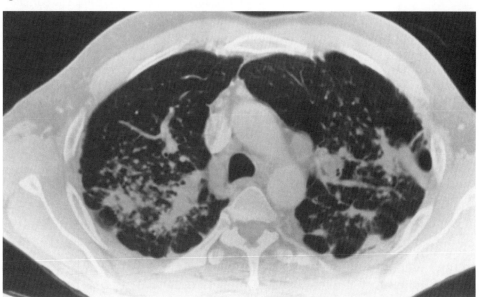

D

FIG. 4-E-16 (*Panels C,D*) Axial CT images (lung window setting) in the patient in case 4-16 show multiple small nodules throughout both upper lobes, as well as a platelike area of conglomerate fibrosis in the right upper lobe (*arrow*). These are typical of silicosis, or coalworker's pneumoconiosis, with progressive massive fibrosis. (*Panel E*) In another patient with silica exposure (a 49-year-old man who shoveled sand in a glass factory), eggshell calcification is visible in nodes in both hila and in the aortopulmonary window (*arrow*). Conglomerate masses in the upper lobes are compatible with progressive massive fibrosis.

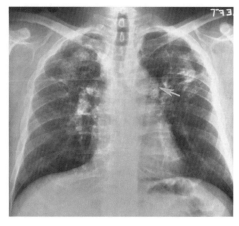

E

The term *asbestosis* is used to refer to the pulmonary fibrosis that may be incited by the presence of the mineral and is not used in reference to the pleural disease. The pulmonary fibrosis is predominantly distributed in the lung bases. When severe, it is detected with plain chest radiography. When it is more subtle, CT is required for its demonstration (Fig. 4-E-15*E*). When confined to the pleura, the process is called *asbestos-related pleural disease*. There are five manifestations of asbestos-related pleural disease: asbestos-related pleural effusion, diffuse pleural thickening, pleural plaques, rounded atelectasis, and malignant mesothelioma. Asbestos-related pleural effusion occurs from 7 to 15 years after exposure. It is self-limited and may resolve without sequelae or result in diffuse pleural thickening. Pleural plaques are fibrous plaques that occur predominately on the parietal pleural surfaces of the lower thoracic wall and diaphragmatic surfaces. Pleural plaques may be up to 8 to 10 mm thick but are not easily visualized when seen en face. Oblique radiographs (Fig. 4-E-15*C*) may show plaques that are projected en face on the PA chest radiograph. The plaques usually occur 10 years or more after exposure. Early in the development of pleural disease, the plaques are not calcified, but with time, the incidence of calcification increases. CT is the most sensitive method of identifying pleural plaques (Fig. 4-E-15*D*). Diffuse pleural thickening may result from the scarring of a previous benign asbestos-related pleural effusion, or it sometimes is due to confluent pleural plaques. Rounded atelectasis is a piece of folded lung tissue that appears as a mass adjacent to the chest wall. The parietal pleura adheres to an area of lung, usually in the posterior lower lobes, and gradually produces a spiraling folded area of lung, which mimics lung cancer. The comet-tail appearance of bronchi and vessels spiraling into the mass may suggest the correct diagnosis, but since there is such a great increase in the risk of lung cancer in the asbestos-exposed individual, the mass should be followed closely. Surgical resection is often necessary to distinguish the mass of rounded atelectasis from lung cancer. The final asbestos-related disease of the pleura is malignant mesothelioma. This is a malignant tumor of the pleura that usually presents as pleural masses or pleural effusion (Fig. 4-E-15*E–G*).

Silicosis is another form of pulmonary fibrosis that occurs after prolonged exposure to silica. Historically, it has developed most often in coal miners. Because of improved ventilation standards and the increased automation of coal mining, silicosis is encountered less commonly today. There is an increased incidence of tuberculosis in coal miners, but no increased risk of lung cancer has been reported. For reasons that are unexplained, silicosis is predominantly an upper lobe process. It appears as small pulmonary nodules, and as the fibrosis progresses, the hila are retracted upward over a period of years. The small granulomatous nodules of simple silicosis coalesce to form larger conglomerate masses. When these reach at least 1 cm in diameter, the disease is called *complicated silicosis,* and as they become larger still, it is designated *progressive massive fibrosis.* Very early disease may be seen only on CT, although in the later stages of the process the small nodules and conglomerate masses are readily seen on either plain films or CT images (Fig. 4-E-16*C,D*). Hilar and mediastinal lymph nodes may calcify in the periphery of the lymph node, a type of calcification known as *eggshell calcification* (Fig. 4-E-16*E*). An acute form of silicosis can occur in sandblasters who inhale a massive amount of sand. This type of silicosis radiographically resembles pulmonary edema. *Coal worker's pneumoconiosis* is a similar process that results from inhalation of coal of a relatively pure carbon content. This dust is relatively more inert than silica and incites less fibrosis. The nodules are less well defined on their periphery, and there is a lesser tendency to develop progressive massive fibrosis. These distinctions are rather artificial, since rock dust is usually not very pure and contains a mixture of silica, carbon, and other minerals.

EXERCISE 4-11: MEDIASTINAL MASSES AND COMPARTMENTS

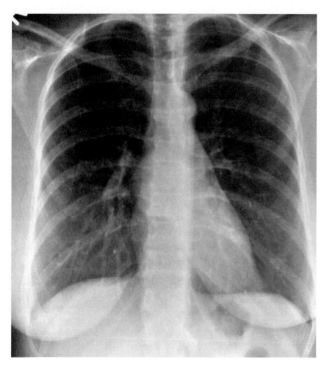

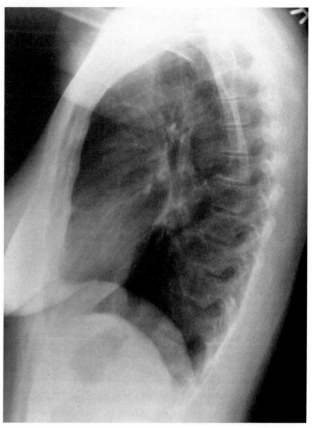

A

FIG. 4-E-17 *(Panels A and B)*

B

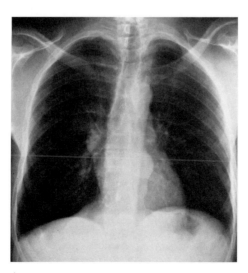

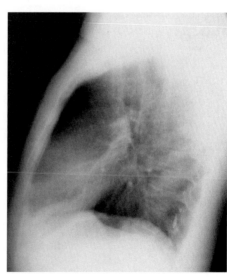

FIG. 4-E-18 *(Panels A and B)*

A

B

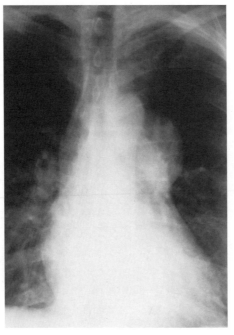 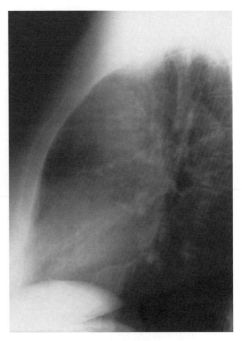

FIG. 4-E-19   (*Panels A and B*)

A   B

Clinical Histories:

CASE 4-17
An asymptomatic 37-year-old woman is seen for a routine chest radiograph (Fig. 4-E-17*A,B*).

CASE 4-18
A 55-year-old man presents with multiple subcutaneous nodules (Fig. 4-E-18*A,B*).

CASE 4-19
A 25-year-old woman presents with a nonproductive cough (Fig. 4-E-19*A,B*).

Questions:

4-17. Match the chest radiographs in Fig. 4-E-17*A,B* with the appropriate radiographic description in Column A and with the best differential diagnosis in Column B of the following table.

4-18. Match the chest radiographs in Fig. 4-E-18*A,B* with the appropriate radiographic description in Column A and with the best differential diagnosis in Column B of the following table.

4-19. Match the chest radiographs in Fig. 4-E-19*A,B* with the appropriate radiographic description in Column A and with the best differential diagnosis in Column B of the following table.

Column A	Column B
I. Anterior mediastinal mass	A. Bronchogenic cyst Lymphoma or lymph node metastasis Esophageal tumor Aortic arch aneurysm
II. Middle mediastinal mass	B. Lymphoma or lymph node metastasis Teratoma Thyroid mass

                                        Thymoma
                                        Ascending aortic aneurysm

III. Posterior mediastinal mass   C. Neural tumor
                                        Paraspinous abscess
                                        Descending thoracic aorta aneurysm
                                        Bochdalek hernia
                                        Lymphoma or lymph node metastasis

---

Radiologic Findings: 4-17. A spherical mass 4 cm in diameter is present in the subcarinal region on the frontal radiograph (Fig. 4-E-17A) and superimposed on the hilar region on the lateral radiograph (Fig. 4-E-17B). CT (Fig. 4-E-17C) shows that the lesion is of fluid attenuation (greater attenuation than the subcutaneous fat but less attenuation than muscle). In an asymptomatic individual, this most likely represents a congenital bronchogenic cyst. These masses can grow to sufficient size to cause symptoms such as dyspnea or dysphagia owing to compression of the trachea or esophagus. Bronchogenic cysts also may occur within the lungs and are often resected surgically because of the likelihood of pulmonary infection (IIA is the correct answer to Question 4-17).

4-18. The frontal radiograph (Fig. 4-E-18A) shows a lobulated mass to the left of the lower thoracic vertebrae. Note that the lateral wall of the descending thoracic aorta remains visible, suggesting that this mass is either anterior or posterior to the aorta, but does not displace lung from the wall of the aorta. The mass is not visible on the lateral radiograph. The residual myelographic contrast material visible within the spinal canal hints at the neural nature of these masses. The axial CT images in Fig. 4-E-18C,D show that the masses are bilateral and paraspinal in location. Neurogenic tumors are the most common cause of posterior mediastinal masses. In this patient with multiple subcutaneous nodules, they most likely are neurofibromas (III,C is the correct answer to Question 4-18).

4-19. In this case, the frontal chest radiographs (Fig. 4-E-19A,C) show a mass projecting over the left hilum (*long arrow*) without obscuration of the interlobar pulmonary artery (*short arrow*). Because the mass does not obliterate the margins of the vessel, it

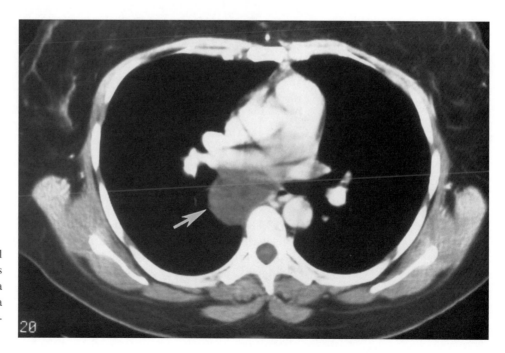

FIG. 4-E-17 (*Panel C*) Axial CT image shows a round mass (*arrow*) of fluid attenuation in a subcarinal position. This is a typical appearance of a bronchogenic cyst.

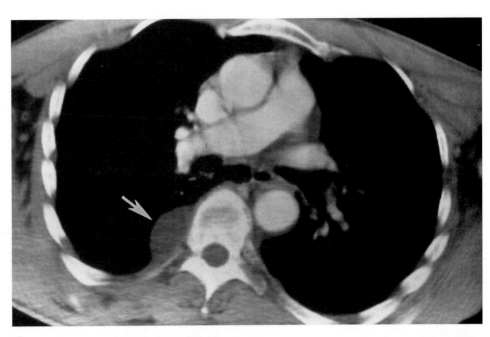

FIG. 4-E-18 (*Panels C,D*) Axial CT images show bilateral paraspinal masses (*arrows*).

C

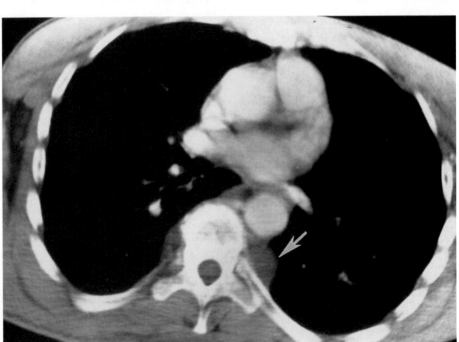

D

must be either anterior or posterior to the hilum. On the lateral view (Fig. 4-E-19*D*), the anterior clear space is somewhat opaque, and there is a suggestion of margins of the mass (*arrows*). The CT scan (Fig. 4-E-19*E*) shows the mass, surrounded by fat, in the anterior mediastinum. The mass is cystic, and the contents have rather low attenuation, suggesting that the mass contains some fat. Notice the thick, irregular wall of the mass. No other abnormalities are present. This mass is a teratoma (I,*B* is the correct answer to Question 4-19).

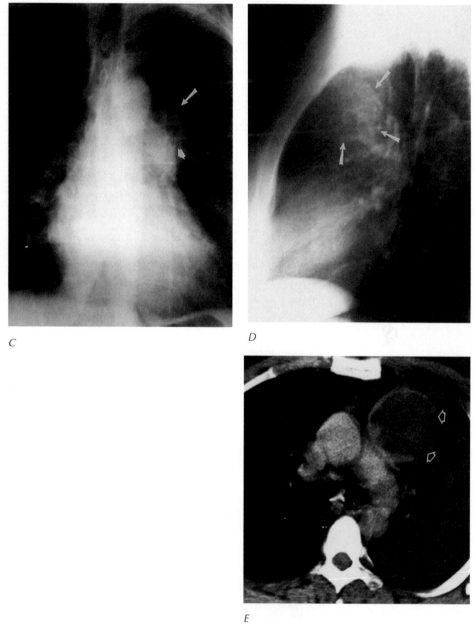

FIG. 4-E-19   Front (*Panel C*) and lateral (*Panel D*) chest radiographs of the same patient. (*Panel E*) CT scan through a level just below the aortic arch shows a mass in the left anterior mediastinum (*arrows*). The mass has a thick, nodular wall, and the central material is relatively radiolucent. The central portion of this mass is fat, and the mass is a teratoma. (*Panel F*) Close-up of the mediastinum in a 75-year-old woman shows a right-sided paratracheal mass with displacement of the trachea to the left. Enlargement of the heart is also seen. (*Panel G*) CT scan through the lung apices at the thoracic inlet shows the right-sided paratracheal mass (*arrow*), which is of soft-tissue density and has a nidus of calcification within it. A soft-tissue mass is also seen adjacent to the left side of the trachea and has an additional calcification (*arrowhead*). These represent regions of enlargement of the thyroid. (*Panel H*) CT scan at a level just above the aortic arch shows the mass (*arrow*) extending into the superior mediastinum just lateral to the trachea and displacing the trachea to the left. (*Panel I*) MRI image shows a mass (*arrows*) at the thoracic inlet from thyroid enlargement. Mass displaces the aorta (Ao) and brachiocephalic artery posteriorly and inferiorly. The left brachiocephalic vein (lbv) is also displaced inferiorly.

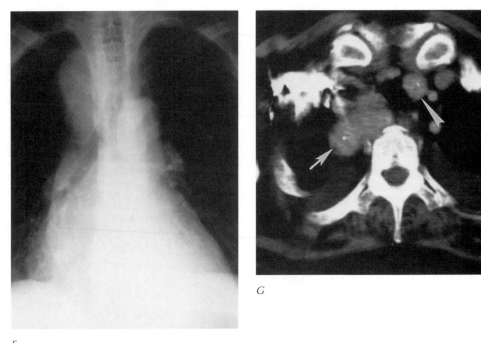

FIG. 4-E-19 *(Continued)*

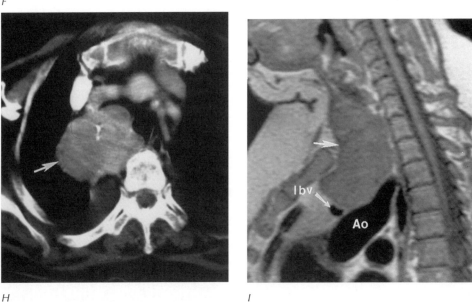

Discussion:

Two methods of dividing the mediastinum for radiographic purposes are in common use. The radiographic divisions are arbitrary and are intended to provide the most appropriate differential diagnosis for abnormalities that occur in these locations. Neither of the divisions follows the divisions used by anatomists. In the older system, the mediastinum is divided into three compartments. The *anterior mediastinum* is that portion of the mediastinum which is anterior to the anterior margin of the trachea and along the posterior margin of the pericardium and inferior vena cava. The *posterior mediastinum* lies behind a plane that extends the length of the thorax behind a line drawn 1 cm posterior to the anterior margin of the vertebral column. The *middle mediastinum* is the region between these two boundaries. This system has been superseded by a four-compartment model, which designates a superior mediastinal compartment as the space that lies above a plane extending from the sternomanubrial junction to the lower border of the fourth thoracic vertebra. The anterior mediastinum is just caudad to the superior compartment and is anterior to a plane extending along the anterior aspect of the tracheal air column and along the anterior pericardium. Note that the heart shifts from the anterior to the middle mediastinum as the system changes. The middle mediastinum occupies the area from the anterior pericardium backward to a plane 1 cm posterior to the anterior margin of the vertebral column. The addition of the fourth compartment occurred when CT was developed and it became easier to identify structures in each compartment.

The differential diagnosis of lesions occurring in each compartment is in part dependent on the structures that exist there. Note that there are vascular structures and lymph nodes in each of the compartments. Therefore, abnormalities of the blood vessels (e.g., aneurysms) and lymph node diseases (e.g., lymphoma) would have to be included in the differential diagnosis of diseases occurring there. The differential diagnosis lists given in Column B include the most common disorders occurring in each region. The most common mass to occur in the superior mediastinum is an enlarged substernal thyroid, which may become large enough to extend into the anterior or middle mediastinum (Fig. 4-E-19*F–I*).

EXERCISE 4-12: PLEURAL ABNORMALITIES

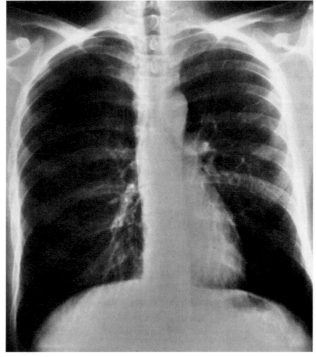

A

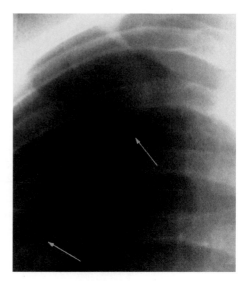

B

FIG. 4-E-20   (*Panels A and B*)

Clinical History: **CASE 4-20**
A tall, 21-year-old man presents when he noted the sudden onset of dyspnea and right-sided pleuritic chest pain (Fig. 4-E-20*A,B*).

Question: **4-20.** The most likely diagnosis in this case is
    A.   pulmonary embolism.
    B.   overinflation associated with asthma.
    C.   pneumothorax.
    D.   normal chest with a skin fold projecting over the right hemithorax.
    E.   left lower lobe atelectasis.

Radiologic Findings: 4-20. In Fig. 4-E-20*A,* there is increased radiolucency in the periphery of the right hemithorax. On the close-up of the right lung (Fig. 4-E-20*B*), there is a thin white line (*arrows*) paralleling, but displaced from, the right lateral chest wall. The thin line represents the visceral pleura. There is air-filled lung medial to this thin white line, and there is air within the pleural space lateral to this line. Note the absence of pulmonary vessels lateral to the pleural line (*C* is the correct answer to Question 4-20). Note the rounded, thin-walled blebs at the apex of the right lung on the close-up view in Fig. 4-E-20*B*.

Discussion: Pneumothorax is the presence of air in the pleural space. The lung collapses away from the chest wall because of its normal elastic recoil. In some instances, a ball-valve mechanism is present, and air continues to enter the pleural space and further collapses the lung and displaces the mediastinum away from the side of the pneumothorax. The relationship of the air in the pleural space to the lung and chest wall can be seen clearly on the CT scan of a patient with a left pneumothorax (Fig. 4-E-20C). Note that air rises to the highest point in the thorax, the anterior thorax in a supine patient and the lung apex in an upright patient. The visceral pleura covering the lung is visible as a thin white line on both chest radiographs and CT scans. No pulmonary vessels may be seen extending beyond the pleural line, and the air in the pleural space appears more radiolucent than the adjacent lung.

The most common mimic of a pneumothorax, particularly in a supine patient, is a skin fold. The film cassette for portable AP chest radiographs is placed behind the patient's back. Skin folds may be pressed between the patient's back and the film cassette. Radiographically, a skin fold produces an interface, or an edge of thick tissue outlined by the greater radiolucency of the superimposed lung. If you can distinguish an edge from a line, then you can distinguish a skin fold from a pneumothorax. The absence of pulmonary markings beyond the pleural line is supporting evidence for a pneumothorax. Since the vessels taper as they approach the lung periphery, the vessels in the extreme periphery of the lung may be too tiny to see.

Pneumothorax is spontaneous if it occurs in the absence of trauma (including barotrauma). Spontaneous pneumothorax may be primary and occur in the absence of significant other lung disease, or it may occur secondarily because of lung disease. Apical blebs are present in a high percentage of patients with primary spontaneous pneumothorax, and their rupture is thought to be the most frequent cause of spontaneous pneumothorax. For unknown reasons, it occurs most frequently in tall young men. Secondary spontaneous pneumothorax may occur in association with any cavitary lesion that lies in the periphery of the lung, as well as in emphysema, in bullous disease, and in pulmonary fibrosis of a variety of etiologies.

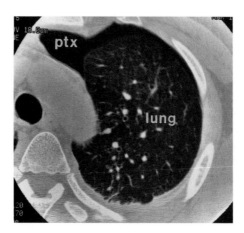

FIG. 4-E-20 (*Panel C*) Axial CT image (lung window settings) shows air in the left pleural space (*ptx*). Note that the pneumothorax in this supine patient rises to the highest part of the thorax. The visceral pleural covering of the left lung is visible as a thin white line.

EXERCISE 4-13: PLEURAL EFFUSION

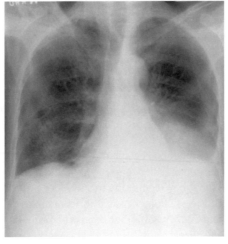 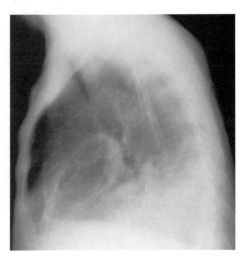

FIG. 4-E-21   *(Panels A and B)*

A   *B*

Clinical History: **CASE 4-21**
A 45-year-old man presents with increasing dyspnea and abdominal swelling of 1 week's duration (Fig. 4-E-21*A,B*).

Question: **4-21.** Which of the following radiographic signs suggest the presence of pleural effusion?

    A. Meniscus-shaped opacity in a posterior costophrenic angle on the lateral projection

    B. Biconvex lens-shaped opacity projecting in the midthorax on the lateral projection

    C. Fluid levels that have different lengths on the PA and lateral views in a hemithorax

    D. Homogeneous increased density in a hemithorax with preservation of the vascular shadows in the lungs

    E. Separation of the gastric air bubble from the inferior lung margin by more than 2 cm

Radiologic Findings: 4-21. The frontal chest radiograph (Fig. 4-E-21*A*) shows opacity at the lower left hemithorax, which has a concave border curving upward laterally adjacent to the chest wall. The overall lung volume is low in both the right and left lungs. There is separation of the gastric bubble from the inferior margin of the lung by several centimeters. On the lateral examination (Fig. 4-E-21*B*), the opacity obscures the posterior heart margin and has a margin curving slightly upward to the posterior chest wall. The findings are those of a pleural effusion on the left. The patient is noted to have a slight abdominal protrusion seen on the lateral examination. This was due to ascites in this patient with cirrhosis.

Discussion: The *visceral pleura* is the outer lining of the lung, and the *parietal pleura* is the lining of the chest cavity. Normally, these surfaces are smooth and are separated by a minimal amount of pleural fluid. This provides a nearly friction-free environment for movement of the lung with the thorax. The pleural space, therefore, is a potential space that, in the normal individual, contains no more than 3 to 5 cc of pleural fluid. Fluid may accumulate within the pleural space as a result of conditions that (1) increase pulmonary capillary pressure, (2) alter thoracic vascular or lymphatic pathways, (3) alter pleural capillary or lymphatic permeability, or (4) affect diaphragmatic peritoneal and pleural surfaces.

Pleural effusions are usually approached clinically according to whether the effusion develops because of alterations of the Starling equation, which controls fluid flow and maintenance in body compartments, or whether the pleura is affected primarily by a disease process. Processes resulting from alterations of the Starling equation include congestive heart failure, hypoproteinemia, fluid overload, liver failure, and nephrosis. These effusions are usually transudates (clear or pale yellow, odorless fluid without elevation of the ratios of pleural fluid to serum protein and lactate dehydrogenase). Processes that alter pleural capillary or lymphatic permeability include infections, inflammation, pulmonary embolism, and neoplasms. These effusions are usually exudates (clear, pale yellow or turbid, bloody, brownish fluid; pleural fluid protein to serum protein ratio greater than 0.5; and pleural fluid lactate dehydrogenase to serum lactate dehydrogenase ratio greater than 0.6). Enlarged lymph nodes or masses within the hila or mediastinum may obstruct lymphatic fluid flow and cause pleural exudates. Abdominal conditions that may produce pleural effusions include pancreatitis, subphrenic abscesses, liver abscesses, ovarian tumors, peritonitis, and ascites.

The most common radiographic sign is a pleural meniscus. The volume of fluid necessary to produce a pleural meniscus within a costophrenic angle varies from individual to individual. Approximately 100 cc of pleural fluid will cause appreciable blunting of the posterior costophrenic angle on the lateral view, and 200 cc will cause blunting of the lateral costophrenic angle on the PA projection in an upright patient (Fig. 4-E-21C–E). A lateral decubitus chest radiograph, with the side containing the pleural effusion placed down (dependent), will demonstrate even smaller amounts of free-flowing pleural effusions (Fig. 4-E-21F). Each millimeter of thickness of pleural fluid in the lateral decubitus projection corresponds to approximately 20 cc of pleural fluid. Large pleural effusions usually may be aspirated without guidance other than the chest radiograph. Small effusions are more difficult to aspirate, and if thoracentesis is planned, additional imaging guidance with ultrasonography or CT may be used. The effusion simply may be marked and aspirated by the clinical physician, or the effusion may be aspirated by a radiologist. If thoracentesis is attempted and fails for a large pleural effusion, it may be loculated, and further imaging guidance is usually helpful.

When pleural adhesions develop, fluid in the pleural space becomes loculated (Fig. 4-E-21G,H) and may be trapped in nondependent areas of the thorax. The appearance of pleural fluid may change and, rather than a meniscus shape, may assume the shape of a convex margin away from the chest wall. If fluid is trapped in the fissures, it will assume a biconvex lens shape. If a bronchopleural fistula develops, the patient will have a hydropneumothorax that may be recognized by air-fluid levels of different lengths on the PA and lateral chest radiographs. When cavities develop in the lung, the fluid levels are usually of the same length (all the options in Question 4-21 are correct).

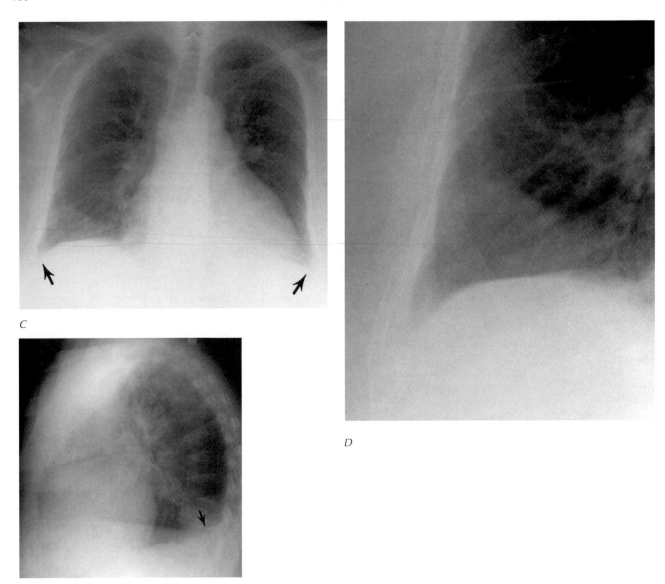

C

D

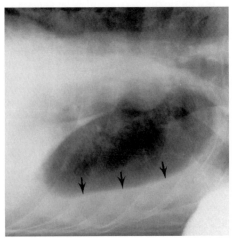

E

F

FIG. 4-E-21　Full (*Panel C*) and close-up (*Panel D*) frontal views of the chest show blunting of both lateral costophrenic angles (*arrows*) caused by small bilateral pleural effusions. (*Panel E*) Lateral chest radiograph shows that the posterior costophrenic angles (*arrows*) are also blunted by fluid in both pleural spaces. (*Panel F*) A left lateral decubitus radiograph shows displacement of the lateral margin of the left lung (*arrows*) from the chest wall by free-flowing pleural effusion. (*Panel G*) Left lateral decubitus shows displacement of the lung away from the ribs by a homogeneous soft-tissue opacity on the left. This represents a pleural effusion. Note that the contour adjacent to the lower thorax wall is convex, away from the chest wall (*arrowheads*). (*Panel H*) Right lateral decubitus view of the same patient shows that the homogeneous opacity along the upper chest wall has moved away and allowed the lung to become adjacent to the ribs. Continued presence of the convex contour adjacent to the costophrenic angle indicates a loculation of pleural fluid at the position (*arrowheads*). Note also the displacement of lung away from the right chest wall and tracking of fluid into the minor fissure (*arrows*) on the right.

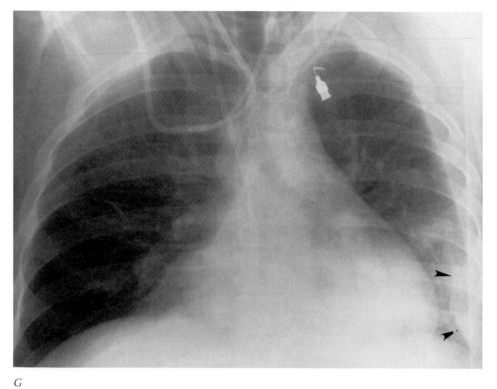

G

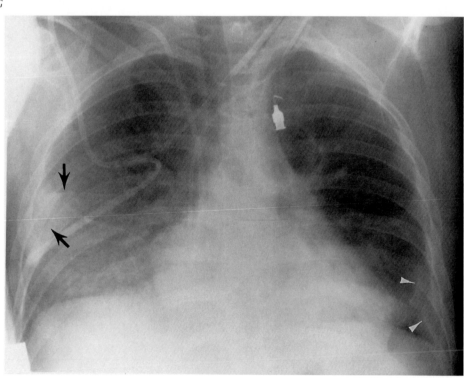

FIG. 4-E-21 *(Continued)*

H

EXERCISE 4-14: PULMONARY VASCULAR DISEASE

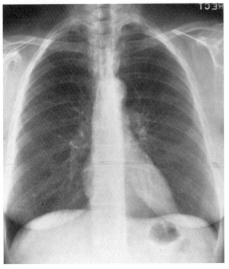

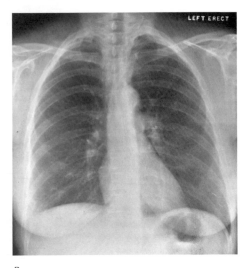

B

A

FIG. 4-E-22   *(Panels A, B, and C)*

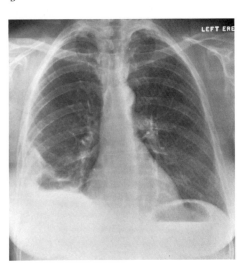

C

Clinical History:

CASE 4-22

A 53-year-old woman presents with leg swelling, right-sided pleuritic chest pain, and dyspnea. You are shown chest radiographs at age 49 (Fig. 4-E-22*A*), at presentation (Fig. 4-E-22*B*), and 4 days later (Fig. 4-E-22*C*).

Question:

4-22. The most appropriate next step in the imaging workup is
    A.   pulmonary arteriogram.
    B.   ultrasonography to look for right pleural effusion.
    C.   radionuclide ventilation-perfusion scan.
    D.   radionuclide gallium scan.
    E.   magnetic resonance angiography.

Radiologic Findings:

    4-22. The chest radiograph in Fig. 4-E-22*A* is normal. In Fig. 4-E-22*B*, there is blunting of the right lateral costophrenic angle, and a faint opacity is present within the adjacent lung. In Fig. 4-E-22*C*, there is a small pleural meniscus at the right costophrenic angle and elevation of the right lung base by subpulmonic pleural effusion. There is a cone-shaped opacity at the right lung base, with the base of the cone against the lateral chest wall and the apex of the cone pointing toward the right hilum. In the clinical setting of pleuritic chest pain, dyspnea, and hypoxemia, these findings should prompt consideration of pulmonary embolism. The next step in the workup of this patient should be a radionuclide $\dot{V}/\dot{Q}$ scan (*C* is the correct answer to Question 4-22) (Fig. 4-E-22*D,E*). The lateral view of the right pulmonary angiogram is shown in Fig. 4-E-22*F*. A saddle embolus is present at the bifurcation of the right descending pulmonary artery.

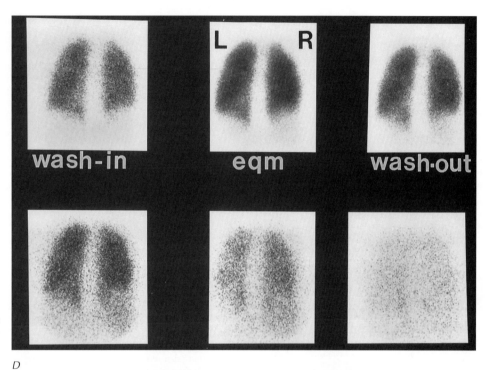

FIG. 4-E-22 (*Panel D*) Ventilation scan shows normal wash-in, a ventilation defect at the right lung base that corresponds to the abnormality seen on the chest radiograph, and normal wash-out, with no evidence of air trapping (*eqm* = equilibrium). (*Panel E*) Perfusion scan shows a defect at the right lateral and posterior costophrenic angle that is larger than the radiographic abnormality and larger than the ventilation defect seen in part *D*. This scan was considered intermediate probability for pulmonary embolism (*ANT* = anterior; *LPO* = left posterior oblique; *RPO* = right posterior oblique; *RAO* = right anterior oblique; *LAO* = left anterior oblique). (*Panel F*) Lateral view of the pulmonary angiogram shows a filling defect (thromboembolus, *arrow*) at the bifurcation of the pulmonary artery to the right lower lobe.

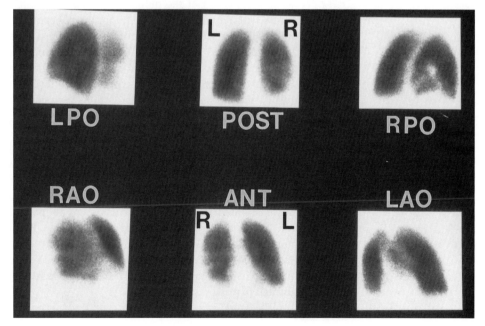

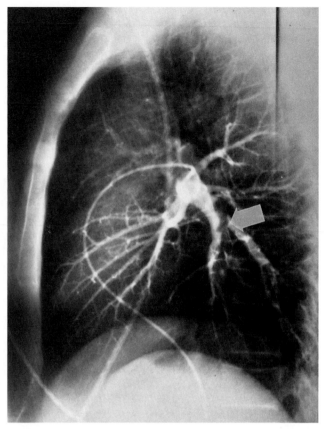

FIG. 4-E-22   (*Continued*)

F

Discussion:
Pulmonary thromboembolism can occur as a result of deep venous thrombosis, typically from the veins of the pelvis and lower extremities. These thrombi dislodge (embolize) and travel via the inferior vena cava and right heart chambers to become trapped in the tapering branches of the pulmonary arterial system. Since pulmonary embolism often occurs without pulmonary infarction, the appearance of the chest radiograph is usually normal. The areas of lung deprived of pulmonary arterial flow are perfused by bronchial arterial collateral vessels. The chest radiograph may demonstrate subtle signs of volume loss or a small pleural effusion. Pulmonary opacities develop because of microatelectasis within the region of lung that has had an embolus or from hemorrhage within a pulmonary infarction. Pulmonary infarction may occur if the pulmonary venous pressure is elevated or the bronchial arterial supply to a region is deficient for some reason. The cone-shaped area of pulmonary infarction has been called a *Hampton's hump* after its original descriptor. An area of radiolucency corresponding to diminished pulmonary vascularity distal to a pulmonary embolism is occasionally seen and is called the *Westermark sign.* There also may be an increase in the size of the pulmonary artery proximal to a large central pulmonary embolus.

The region of decreased perfusion due to the embolus is most easily demonstrated as a defect on a radionuclide perfusion lung scan. Regions of pneumonia, emphysema, or bronchial obstruction may result in diversion of blood flow away from the involved area. Because of this, ventilation scans are also performed to demonstrate that the ventilation to the involved areas is normal. These disorders result in matched defects on the ventilation and perfusion scans.

The study is interpreted as normal if no perfusion defects are present. The probability of pulmonary thromboembolism is considered to be low if the perfusion defects involve only a single segment of lung and the chest radiograph is normal, or if no more than four segments of one lung are involved on the perfusion scan with matching ventilation defects equal to or larger than the perfusion defects. Pulmonary embolism is considered a high probability if there are at least two segmental perfusion defects without corresponding ventilation or radiographic abnormalities. Probability is intermediate or indeterminate if it falls between these high- and low-probability categories. A scan with matched defects is likely to be interpreted as indeterminate for the diagnosis of pulmonary embolism. When both pulmonary arteriograms and $\dot{V}/\dot{Q}$ scans are performed, patients with a high-probability scan have an 88 percent incidence of pulmonary thromboembolism; patients with an intermediate-probability scan have a 33 percent incidence of pulmonary thromboembolism; patients with a low-probability scan have a 12 percent incidence of pulmonary thromboembolism, based on the results of the Prospective Investigation of Pulmonary Embolism Diagnosis (PIOPED) study.

Clinical criteria have been developed that enhance the value of the $\dot{V}/\dot{Q}$ scan. These include the presence of chest pain, dyspnea, hypoxemia, known venous thrombosis, and hypercoagulable state. In patients with 80 to 100 percent likelihood of pulmonary embolism by clinical criteria, a high-probability $\dot{V}/\dot{Q}$ scan means a 96 percent probability of pulmonary embolism. In a patient with a low clinical probability (0 to 20 percent) of having pulmonary embolism, a low-probability $\dot{V}/\dot{Q}$ scan is associated with a 4 percent incidence of pulmonary embolism. Therapeutic decisions are often based on the concordant clinical and $\dot{V}/\dot{Q}$ scan likelihoods of pulmonary embolism. If there is a high index of suspicion based on clinical data and the radionuclide scan is interpreted as indicating high probability, then anticoagulation therapy is warranted without further evaluation. If there is a clinical contraindication to anticoagulant therapy, or if the clinical assessment and the $\dot{V}/\dot{Q}$ scans are discordant (e.g., high clinical likelihood and low-probability $\dot{V}/\dot{Q}$ scan, or vice versa), then confirmation of the diagnosis with pulmonary angiography is standard practice.

When CT scanning was first developed, the machines were not fast or powerful enough to be reliable for diagnosing pulmonary emboli. CT scanners today are more powerful and sophisticated. With these machines and power injectors for delivery of intravascular contrast material, large, central emboli can be identified in about 90 percent of the cases in which they are demonstrated by means of pulmonary angiography.

GLOSSARY OF TERMS IN CHEST ROENTGENOLOGY*

Acinar pattern (synonyms: *alveolar pattern, airspace disease, consolidation*)   A collection of round or elliptic, ill-defined, discrete or partly confluent opacities in the lung, each measuring 4 to 8 mm in diameter and together producing an extended, inhomogeneous shadow.

Air bronchogram   A branching lucency that represents the roentgenographic shadow of an air-containing bronchus peripheral to the hilum and surrounded by airless lung (whether by virtue of absorption of air, replacement of air, or both), a finding generally regarded as evidence of the patency of the more proximal airway.

Air-fluid level   A local collection of gas and liquid that, when traversed by a horizontal x-ray beam, creates a shadow characterized by a sharp horizontal interface between a gas density above and liquid density below.

Airspace   The gas-containing portion of lung parenchyma, including the acini and excluding the interstitium and purely conductive portions of the lung.

Anterior junction line   A vertically oriented linear opacity approximately 1 to 2 mm wide produced by the shadows of the right and left pleural surfaces in intimate contact between the aerated lungs anterior to the great vessels. It is usually obliquely oriented, projected over the tracheal air column, below the level of the clavicles.

Aortopulmonary window   A zone of relative lucency seen on both the PA and lateral chest radiographs bounded medially by the left side of the trachea, superiorly by the inferior surface of the aortic arch, and inferiorly by the left pulmonary artery. The pleural surface of the aortopulmonary (AP) window is normally concave; convexity of the AP window suggests lymphadenopathy.

Atelectasis   Less than normal inflation of all or a portion of lung with corresponding diminution in volume. Qualifiers are often used to indicate extent and distribution (linear or platelike, subsegmental, segmental, lobar) as well as the mechanism (resorption, relaxation, compressive, passive, cicatricial, adhesive).

Azygoesophageal recess   On the frontal chest radiograph, a vertically oriented interface between air in the right lower lobe and the adjacent mediastinum containing the azygos vein and esophagus. It projects in the middle of the heart and spine on the frontal view.

Bleb   A thin-walled lucency within or contiguous with the visceral pleura.

Bulla   A sharply demarcated area of avascularity (lucency) within the lung measuring 1 cm or more in diameter and possessing a wall less than 1 mm in thickness.

Carina   The bifurcation of the trachea into right and left main bronchi.

Cavity   A gas-containing space within the lung surrounded by a wall whose thickness is greater than 1 mm, and often irregular in contour.

Fissure   The infolding of visceral pleura that separates one lobe, or a portion of a lobe, from another. Radiographically visible as a linear opacity normally 1 mm or less in width. Qualifiers: minor (horizontal), major, accessory, azygos, anomalous.

Ground-glass pattern   A finely granular pattern of pulmonary opacity such that pulmonary vessels remain visible. The degree of opacity is not sufficient to result in air bronchograms.

Hilum (plural: hila)   Anatomically, the depression or pit in that part of an organ where the vessels and nerves enter. On chest radiographs, the term *hilum* represents the composite shadow of the bronchi, pulmonary arteries and veins, and lymph nodes on the medial aspect of each lung.

Honeycomb pattern   A number of ring shadows or cystic spaces within the lung representing airspaces 5 to 10 mm in diameter with walls 2 to 3 mm thick that resemble a true honeycomb. The finding implies interstitial fibrosis and "end-stage" lung disease.

---

*Adapted from Glossary of words, terms and symbols in chest medicine and roentgenology, in *Diagnosis of Diseases of the Chest,* edited by RG Fraser, JAP Pare, PD Pare, RS Fraser, GP Genereux. Philadelphia, Saunders, 1988, pp xiii–xxx.

Interface (synonyms: *edge, border*)   The boundary between the shadows of structures of different opacity (e.g., the lung and the heart).

Interstitium   A continuum of loose connective tissue throughout the lung consisting of three subdivisions: (1) bronchoarterial (axial), surrounding the bronchoarterial bundles; (2) parenchymal (acinar), between the alveolar and capillary basement membranes; and (3) subpleural, between the pleura and lung parenchyma and continuous with the interlobular septa and perivenous interstitial space.

Line   A longitudinal opacity no greater than 2 mm in width.

Lobe   One of the principal divisions of the lungs (usually three on the right, two on the left) enveloped by the visceral pleura except at the hilum. The lobes are separated in whole or in part by pleural fissures.

Lucency (synonym: *radiolucency*)   The shadow of tissue that attenuates the x-ray beam less effectively than surrounding tissue. On a radiograph, the area that appears more nearly black, usually applied to areas of air density or fat density.

Lymphadenopathy (synonym: *adenopathy*)   Enlargement or abnormality of lymph nodes.

Mass   Any pulmonary or pleural lesion greater than 3 cm in diameter.

Miliary pattern   A collection of tiny (1 to 2 mm in diameter), discrete opacities in the lungs, generally uniform in size and widespread in distribution.

Nodular pattern   A collection of innumerable small, discrete opacities (2 to 10 mm in diameter), generally widespread in distribution.

Nodule   A sharply defined, discrete, circular opacity up to 3 cm in diameter within the lung.

Opacity   The shadow of tissue that attenuates the x-ray beam more than surrounding tissue. On a radiograph, areas that are more white than the surrounding area are said to be more opaque.

Peribronchial cuffing   Widening of the normal thickness of the bronchial walls seen as ring-shaped structures near the hila or as tram lines. The edge definition is less distinct than normal.

Posterior junction line   A vertically oriented, linear opacity approximately 2 mm wide produced by the shadows of the right and left pleurae in intimate contact between the aerated lungs, representing the plane of contact between the lungs posterior to the trachea and esophagus and anterior to the spine; the line may project above and below the suprasternal notch.

Posterior tracheal stripe   A vertically oriented linear opacity 2 to 5 mm wide extending from the thoracic inlet to the bifurcation of the trachea, visible on the lateral radiograph, representing the posterior tracheal wall and contiguous mediastinal tissue (anterior, and often posterior, walls of the esophagus).

Primary complex   The combination of a focus of pneumonia due to a primary infection (e.g., tuberculosis or histoplasmosis) with granulomas in the draining hilar or mediastinal lymph nodes. (Synonym: *Ranke complex.* The term *Ghon focus* describes the pulmonary lesion that has calcified. *Ranke complex* is the term to describe the combination of the Ghon focus and calcified hilar lymph nodes.)

Reticular pattern   A collection of innumerable small, linear opacities that together produce the appearance of a net.

Reticulonodular pattern   A collection of innumerable small, linear, and nodular opacities that together produce the appearance of a net and superimposed small nodules.

Right paratracheal stripe   A vertically oriented linear opacity 2 to 3 mm wide, extending from the thoracic inlet to the right tracheobronchial angle. It represents the right tracheal wall and contiguous mediastinal tissue (visceral and parietal pleurae of the right lung).

Secondary pulmonary lobule   A unit of lung structure supplied by three to five terminal bronchioles.

Septal line (synonym: *Kerley line*)   A linear opacity, usually 1 to 2 mm in width, produced by thickening of the interlobular septa and often due to either edema or cellular infiltration.

Silhouette sign   The effacement of an anatomic soft-tissue border by either a normal anatomic structure or a pathologic state, such as airlessness of adjacent lung or accumulation of fluid in the contiguous pleural space.

Stripe   A longitudinal opacity 2 to 5 mm in width.

Tram line shadow   Parallel or slightly convergent linear opacities that suggest the projection of tubular structures, generally representing thickened bronchial walls.

BIBLIOGRAPHY

Blank N: *Chest Radiographic Analysis.* New York, Churchill-Livingstone, 1989.

Felson B: *Chest Roentgenology.* Philadelphia, Saunders, 1973.

Freundlich IM, Bragg DG: *A Radiologic Approach to Diseases of the Chest.* Baltimore, Williams & Wilkins, 1992.

Groskin SA: *Heitzman's The Lung: Radiologic-Pathologic Correlations,* 3d ed. St. Louis, Mosby, 1993.

Heitzman ER: *The Mediastinum: Radiologic Correlations with Anatomy and Pathology,* 2d ed. New York, Springer-Verlag, 1988.

Reed JC: *Chest Radiology: Plain Film Patterns and Differential Diagnoses,* 2d ed. St. Louis, Mosby–Year Book, 1991.

5

RADIOLOGY OF THE BREAST

Rita I. Freimanis

Imaging of the breast is undertaken as part of a comprehensive evaluation of this organ, integrating the patient's history, clinical signs, and symptoms. Radiography of the breast is known as *mammography* or *radiomammography.* When used periodically in asymptomatic patients, this is called *screening mammography.* When imaging is targeted to symptomatic patients, it is referred to as *diagnostic breast imaging* and usually is a tailored evaluation consisting of some combination of mammography and other techniques described below. Using the integrated approach, it is often possible to make an accurate diagnosis nonoperatively, and treatment may be individualized according to each patient's needs. The primary purpose of breast imaging is to detect breast carcinoma. A secondary purpose is to evaluate benign disease, such as cyst formation, infection, and trauma.

Before the 1980s, when breast imaging was used much less widely, the proportion of surgery for benign breast disease was higher, and treatment for breast carcinoma was initiated at later stages of the disease than at present. Breast imaging has increased the detection of tumors smaller than those found on clinical breast examination and has enabled patients to avoid unnecessary surgery.

The outcome of earlier diagnosis and treatment, however, is yet to be proven. Mortality from breast cancer has remained fairly stable for several decades despite the introduction and popularization of screening mammography. Debate continues as to the efficacy of routine breast screening in certain age groups. It is universally acknowledged that women over 50 years of age benefit from periodic screening mammography. Several large population studies have shown a decrease in mortality of around 30 percent in this group. The greatest current controversy concerns the value of screening mammography for women under age 50. Since breast cancer has a lower prevalence in this age group, the impediment to mass screening is largely economic; i.e., the number of lives saved relative to dollars spent must be justified. Another difference is that in younger women the breast parenchyma is more often dense and nodular. This condition decreases the sensitivity for detection for carcinoma and leads to more false-negative and false-positive results.

Besides a decrease in mortality, a second benefit of earlier diagnosis is that patients with breast carcinoma are afforded more treatment options; lumpectomy with radiation therapy is now being presented as an option to mastectomy in selected patients.

Mammography has been in common use since about 1980, and breast ultrasonography has been the most often used adjunctive technique during this time. The major contribution of ultrasonography has been its effectiveness in distinguishing cystic lesions from solid masses. Sonography has therefore helped to avoid unnecessary surgery, since asymptomatic simple cysts do not require intervention.

In the 1990s, magnetic resonance MR imaging of the breast has been used in selected patients. Current applications include evaluation of masses, both mammographically and clinically detected, differentiation of dense breast tissue or fibrosis from tumor, and evaluation of breast implants for possible complications. Because of its present investigational status, cost, and inaccessibility, however, MR imaging is used infrequently.

Also in the 1990s, image-guided needle biopsy of the breast has been popularized in this country. Stereotactic mammographic guidance for needle aspiration of the breast has been used heavily in Sweden since the 1970s and is now increasingly available elsewhere. This technique has contributed to a reduction in the number of surgical biopsies for benign and malignant disease.

Computed tomography (CT), nuclear medicine, and contrast injection studies (ductography) are used occasionally under special circumstances with specific indications.

TECHNIQUE AND NORMAL ANATOMY

Film-Screen Radiography (Radiomammography)

At present in the United States, the mammogram is created with x-rays, radiographic film, and intensifying screens adjacent to the film within the cassette, hence the term *film-screen mammography*. The examination consists of two views of each breast, the craniocaudal (CC) view and the mediolateral oblique (MLO) view, with a total of four films. The CC view can be considered the "top down" view and the MLO an angled view from the side (Fig. 5-1). The patient undresses from the waist up and stands for the examination, leaning slightly against the mammography unit. The technologist must mobilize, elevate, and pull the breast to place as much breast tissue as possible on the surface of the film cassette holder. A flat, plastic compression paddle is then gently but firmly lowered onto the breast surface to compress the breast into as thin a layer as possible. This compression achieves both immobilization during film exposure and dispersion of breast tissue shadows over a larger area of film, thereby permitting better visual separation of imaged structures. Compression may be uncomfortable and may even be painful in a small proportion of patients. However, most patients accept this level of discomfort for the few seconds required for each exposure, particularly if they understand the need for compression and know what to expect during the examination. Film-screen technique has proved to be more cost-effective, while maintaining resolution high enough to demonstrate

early malignant lesions, than any other breast imaging technique. In its present state of evolution, however, the sensitivity of radiomammography ranges from 85 to 95 percent.

LIMITATIONS

Sensitivity is limited by three factors: (1) the nature of breast parenchyma, (2) the difficulty in positioning the organ for imaging, and (3) the nature of breast carcinoma.

The Nature of Breast Parenchyma. Very dense breast tissue may obscure masses lying within adjacent tissue. Masses are more easily detected in a fatty breast.

Positioning. A technologist performing mammography must include as much breast tissue as possible in the field of view for each image. The x-ray beam must pass through the breast tangentially to the thorax, and no other part of the body should intrude into the field of view so as to not obscure any part of the breast. This requires both a cooperative patient and a skilled technologist. If a breast mass is located in a portion of the breast that is difficult to include in the image, mammography may fail to demonstrate the lesion. Also, because of these practical considerations, routine mammography is not performed in markedly debilitated patients.

The Nature of Breast Carcinoma. Some breast carcinomas are seen as well-defined, rounded masses or as tiny, but bright calcifications and are easily detected. Others, however, may be poorly defined and irregular, mimicking normal breast tissue. Rarely, still others may have no radiographic signs at all.

For these reasons, it must be remembered that mammography has significant limitations in detection of carcinoma. It cannot be overemphasized that any suspicious finding on breast physical examination should be evaluated further, even if the mammogram shows no abnormality. Occasionally, additional imaging may reveal an abnormality, but if not, short-term close clinical follow-up or biopsy is warranted.

NORMAL STRUCTURES

Radiomammography uses lower-energy x-rays than do other radiographic procedures. For this reason, there is greater contrast of soft-tissue elements. A breast shadow on a chest radiograph is uniformly white, but breast densities as seen on mammograms range from nearly black to white (Fig. 5-2).

Normal breast is composed mainly of parenchyma (lobules and ducts), connective tissue, and fat. Lobules are drained by ducts, which arborize within lobes. There are about 15 to 20 lobes in the breast. The lobar ducts converge on the nipple.

Parenchyma. The lobules are glandular units and are seen as ill-defined, splotchy opacities of medium density. Their size varies from one to several millimeters, and larger opacities result from conglomerates of lobules with little interspersed fat. The breast lobes are intertwined and

FIG. 5-1 (*A*) Positioning of the patient for the craniocaudal view of the mammogram. (*B*) Positioning of the patient for the mediolateral oblique view of the mammogram. (*C*) Normal bilateral craniocaudal views. (*D*) Normal bilateral mediolateral oblique views. This patient shows a moderate amount of residual fibroglandular density, having a mixed pattern of dense and fatty areas of the breast.

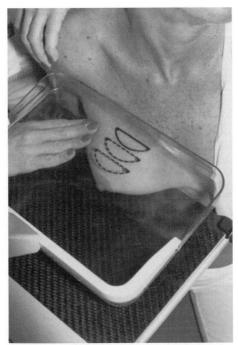

A

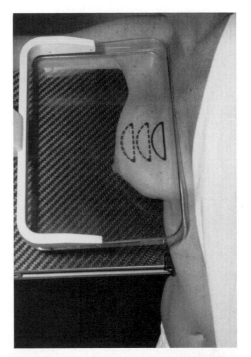

B

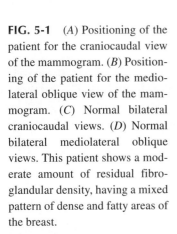

C

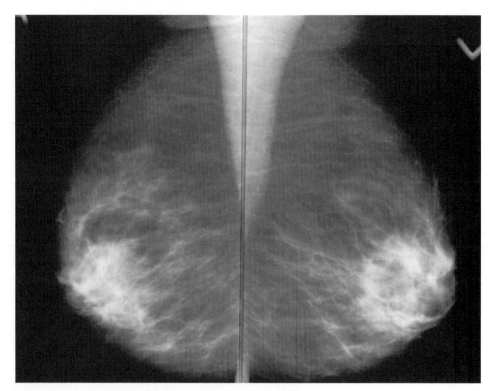

FIG. 5-1 (*Continued*)

D

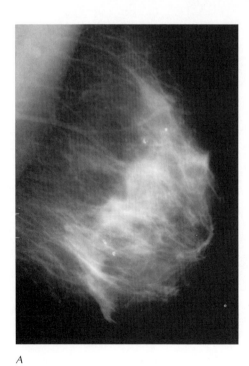

A

FIG. 5-2 (*A*) Mediolateral oblique view of
normal breasts. (*B*) Line drawing with identification of normal structures visible in part *A*.

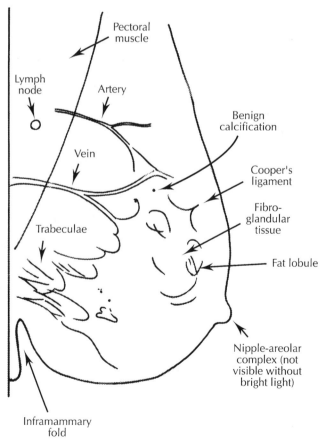

B

are therefore not discretely identifiable. This parenchymal tissue is contained between the premammary and retromammary fasciae, which are best seen on sonographic images (Fig. 5-3).

The amount and distribution of glandular tissue are highly variable. Younger women tend to have more glandular tissue than do older women. Glandular atrophy begins inferomedially, and residual glandular density persists longer in the upper outer breast quadrants. However, any pattern can be seen at any adult age (Fig. 5-4).

Along with glandular elements, the parenchyma consists of ductal tissue. Only major ducts are visualized mammographically, and these are seen in the subareolar region as thickened linear structures of medium density converging on the nipple.

Connective Tissue. Trabecular structures, which are condensations of connective tissue, appear as thin (<1 mm) linear opacities of medium to high density. Cooper's ligaments are the supporting trabeculae over the breast that give the organ its characteristic shape and are thus seen as curved lines around fat lobules along the skin-parenchyma interface within any one breast (see Fig. 5-2).

Fat. The breast is composed of a large amount of fat, which is lucent, or blackish, on mammograms. Fat is distributed in the subcutaneous layer, in among the parenchymal elements centrally, and in the retromammary layer anterior to the pectoral muscle (see Figs. 5-2 and 5-3).

Lymph Nodes. Lymph nodes are seen in the axillae and occasionally in the breast itself (see Fig. 5-2).

Veins. Veins are seen traversing the breast as uniform, linear opacities about 1 to 5 mm in diameter (see Fig. 5-2).

Arteries. Arteries appear as slightly thinner, uniform linear densities and are best seen when calcified, as in patients with atherosclerosis, diabetes, or renal disease (see Fig. 5-2).

Skin. Skin lines are normally thin and are not easily seen without the aid of a bright light. On a well-exposed mammogram, the margins of the breast are often overpenetrated.

SCREENING MAMMOGRAPHY

The standard mammogram (along with appropriate history taking) makes up the entire screening mammogram. The indication for this examination is the search for occult carcinoma in an asymptomatic patient. Physical examination by the patient's physician, known as the *clinical breast examination* (CBE), and breast self-examination (BSE) are the other two indispensable elements in complete breast screening. Table 5-1 includes guidelines for frequency.

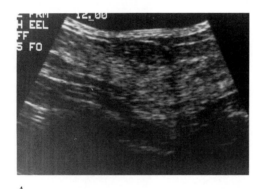

A

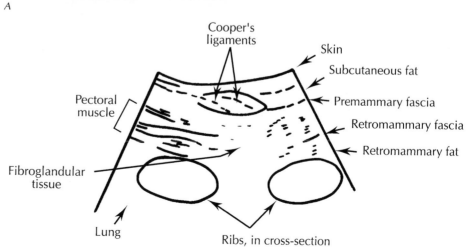

FIG. 5-3 (*A*) Ultrasonographic image of a portion of normal breast. (*B*) Line drawing identifying normal structures visible on the sonographic image.

B

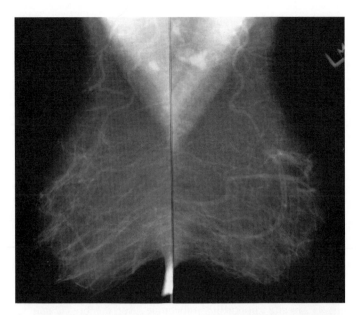

A

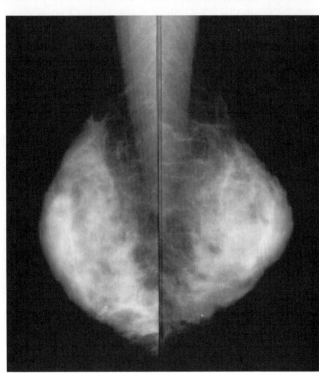

B

FIG. 5-4 (*A*) Normal mammograms of fatty breasts. (*B*) Normal mammograms of dense breasts. Note the extreme variation of the normal breast parenchymal pattern between patients. A small carcinoma would be much more difficult to detect in the patient with dense breasts (*B*) than in the patient with fatty breasts (*A*).

DIAGNOSTIC MAMMOGRAPHY

The diagnostic mammogram begins with the two-view standard mammogram. Additional maneuvers are then used as appropriate in each case, dictated by history, physical examination, and findings on initial mammography. Indications for diagnostic mammography are (1) a palpable mass or other symptom or sign (e.g., skin dimpling, nipple retraction, or nipple discharge that is clear or bloody), and (2) a radiographic abnormality on a screening mammogram.

Other Projections. The angle of the x-ray beam and position of the breast are changed to include areas not otherwise imaged and to view a structure or opacity within the breast from a different perspective so as to gain a better three-dimensional perception.

Magnification. Small opacities are better evaluated by means of magnification views for improved detail (see Exercise 5-7). This is achieved by positioning the breast farther from the film and closer to the x-ray tube during exposure.

TABLE 5-1   AMERICAN CANCER SOCIETY RECOMMENDATIONS FOR BREAST CANCER DETECTION IN ASYMPTOMATIC WOMEN

Age Group (years)	Examination	Frequency
20–40	Breast self-examination (BSE)	Every month
	Clinical breast examination (CBE)	Every three years
40–50	Breast self-examination	Every month
	Mammography	*Every 1 to 2 years*
	Clinical breast examination	Every year
50 and older	Breast self-examination	Every month
	Mammography	*Every year*
	Clinical breast examination	Every year

Spot Compression.   When localized opacities are not well seen because of overlapping breast tissue or insufficient compression, a smaller compression paddle targeting only a portion of the breast is used to better compress and disperse the tissue in the area of interest (see Exercise 5-1, Case 5-3).

Implant Views.   Patients with breast implants require specialized views to best image residual breast tissue because the implants obscure large areas of the breast tissue with routine mammography. These specialized views, Eklund or "pinch-back" views, displace the implants posteriorly while the breast tissue is pulled anteriorly as much as possible.

Ultrasonography

The indications for ultrasonography are (1) a mammographically detected mass, the nature of which is indeterminate, (2) a palpable mass that is not seen on mammography, and (3) a palpable mass in a patient below the age recommended for routine mammography. Ultrasonography is a highly reliable technique for differentiating cystic from solid masses. If criteria for a simple cyst are met, the diagnosis is over 99 percent accurate. Although certain features have been described as indicative of benign or malignant solid masses, this determination is much more difficult to make and less accurate than determination of the cystic nature of a mass.

A limitation of ultrasonography is that it is very operator-dependent. Also, it images only a small part of the breast at any one moment. Therefore, an overall inclusive survey is not possible in one image, and lesions may easily be missed.

The patient normally lies in the supine position for ultrasonography. A hand-held probe (transducer) is moved over the skin of the breast as real-time images are generated and observed. Coupling gel is applied to the skin to improve contact and signal transmission.

NORMAL STRUCTURES

In the breast, as elsewhere in the body, sonographic images are created by echoes of reflective surfaces. Therefore, the skin, premammary and retromammary fasciae, trabeculae, walls of ducts and vessels, and pectoral fasciae are well seen as linear structures. The glandular and fat lobules are oval, of varying sizes, and hypoechoic relative to the surrounding connective tissue (see Fig. 5-3).

Simple cysts are anechoic (echo-free) and have thin, smooth walls. Increased echogenicity is seen deep to cysts (enhanced through-transmission). Most solid masses are hypoechoic relative to surrounding breast tissue.

MR Imaging

MR imaging is the best technique to evaluate soft tissue but is at present infrequently used in breast evaluation. However, it may prove to be indicated in certain patients to help distinguish postoperative change from tumor or normal dense breast tissue from neoplasms. MR imaging is also used to evaluate the integrity of breast implants when the specialized mammographic views (Eklund views) are insufficient. Selection of pulse sequences and intravenous contrast administration is based on the indication.

The patient lies prone on the scanner table, and a specialized coil surrounds the breast. The patient must remain motionless in the scanner for several minutes at a time. The entire procedure time varies from 20 min to 1 h. Some patients experience claustrophobia in the scanner and may require sedation. Intravenous contrast material is administered if carcinoma is to be ruled out.

NORMAL STRUCTURES

Tissues are differentiated by their pattern of change on different pulse sequences. The skin, nipple and areola, mammary fat, breast parenchyma, and connective tissue are normally seen, in addition to the anterior chest wall, including musculature, ribs, and their cartilaginous portions, and portions of internal organs. Small calcifications are not visible, and small solid nodules may not be detected. Cystic structures are well seen. Normal implants appear as cystic structures with well-defined walls. Their location is deep to the breast parenchyma or subpectoral, depending on the surgical technique that was used to place the implants. Internal signal varies and depends on implant contents, either silicone or saline.

Computed Tomography (CT)

CT is an infrequently used breast imaging technique. Indications for breast CT are (1) inability to localize and evaluate a structure with other imaging and (2) guidance for needle placement in selected patients for needle aspiration or excisional biopsy.

The appearance of the breast on CT is similar to that on MR imaging, but CT has slightly greater spatial resolution and less soft-tissue differentiation.

Ductography

Ductography, or galactography, uses mammographic imaging with contrast injection into the breast ducts. The indication for use is a profuse spontaneous nonmilky nipple discharge from a single duct orifice. If these conditions are not present, the ductogram is likely to be of little help. The purpose is to reveal the location of the ductal system involved. The cause of the discharge is frequently not identified. Occasionally, an intraluminal abnormality is seen, but findings have low specificity.

The patient lies in supine position while the discharging duct is cannulated with a blunt-tipped needle under visual inspection and with the aid of a magnifying glass. A small amount of contrast material (usually not more than 1 cc) is injected gently by hand into the duct. Several mammographic images are then made. The procedure requires about 30 minutes and is not normally painful.

NORMAL STRUCTURES

Just deep to the opening of the duct on the nipple, the duct expands into the lactiferous sinus. After a few millimeters, the duct narrows again and then branches as it enters the lobe containing the glands drained by this ductal system. The normal caliber of the duct and its branches is highly variable, but normal duct walls should be smooth, without truncation or abrupt narrowing (see Exercise 5-3). With high-pressure injection, the lobules, as well as cystically dilated portions of ducts and lobules, may opacify.

Image-Guided Needle Aspiration

The indications for needle aspiration of breast lesions are varied and are variably interpreted by radiologists and referring physicians. Two categories are discussed here. The first indication is aspiration of cystic lesions to confirm di-

agnosis, to relieve pain, or both. Nonpalpable cysts require guidance with either ultrasound or mammography. A fine needle (20 to 25 gauge) usually suffices. The cystic fluid is not routinely sent for cytology unless it is bloody.

The second indication concerns solid lesions. Aspiration is used in this case to (1) confirm benignity of a lesion carrying a low suspicion of malignancy mammographically, (2) to confirm malignancy in a highly suspicious lesion prior to initiating further surgical planning and treatment, and (3) to evaluate any other relevant mammographic lesion for which either follow-up imaging or surgical excision is a less desirable option for further evaluation. Both fine-needle and core-needle (14 to 18 gauge) techniques can be used. Fine needles yield cytologic information, whereas core needles yield histologic information.

The imaging modality for needle guidance is selected on the basis of lesion characteristics, availability of technology, and personal preference of the radiologist. Ultrasound and mammography are most commonly used.

Mammographic guidance is most easily and accurately performed with a stereotactic table unit. Lesions of only a few millimeters can be biopsied successfully. With stereotactic tables, the patient lies prone with the breast protruding through an opening in the table surface. A needle is guided mechanically to the proper location in the breast with computer assistance (Fig. 5-5). The entire procedure requires 30 min to 1 h.

Image-Guided Needle Localization

When a nonpalpable breast lesion must be excised, imaging is used to guide placement of a needle into the breast, with the needle tip traversing or flanking the lesion. Either ultrasonographic or mammographic guidance can be used, and the choice again depends on lesion characteristics and personal preference. Once the needle is in the appropriate position, a hook wire is inserted through the needle to anchor the device in place. This prevents migration during patient transport and surgery. After needle placement, the patient is taken to the operating area for excision of the lesion by the surgeon.

Infrequently, the guidance for localization of some lesions is CT or MR imaging. These techniques are used when the lesions are not seen with ultrasonography or radiomammography or when they are located in a portion of the breast that is difficult to access.

Biopsy Specimen Radiography

When a lesion is excised from the breast, a surgical specimen can be radiographed to document that the mammographic abnormality was removed. This practice is followed routinely with needle-localized lesions, but palpable lesions that are excised also may be radiographed to confirm that the specimen contains an abnormality that may have been present on the mammogram.

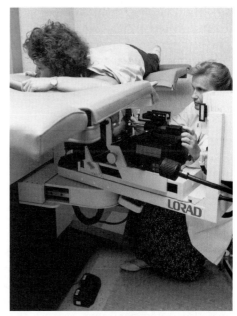

FIG. 5-5 Stereotactic biopsy table (*A*) with patient undergoing core needle biopsy of the breast. The needle is mechanically guided into the breast (*B*) with the aid of computer targeting on mammographic images.

A

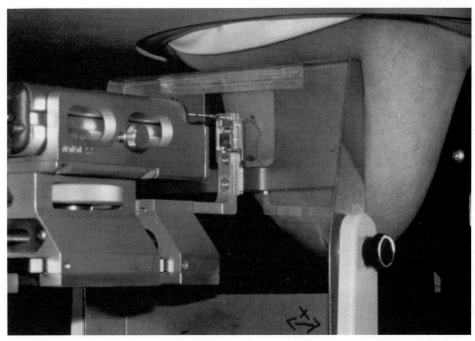

B

TECHNIQUE SELECTION

As with other organ systems, the task of the referring physician with regard to breast imaging is to determine which patients may benefit from these studies and which are the appropriate studies to order. To do this, the physician first categorizes the patient as asymptomatic or symptomatic. As a group, *asymptomatic patients* will benefit from routine screening mammography performed according to published national guidelines. A particular patient may require an individualized program for specific reasons; for example, a 30-year-old asymptomatic woman whose mother died of breast cancer at age 35 may justifiably begin yearly screening mammography. *Symptomatic patients* are women who have any of the following signs or symptoms: a new or enlarging breast lump, skin changes (primarily dimpling), nipple retraction, eczematoid nipple changes, bloody or serous nipple discharge, and focal pain or tenderness. Diagnostic mammography is indicated in these patients. If the patient is under 35 years of age, the examinations may be tailored differently than for older patients. A telephone call to the radiologist may be helpful in determining a suitable evaluation plan in any patient for whom the usual guidelines are not helpful.

If a diagnostic study is needed, a standard two-view mammogram is obtained first. The need for further studies will be determined by the results of the mammogram. Whether ultrasonography or another modality is needed is best decided by the person interpreting the films, provided that he or she has the necessary clinical information available. For example, it is imperative that the location and description of a suspected mass be made known to the radiologist so that a specific search can be made for a lesion.

Also, knowledge of prior surgery, inflammation, or trauma to the breast is a requirement for accurate image interpretation. The different disease processes may have overlapping appearances on breast images, and refining the differential diagnosis, therefore, depends on accurate breast physical examination and the patient's history.

When it has been determined that an abnormality is present, then the decision as to whether close follow-up, needle biopsy, or excision is warranted is best made by integrating the image-based diagnosis and clinical considerations. Good communication between the radiologist and referring physician is needed to optimize management of breast lesions.

Patient Preparation

For the mammogram, two-piece clothing is most convenient because the patient will need to undress from the waist up. Patients should not apply antiperspirant to the breast or axilla, since it may cause artifacts. Patients with tender breasts may minimize their discomfort by planning the mammogram for the 2-week period following onset of menses and by abstaining from all sources of caffeine for the preceding few days.

Mammography is generally limited to ambulatory, cooperative patients because of the difficulties in proper positioning and because mammography units are not portable. If a debilitated patient has a palpable mass, then ultrasound would be a reasonable first step, followed by bedside needle aspiration or biopsy if the mass is solid. Screening mammography in markedly debilitated patients rarely has clinical utility.

If MRI is planned, patients should be informed that claustrophobic people have difficulty remaining in the scanner long enough to complete the procedure. Antianxiety medications are usually helpful.

Patients undergoing CT or MRI also should be advised that contrast material injection may be needed. Establishing venous access prior to the appointment time may be advisable in those patients in whom vascular access is a known problem. Patients for whom stereotactic biopsy is being considered should be able to lie in a prone position without moving for about 1 hour.

Conflict with Other Procedures

Coordinating with other techniques is an infrequent problem with breast imaging. One situation that does occasionally cause difficulty occurs in the patient with a palpable mass that is aspirated with a needle prior to imaging. Aspiration of a simple cyst may cause bleeding into the lesion. Subsequent ultrasonography then shows a complex lesion with debris or some apparently solid elements rather than a simple cyst. A complex lesion requires more aggressive management than does a simple cyst. Therefore, imaging is best performed prior to aspiration.

THE SYMPTOMATIC PATIENT

EXERCISE 5-1: THE PALPABLE MASS

(Please answer questions for this exercise before looking at the images, which are presented with the discussion.)

Clinical Histories:

CASE 5-1
A 34-year-old woman is seen who noticed a new lump in her breast.

CASE 5-2
A 60-year-old woman is seen who, upon the insistence of her children, went for her first routine physical examination in many years. A mass was found in her breast.

CASE 5-3
A 53-year-old woman presents who thinks she feels a hard nodule deep in her breast. Her breasts have always been difficult to examine because of their dense nodular texture.

CASE 5-4
A 78-year-old woman presents with a soft, rounded mass discovered during physical examination.

Questions:

5-1. What test should be ordered first in Case 5-1?
  A. Screening mammography
  B. Excisional biopsy
  C. Ultrasonography
  D. Diagnostic mammography
  E. Needle aspiration

5-2. What test should be ordered first in Case 5-2?
  A. Screening mammography
  B. Excisional biopsy
  C. Ultrasonography
  D. Diagnostic mammography
  E. Needle aspiration

5-3. What test should be ordered first in Case 5-3?
  A. Screening mammography
  B. Excisional biopsy
  C. Ultrasonography
  D. Diagnostic mammography
  E. Needle aspiration

5-4. With respect to the patient in Case 5-4, which one of the following statements is true?
  A. A 78-year-old will not likely benefit from mammography.
  B. Soft, rounded masses are benign and do not require biopsy.
  C. This mass should be aspirated initially with a needle.
  D. If this mass is carcinoma, the patient will probably die of this disease.
  E. Her physical findings could easily be caused by a lipoma.

Approach to the Palpable Lump

When a breast lump is found, several questions must be answered before proceeding with breast imaging. First, given that lumpy breasts are a normal variant, when is a lump significant? Experts in CBE advise palpation with the flat surface of two to three fingers, not with the fingertips. With this technique, nonsignificant lumps will disperse into background breast density, but a significant lump will stand out as a dominant mass.

Second, is the lump new or enlarged? A new lump is more suspicious than a lump that has not changed over a few years.

Third, how big is the lump? Tiny pea-sized or smaller lumps, particularly in young women, are often observed closely with repeated CBE, since small breast nodules are extremely common, frequently resolve spontaneously, and usually are benign. Repeating CBE in 6 weeks allows for interval menses, which frequently causes waning or resolution of the lump. If the lump persists, diagnostic mammography is indicated.

Fourth, how old is the patient? If the patient is under 40 years of age, then radiation is avoided unless specifically indicated, since the younger breast is more sensitive to radiation. For patients over age 40, breast imaging begins with a diagnostic mammogram at the time a lump is deemed to be significant. The mammogram provides a view of the lump, as well as of the remainder of the involved breast and the opposite breast, where associated findings may aid in diagnosis and treatment planning.

If the patient is below age 40, a significant lump is usually first examined with ultrasonography to determine whether a simple cyst is present. If there is no cyst and the patient is below age 30, a single lateral view of the involved breast may be obtained. The density of the breast in such a young patient usually limits the usefulness of radiomammography except as a baseline image.

For women between the ages of 30 and 40, judgment is needed as to whether other imaging is indicated. Several factors should be weighed, including age, family history of breast carcinoma, reproductive history, and findings at CBE. If the primary care physician is uncertain of the significance of the findings of CBE, evaluation by a breast specialist may be helpful prior to requesting radiologic tests.

Discussion:

The 34-year-old woman in Case 5-1 indeed has a dominant mass 2 cm in diameter on CBE. She says it was definitely not present until recently. She has no risk factors for breast cancer. The mass most likely is a fibroadenoma or a cyst, but carcinoma cannot be excluded. The patient now needs breast ultrasonography (C is the correct answer to Question 5-1).

Ultrasonography is best ordered before attempted needle aspiration because aspiration can alter the appearance of simple cysts, giving a misleading suspicious appearance. Therefore, answer E, needle aspiration, is incorrect.

Figure 5-E-1A shows an image from the ultrasound study that represents the area precisely in the location of the palpable mass. This area is echo-free, with sharply delineated walls and posterior acoustic enhancement (increased echogenicity deep to the anechoic area) consistent with a simple cyst. If these three features are seen, the probability of a simple cyst is greater than 99 percent, and no further treatment is indicated unless the patient has pain and needs cyst drainage for symptomatic relief. Therefore, option B, excisional biopsy, is inappropriate because biopsy can be avoided by showing a simple cyst. No further imaging is needed. The patient is under age 40, not yet of screening age, and radiation should be avoided in young patients. Therefore, answers A and D, screening and diagnostic mammography, are not viable options until ultrasound is performed. Figure 5-E-1B illustrates the mammographic features of a cyst in another patient. The shape is round or oval, and the margins are smooth and sharply delineated.

Simple cysts are very common in the premenopausal patient and in patients who are being treated with replacement hormone therapy. A complex cyst is one that has internal debris—either blood, pus, or tumor. A complex cyst requires further evaluation, and a short-term follow-up (6 to 8 weeks) ultrasound may be sufficient. If the debris is due to

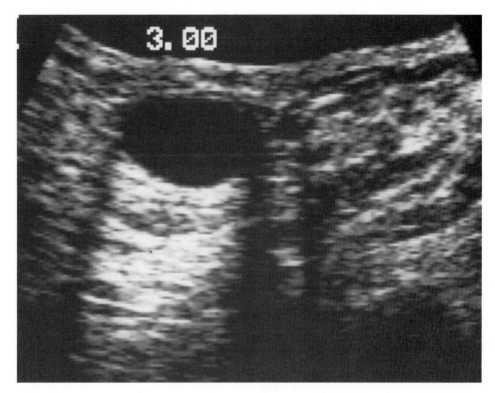

A

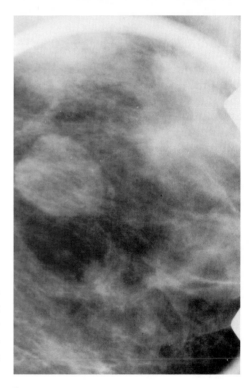

FIG. 5-E-1 (*Panel A*) Ultrasonographic image of the patient in Case 5-1. The anechoic, uniformly black area represents a simple cyst. Note that the walls of the cyst
are sharp, and there is a brighter echo pattern deep to the cyst (enhanced through-
transmission). (*Panel B*) Detail of a mammogram of a patient with a simple cyst.
The smoothly circumscribed margin and the round to oval opacity, through which
normal breast structures are visible, are characteristic of a simple cyst.

B

attempted aspiration, it may clear on follow-up ultrasonography. Otherwise, excision or needle biopsy is indicated.

The 60-year-old woman in Case 5-2 has a 1.5-cm dominant mass on CBE. It is irregular and not freely mobile. The patient has never had a mammogram. Since she has a palpable mass, however, a screening mammogram is inappropriate, and option *A* is incorrect. Although the mass feels suspicious, she still needs a diagnostic mammogram prior to biopsy (option *B,* excisional biopsy, is incorrect) to exclude other lesions such as multifocal carcinoma (*D* is the correct answer to Question 5-2). The need for ultrasonography in a patient of this age is dictated by the mammographic appearance; therefore, option *C,* ultrasonography, is incorrect.

A detail of her mammogram (Fig. 5-E-2) shows a fatty breast, making any abnormal findings readily apparent. There is a mass measuring 1 cm in the upper outer quadrant that corresponds to the area of the palpated mass. The mass is of high density, being white on the mammogram. There is abundant spiculation and stranding around the mass, which is represented by the radiating linear densities around the periphery of the mass. There is also retraction of the linear patterns of the normal breast tissue; this retraction is known as *architectural distortion.* These findings represent the classic features of a malignant lesion on mammography, and this mass must be biopsied. A spiculated mass such as this is the most common appearance of invasive breast carcinoma. Less common signs are a circumscribed mass, asymmetrical density, and architectural distortion alone. Intraductal (noninvasive) carcinoma more commonly appears as calcifications.

Spiculation around an invasive carcinoma corresponds to fingers of tumor, as well as to a desmoplastic reaction of adjacent normal breast tissue responding to the presence of tumor. This patient has an invasive ductal carcinoma. About 90 percent of primary breast carcinomas are ductal carcinomas, and the other 10 percent are lobular carcinomas.

Besides carcinoma, the primary differential diagnosis for a spiculated mass includes postoperative change, other trauma with hematoma, fat necrosis, infection, and radial scar (a complex, spontaneous, benign lesion involving ductal proliferation, elastosis, and fibrosis).

There are no other lesions in our patient's breast, and the other breast appears normal. By mammographic criteria, then, the patient is a good candidate for treatment with

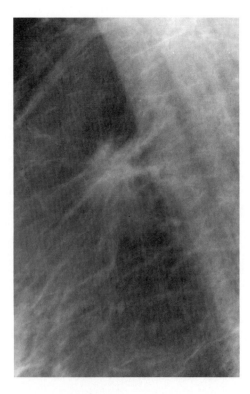

FIG. 5-E-2 Detail of a mammogram of the patient in Case 5-2. Note the spiculated mass adjacent to the pectoral muscle in the upper outer quadrant of this otherwise fatty breast. Diagnosis: invasive ductal carcinoma.

lumpectomy and radiation therapy rather than mastectomy. Her tumor is solitary and localized to one quadrant, and her breast tissue is otherwise easy to evaluate mammographically. Recurrent tumor or additional lesions therefore should be readily seen on post-treatment follow-up mammograms.

For a mass that feels malignant and appears suspicious on a mammogram, fine-needle aspiration (FNA) at the bedside may provide a rapid cytologic diagnosis of carcinoma. Since FNA best follows mammography, option *E,* needle aspiration, is incorrect. FNA may then be followed by definitive surgical treatment at a later date, after the patient has had time to consider the treatment options available. If FNA fails to disclose carcinoma, then excisional biopsy is required because of the suspicious findings on mammography and CBE. The occasional false-negative FNA occurs with tumors that do not shed cellular material readily.

Cytology of this palpable mass revealed ductal carcinoma, and this patient chose to have a lumpectomy.

The 53-year-old patient in Case 5-3 has an ill-defined 1.5-cm hardened nodular area in her breast. Results of screening mammography less than 1 year ago were normal. Her breast tissue is not fatty, as in Case 5-2, but she has quite dense, nodular, fibroglandular tissue, which may obscure small masses. The average doubling time of breast carcinoma makes it unlikely that she has a palpable carcinoma that is entirely new since her last mammogram. It is quite possible, however, that she has had a smaller cancer for a few years and that it has now grown large enough to be palpated. Breast tumors are typically not palpable unless they are at least 1 cm in diameter. Before this stage, in the preclinical phase, the tumor may be visible up to 2 to 3 years earlier on the mammogram if the breast is fatty. In dense breasts, as discussed previously, tumors may not be seen on the mammogram until later stages. For this reason, regular BSE and CBE are important. Mammography will miss some cancers, regardless of the situation, at a rate variably reported to be between 5 and 15 percent.

With a new area of abnormality on physical examination, being in a high-risk age group (over 50 years old), and having a dense parenchymal pattern, the patient needs another mammogram, this time a diagnostic mammogram of the involved breast only (*D* is the correct answer to Question 5-3). Option *A,* screening mammogram, is incorrect, because it is too soon to repeat screening mammography at this time, and the woman does have a palpable finding as a contraindication for a screening study.

Figure 5-E-3*A* shows a vague, rounded opacity within dense fibroglandular tissue. This is in the area of the palpable mass, as indicated by a small BB placed on the skin over the abnormality. Detail is not adequate to make a judgment as to the possibility of malignancy here or even to confirm that a real lesion is present. The appearance may merely be due to superimposed normal breast shadows. Compression spot films are needed to confirm the presence of a mass and to better define its borders.

Figure 5-E-3*B* shows spot compression of the questioned opacity seen on initial images. This localized compression with a smaller paddle placed directly over the abnormality achieves two things. First, it separates the opacity from adjacent breast tissue, demonstrating this to be a discrete mass with high density and not merely superimposition of normal shadows. Second, it elicits clear spiculation and architectural distortion around the mass. These features are classic for breast carcinoma, and biopsy is therefore required. Biopsy of this lesion showed invasive ductal carcinoma.

The 78-year-old patient in Case 5-4 has a soft mass in her breast and clearly needs a diagnostic mammogram because of her age and the palpable findings. Soft, rounded masses on physical examination are often benign fibroadenomata or cysts, but carcinoma also may present this way (statement *B* is false).

Other benign causes of these physical findings include hematoma, abscess, and lipoma (statement *E* is true and the correct answer to Question 5-4). Therefore, a mammogram may be beneficial for two reasons: (1) if a benign finding is revealed, biopsy may be avoided, and (2) if findings suggest malignancy, optimal treatment can be planned on the basis of extent of the lesion and presence or absence of additional lesions (statement *A* is false).

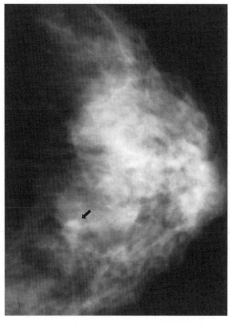

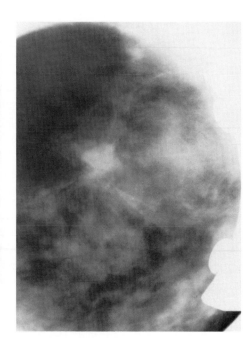

FIG. 5-E-3 (*Panel A*) Detail of a mammogram of the patient in Case 5-3. There is a dense nodular breast pattern with a vague, small, rounded opacity (*arrow*). (*Panel B*) Spot-compression view of the region of suspected abnormality in part *A*. Note how much easier it is to see the lesion and the spiculation (around it) with spot compression. Note also the difficulty in detecting and evaluating this tumor within dense glandular tissue compared with the fatty breast in Case 5-2.

A   *B*

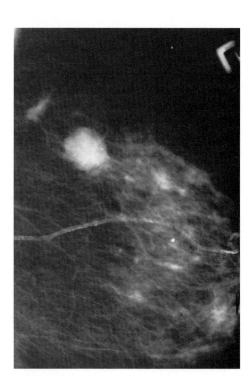

FIG. 5-E-4 Detail of a mammogram of the patient in Case 5-4.

Her mammogram (Fig. 5-E-4) shows two findings. There is a rounded mass with multiple lobulations and circumscribed borders. The fact that the borders are not sharply outlined on all sides raises the suspicion level for this finding. Masses that are sharply delineated may be followed with serial mammograms at 6-month intervals if they are not known to be new, are nonpalpable, and show no other features of malignancy. This is not the case with the patient in Case 5-4. Note the fading margin along portions of the mass. This mass corresponds to the palpable finding. Ultrasonography would be useful to exclude a multiloculated cyst and show the lesion to be solid. Biopsy is indicated, but needle aspiration without imaging would have been inappropriate (statement C is false).

A circumscribed mass representing carcinoma is seen less often than a spiculated mass. About 10 percent of invasive ductal carcinomas represent the better-differentiated subtypes, including medullary carcinoma, mucinous (colloid) carcinoma, and papillary carcinoma, all of which are frequently seen as circumscribed masses. They tend to have a better prognosis than the less well-differentiated garden-variety ductal carcinomas.

The differential diagnosis for the circumscribed mass on mammography includes carcinoma (primary as well as metastatic), fibroadenoma, and cysts; hematoma, abscess, and miscellaneous benign lesions are seen much less often. Correlation with clinical history and physical examination can help to narrow the differential diagnosis. When carcinoma cannot be excluded, either needle aspiration or excisional biopsy is required.

This patient had a needle biopsy. Since palpation alone could not reliably localize this lesion for needle biopsy because of its soft nature and the difficulty in fixing its position, stereotactic mammographic guidance was used in localizing the lesion for this procedure. The diagnosis of mucinous carcinoma was made by microscopic inspection of the specimen.

Now, were you astute enough to perceive the second lesion? Above and to the left of the large mass is a smaller, dense spiculated area. This also was biopsied and proved to be a carcinoma of the very well-differentiated tubular type. Even though the patient has two lesions now, both carry an excellent prognosis, and she will be unlikely to die from breast carcinoma (statement D is false). In fact, although mastectomy is certainly a reasonable treatment for her, local excision also would be an option with these nonaggressive lesions.

EXERCISE 5-2: LUMPINESS

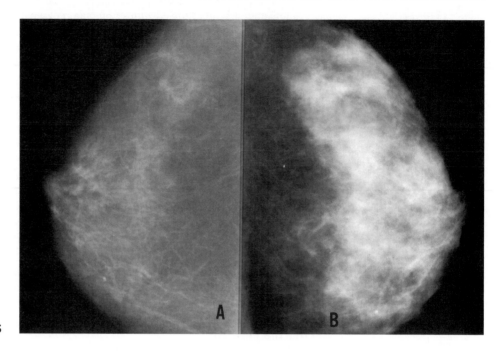

FIG. 5-E-5

Clinical History:

CASE 5-5

An 82-year-old woman complains of newly lumpy, painful breasts. Figure 5-E-5 is the same breast; part *A* was taken 1 year before part *B*.

Question:

5-5. The most likely explanation for this patient's symptoms and mammographic change is

   A. hormone effect.
   B. infectious mastitis.
   C. carcinoma.
   D. congestive heart failure.
   E. cystic disease.

Radiologic Findings:

5-5. These mammograms show a diffuse marked increase in mammographic density with a nodular character.

Discussion:

Lumpy breasts are a variant of normal and, as such, require careful physical examination and mammography to avoid unnecessary surgery, as well as to avoid missing a carcinoma. Diffuse lumpiness is not a contraindication to screening mammography, but when a particular lump becomes dominant, a diagnostic study is indicated.

The two mammograms of the patient in Fig. 5-E-5 were obtained 1 year apart. Between these two examinations, the patient was started on hormonal replacement therapy (*A* is the correct answer to Question 5-5). The breasts, which were previously largely fatty (part *A*), have become moderately dense and very lumpy on palpation 1 year later (part *B*). This change also can be seen, although not usually as dramatically, in the perimenopausal time of estrogen flare.

Such changes can be seen asymmetrically or unilaterally, and it is useful to remember the estrogen effect when evaluating mammograms with interval changes. Correlation with clinical history is then needed.

Option *B*, infectious mastitis, and option *C*, carcinoma, are incorrect because both these entities are usually unilateral and focal. Option *D*, congestive heart failure (CHF), is incorrect because CHF causes changes that have a more linear pattern of trabecular thickening on mammography rather than the patchy, ill-defined nodular pattern characteristic of glandular and cystic densities seen here. Option *E*, cystic disease, is incorrect. Cysts are seen as a component of hormone-related breast changes, but spontaneous cystic disease alone does not occur at this age.

EXERCISE 5-3: DISCHARGE

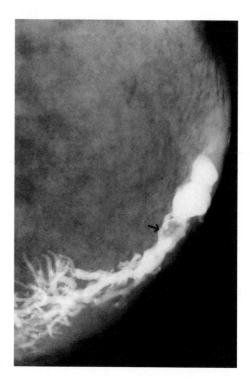

FIG. 5-E-6

Clinical History:

CASE 5-6
A 45-year-old woman presents with a profuse, serous nipple discharge. Ductography was performed (Fig. 5-E-6).

Question:

5-6. With respect to ductography and this patient's condition, is each of the following statements true or false?
  A. Ductography should be performed in all patients with nipple discharge.
  B. This patient's discharge is more likely to be caused by a benign condition than by a malignancy.
  C. This ductogram shows an intraluminal filling defect.
  D. Ductography has a high specificity for malignant lesions.
  E. Ductography is helpful in guiding the surgeon's approach.

Radiologic Findings:

In this ductogram, contrast material has been injected into a portion of a single ductal system with opacification of the lactiferous sinus and larger branching ducts. Most of the walls are smooth, as they should be. However, there is a filling defect in one of the major branches, as exhibited by the lucency outlined by contrast material on all sides and indicated by the arrow (statement *C* is true).

Discussion:

In this patient, there is a single intraluminal filling defect on ductography. However, we cannot determine from these findings alone whether the defect is due to a benign or a malignant nodule (statement *D* is false), although approximately 90 percent of nipple discharges are due to benign causes (statement *B* is true). The filling defect in this woman was a benign papilloma, the most common cause of bloody or serous discharge. Mammograms usually do not show these small, intraductal nodules.

Whether or not a filling defect is seen on a ductogram, biopsy is needed to rule out carcinoma, and the ductogram may be helpful in showing the surgeon which area of the breast harbors the cause of discharge (statement *E* is true). However, many surgeons are able to identify the lobe(s) involved by the pathology by inspecting the nipple, noting the location of the discharging duct, and by palpation, observing which portion of the breast produces discharge when compressed. Usually, ductography is not easily performed and is of limited usefulness when discharge is not spontaneous, profuse, and confined to a single duct. Therefore, statement *A* is false; ductograms should not be performed on all patients with nipple discharge. Furthermore, only bloody or serous discharges are of concern. A large portion of patients with discharge have secretions typical of fibrocystic change (i.e., a dark brownish or greenish fluid rather than a truly bloody or serous discharge). Milky discharge is normal.

EXERCISE 5-4: PAIN

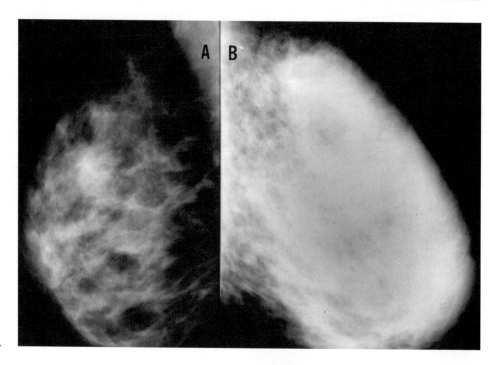

FIG. 5-E-7 *Panel A.*

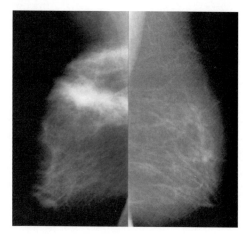

FIG. 5-E-8

Clinical Histories:

CASE 5-7
A 37-year-old woman comes to the emergency department with a reddened, swollen, painful left breast. The right (*A*) and left (*B*) breasts are shown in Fig. 5-E-7*A*.

CASE 5-8
A 52-year-old woman presents with soreness in the right breast, the mammogram of which is seen in Fig. 5-E-8.

Questions:

5-7. With respect to Case 5-7, is each of the following statements true or false?
A. There is diffuse abnormality on the left.
B. Inflammatory carcinoma is high on the differential diagnostic list.
C. Infectious mastitis is unlikely to be the cause in this nonlactating patient.
D. The mammographic appearance is nonspecific.
E. Follow-up imaging after a course of antibiotics would be appropriate.

5-8. With respect to Case 5-8, which one of the following statements is true?
A. The soreness indicates a benign process.
B. The appearance is malignant, and biopsy is necessary.
C. Findings on physical examination and history may radically alter our management decision.
D. Bleeding, such as that due to anticoagulation therapy, would not have this appearance.
E. The most likely diagnosis is fibrocystic change.

Radiologic Findings:

5-7. Views of the right and left breast of the patient in this case show that the entire left breast (*B*) is abnormally dense.

5-8. Mammogram of the patient in this case shows a large band of high density with markedly spiculated margins in the upper part of the breast.

Discussion:

In Case 5-7, the patient's entire left breast is abnormally dense (statement *A* is true). There is skin thickening as well. This is a nonspecific appearance (statement *D* is true); infection and inflammatory carcinoma are both high on the differential diagnostic list (*B* is true and *C* is false). Breast carcinoma may incite an inflammatory response in the breast, mimicking a benign infectious process both clinically and radiographically. The patient turns out to have an elevated white blood cell count and fever with marked pain. This information now makes infection more likely than tumor, and a course of antibiotics with follow-up imaging to monitor resolution is appropriate (statement *E* is true).

Figure 5-E-7*B* shows the follow-up mammogram after significant clinical resolution. The mammographic findings have resolved, and the left breast now appears very similar to the right one.

Infectious mastitis occurs more frequently in lactating women but is not uncommon in nonlactating women, particularly in diabetic patients. Imaging (mammography or ultrasound) is useful to exclude a drainable abscess collection and to provide a baseline for monitoring resolution to exclude carcinoma.

Case 5-8 illustrates the importance of correlation with history and physical examination. This patient has pain, as in the last case, but her mammographic abnormality is much more localized and appears more like a malignant mass, being a high-density opacity with excessive spiculation. However, this, too, is a benign process. The patient was in a motor vehicle accident 2 months earlier and sustained a severe injury to the right side of her chest. Physical examination shows a resolving laceration and contusion that extends in a linear fashion over the right breast (no wonder she is sore!). A CT scan performed at the time of trauma showed the acute injury precisely in the area indicated on the mammogram. These mammographic features are consistent with resolving (or acute) trauma. Therefore, no further action is warranted at this time other than follow-up (statement *C* is true and is the correct answer to Question 5-8). Although pain is not a prominent feature of carcinoma, patients with cancer may be symptomatic. Therefore, pain does not always mean benignancy (statement *A* is false).

The mammographic appearance would certainly be highly suspicious for invasive carcinoma in the absence of clinical information, but with careful correlation, we are able to avoid biopsy in this case (statement *B* is false).

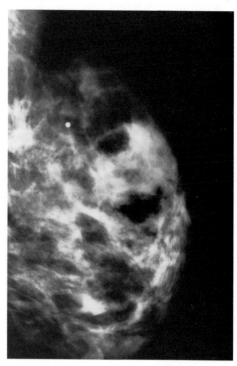

FIG. 5-E-7   (*Panel B*) Follow-up mammogram of the patient in Case 5-7 after a short course of antibiotics. Note the resolution of abnormal findings and the resultant symmetrical appearance compared with that of the opposite breast.

B

Anticoagulation therapy with resultant bleeding also could have this appearance (statement *D* is false). Fibrocystic change, although very common, is an unlikely diagnosis. Fibrocystic change appears as increased cloudy densities, nodular densities, and occasionally some thickened linear densities but rarely as a spiculated mass (statement *E* is false).

THE ASYMPTOMATIC PATIENT

EXERCISE 5-5: THE FIRST MAMMOGRAM

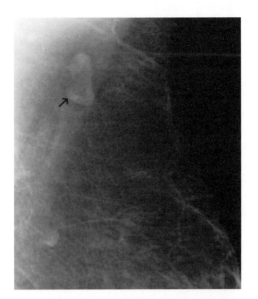

FIG. 5-E-9

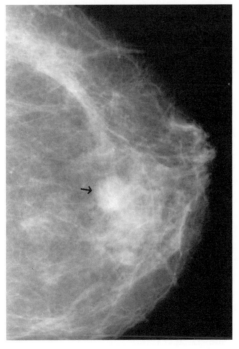

FIG. 5-E-10

FIG. 5-E-11 *Panel A.*

A

Clinical Histories:

CASE 5-9
A 40-year-old woman presents whose mother died of breast carcinoma (Fig. 5-E-9).

CASE 5-10
A 42-year-old woman presents with no risk factors for breast carcinoma. She has no symptoms (Fig. 5-E-10).

CASE 5-11
A 45-year-old asymptomatic woman presents with no risk factors (Fig. 5-E-11*A*).

Questions:

5-9. According to the American Cancer Society, the best program of breast screening for the woman in Case 5-9 includes all the following except
A.   monthly breast self-examination.
B.   yearly mammograms from age 40.
C.   cessation of routine mammograms at age 65.
D.   annual clinical breast examination.

5-10. The most likely diagnosis in Case 5-10 is
A.   complex cyst.
B.   fibroadenolipoma.
C.   galactocele.
D.   ductal carcinoma.
E.   oil cyst.

5-11. The differential diagnosis in Case 5-11 includes all the following except
A.   invasive ductal carcinoma.
B.   cyst.
C.   intraductal comedocarcinoma.
D.   fibroadenoma.
E.   mucinous carcinoma.

Radiologic Findings:

5-9. Detail of mammogram of the patient in this case shows a smooth, marginated small mass with a lucent center (*arrow*).

5-10. The mammogram in this case shows a circumscribed mass with lucency as well as medium-density internal opacity.

5-11. The mammogram of the patient in this case shows a nodular density (*arrow*) partially obscured by adjacent glandular tissue.

Discussion:

In Case 5-9, this 40-year-old woman has a strong family history of breast cancer, which puts her at high risk for developing the disease. As was stated earlier in this chapter, great controversy exists concerning when mammographic screening should be initiated and the appropriate frequency of examinations in different groups. Most experts agree, however, that patients with a strong family history will benefit from screening beginning at age 40. The American Cancer Society (ACS) recommends annual screening above age 40 in high-risk patients; therefore, *B* is not the correct answer.

Although the upper age limit for mammographic screening has not been defined, we certainly cannot recommend cessation over age 65, since the prevalence of breast cancer is greatest in women in their fifties and sixties (*C* is the correct answer to Question 5-9). Current ACS guidelines recommend yearly mammograms for all women over age 50. Appropriate age for termination of screening is best judged by the patient's physician, weighing life expectancy against potential benefits from screening.

ACS also recommends yearly physical examination by the physician and monthly BSE by the patient to detect tumors missed by mammography, as well as those which become detectable between routine mammograms (interval cancers). Therefore, *A* and *D* are not correct answers to Question 5-9.

This patient's mammogram is normal and demonstrates a typical normal lymph node. The node is smoothly marginated and has a fatty hilum, indicated by the darker center.

In Case 5-10, there is a circumscribed mass in the axillary tail of this breast. The key to diagnosis is the mixture of densities within the lesion. There are medium-density opacities interspersed with lucencies within a smoothly marginated mass. This appearance is pathognomonic for a fibroadenolipoma, sometimes known by the misnomer *hamartoma* (*B* is the correct answer to Question 5-10). Being composed of elements of normal breast (fatty, glandular, and fibrous tissues) organized within a thin capsule, a fibroadenolipoma forms a "breast within a breast." As such, it is benign and needs no further evaluation. It may be palpable as a soft mass.

The point to remember here is that fat-containing masses are always benign. Answer *D,* ductal carcinoma, is incorrect. The differential diagnosis of a fatty mass, besides fibroadenolipoma, includes lymph node, as in Case 5-9, galactocele, lipoma, and oil cyst. Galactoceles are usually smaller and are seen in lactating women (answer *C* is incorrect).

Oil cysts result from fat necrosis and are usually smaller. Typically, they are entirely lucent, since they are filled with oil, except for a thin wall (answer *E* is incorrect).

Option *A,* complex cyst, is incorrect because this entity would not contain fat. A cyst, whether it contains serous fluid, blood, or pus, is always opaque and of low to high density, not lucent.

In Case 5-11, an asymptomatic 45-year-old woman's first mammogram shows a 1.5-cm nodule centrally located in this breast. It is somewhat well marginated, but adjacent glandular tissue obscures some of the margins. The differential diagnosis remains broad without further studies to help characterize this nodule. All choices except option *C,* intraductal comedocarcinoma, may have this appearance. Intraductal carcinoma, when not mammographically occult, usually appears as microcalcifications.

Since this patient has had no previous mammograms, we cannot use stability over time as an indicator of benignity. If this nodule had not changed over a period of 1 to 2 years, we would have continued routine screening, deferring additional evaluation at this time. In this case, however, the patient must be recalled to rule out carcinoma.

At ultrasonography, a solid lesion is seen, ruling out a simple cyst. Spot compression is then used to evaluate the borders. If all margins appear smooth, one acceptable course of action is serial 6-month follow-up mammograms for a period of 2 years to demonstrate stability. If any change occurs during this time, biopsy is indicated.

Spot compression (Fig. 5-E-11*B*) separates the nodule from adjacent tissue and reveals that a portion of the border is not smooth, raising the level of suspicion for malignancy. To exclude carcinoma, biopsy is needed.

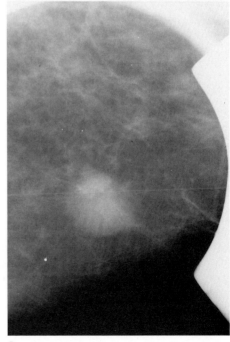

FIG. 5-E-11 (*Panel B*) Spot compression of nodular density seen in *Panel A*. Note that although spot compression separates the nodule from adjacent breast tissue, the margins are not completely smooth. Biopsy is recommended. (*Panel C*) Mammographic image obtained during stereotactic needle biopsy of the nodule in Case 5-11. The needle tip is about to pierce the nodule (*arrows*). (*Panel D*) Characteristic appearance of heavily calcified involuting fibroadenoma.

B

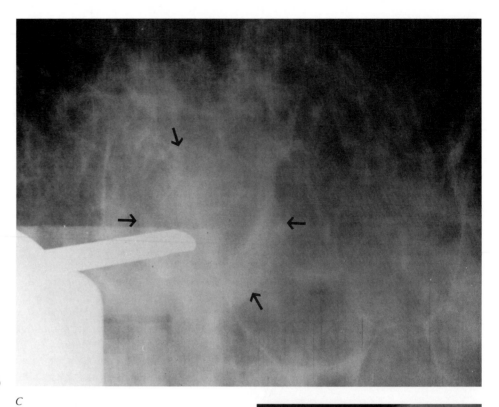

FIG. 5-E-11 (*Continued*)

C

D

Biopsy may be accomplished with excision or with needle aspiration. Excision would require needle localization of the nodule for the surgeon, since this is a nonpalpable lesion. Stereotactic needle biopsy is preferable because it is minimally invasive, causes less morbidity to the patient, leaves no distortion in the breast or on the skin, and is often less expensive than surgical excision. Accurate needle biopsy devices, however, are expensive and are not universally available.

This nodule was diagnosed as a fibroadenoma with stereotactic needle aspiration biopsy (Fig. 5-E-11C). Fibroadenomas are very common and are frequently the cause of benign breast biopsy. They occur in very young women (teenagers and women under age 30) and persist into the age at which the first mammogram is obtained, to the great concern of both physician and patient. They also may become palpable or mammographically visible in older women after previously normal mammograms. They continue to be a management problem because fibroadenoma and carcinoma have overlapping mammographic features and both are common lesions in middle-aged women. With age, fibroadenomas become involuted and heavily calcified, thereby revealing their true identity (Fig. 5-E-11D). Without this appearance, however, biopsy is often necessary.

A high index of suspicion and careful evaluation, together with either close follow-up or liberal use of needle biopsy, are needed to minimize both false-negative impressions and excessive breast surgery.

EXERCISE 5-6: ASYMMETRIC DENSITY

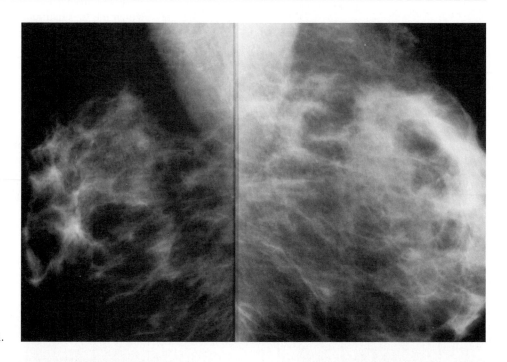

FIG. 5-E-12 *Panel A.*

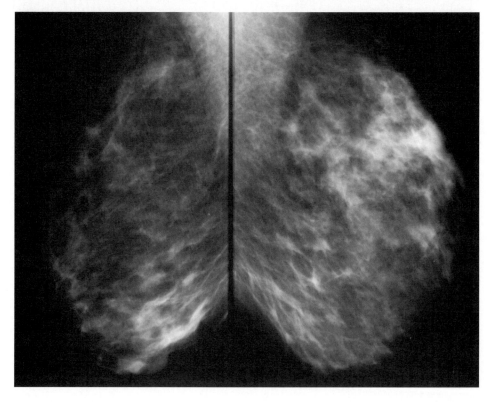

FIG. 5-E-13

Clinical Histories:

CASE 5-12

A 51-year-old woman is evaluated with screening mammography (Fig. 5-E-12*A*).

CASE 5-13

A 61-year-old woman is evaluated with screening mammography (Fig. 5-E-13).

Questions:

5-12. Concerning the asymmetric lacy pattern of density in the left breast, which statement is false?
  A. Without symptoms, infection is unlikely.
  B. Previous mammograms would have been very helpful.
  C. It is probably nonmalignant because the patient does not complain of a mass.
  D. Invasive lobular carcinoma commonly has this appearance.
  E. It may represent an asymmetric response to hormone therapy.

5-13. The mammographic appearance is least likely to be caused by
  A. normal breasts.
  B. postoperative change.
  C. trauma.
  D. cystic disease.
  E. tumor.

Radiologic Findings:

5-12. Bilateral mediolateral oblique views of the patient in this case show asymmetric density in the left breast without a discrete dominant mass. There is subtle spiculation in some areas and the suggestion of architectural distortion.

5-13. Bilateral mediolateral oblique views of patient in this case show areas of asymmetric density in the left upper and right lower breasts. The densities are interspersed with fat. Margins are generally concave, and there is no architectural distortion.

Discussion:

Although normal breast tissue is remarkably symmetrical, it is never exactly the same on both sides. The challenge in mammography is to recognize normal variation and to be able to distinguish nonpathologic asymmetry from disease. This is not always possible, particularly in the asymptomatic group. A high index of suspicion is needed in evaluating the screening mammogram, just as in the baseline clinical breast examination. Once asymmetry is noted mammographically, a careful, focused breast examination is needed. If no suspicious areas are detected, and if the radiographic features suggest fibroglandular tissue, then follow-up alone is adequate. Radiographically, we look for a homogeneous, nondistorted pattern of fat interspersed with lobular densities. Any dominant mass or architectural distortion should cause concern.

In Case 5-12, one area is denser than the others, and surrounding it are subtle architectural distortion and spiculation. Because of the subtlety of the findings, the mammogram is shown again with a line diagram (Fig. 5-E-12*B,C*). This is a classic appearance of invasive lobular carcinoma. Remember that 90 percent of breast cancers are ductal in origin, and the other 10 percent are lobular, as in this case. This type of carcinoma shows a subtle infiltrating pattern much more often than does ductal carcinoma (statement *D* is true).

One of the problems with this disease is that it is difficult to describe the extent of tumor mammographically. There is a large area of asymmetric opacity in this patient, but where tumor ends and stromal reaction or lymphatic congestion begins are unclear. This patient had a carcinoma that measured 4 × 3.5 × 3 cm.

A correlated clinical examination often reveals abnormalities not detected without the guidance of mammographic findings (statement *C* is false and is the correct answer

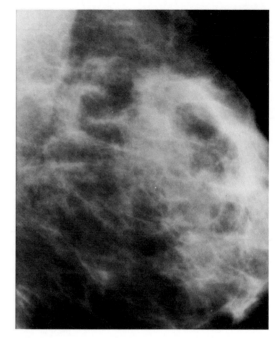

B

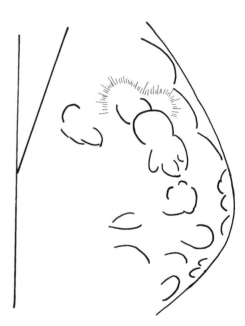

FIG. 5-E-12 (*Panel B*) Left breast of the patient in Case 5-12 showing ill-defined area of asymmetrical density. (*Panel C*) A line diagram outlines the area of most suspicious density, with slight spiculation and architectural distortion. Note the subtlety of the mammographic findings.

C

to Question 5-12). Biopsy of any suspicious-feeling area is strongly recommended. Studies have shown that a high percentage of carcinomas "missed" at mammography appear as asymmetric density. This patient did have a large area of hardening in the upper aspect of this breast, confirming the suspicious nature of the mammographic findings.

Previous mammograms are definitely useful in evaluating asymmetric density. If the density is unchanged over time and has features of glandular tissue, no further action is needed (option *B* is true). If the density is new or is increasing, it becomes suspicious. Hormonal therapy may indeed have an asymmetrical effect (statement *E* is true), but we would need to confirm this history and verify that the density has characteristics of breast tissue with additional spot films.

Although even large breast carcinomas may present without physical findings, infection is, by its nature, symptomatic. Without pain, tenderness, redness, or swelling, infection would not be considered with this appearance (statement *A* is true).

Unlike the previous patient, this woman in Case 5-13 has multiple areas of breast asymmetry. There is a large area in the upper part of the left breast and a smaller area in the lower part of the right breast. Both areas show fat interspersed with fibroglandular densities. There is no architectural distortion. Margins of the larger opacities are generally concave—a sign of benignity. There are no dominant or circumscribed masses, and cystic disease therefore would not be part of the differential diagnosis, since cysts are rounded masses (*D* is the correct answer to Question 5-13).

Having learned from the preceding case that missed carcinoma often presents as asymmetric density, tumor must remain in the differential diagnosis, and answer *E* is incorrect.

Both trauma and postoperative change can lead to ill-defined asymmetric density. With trauma there may be bleeding, contusion, or actual deformity, if severe. With surgery, asymmetry results both from removal of normal tissues, having less density on the operated side, and from surgical trauma (hematoma and distortion), which causes increased localized densities. Therefore, options *B* and *C* are both incorrect. The most likely cause of this woman's mammographic appearance is normal breast tissue, and answer *A* is incorrect. The multiplicity and bilaterality of areas of asymmetry, the lack of signs or symptoms of breast cancer, and the fibroglandular characteristics of the densities all support this diagnosis.

EXERCISE 5-7: THE FOLLOW-UP MAMMOGRAM

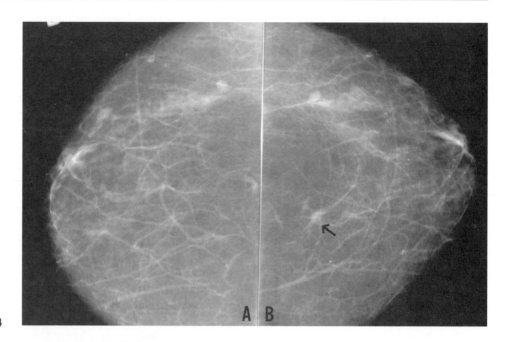

FIG. 5-E-14

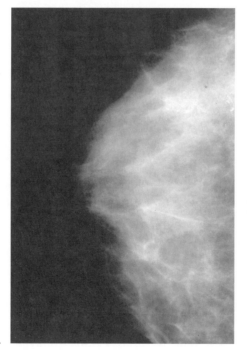

FIG. 5-E-15 *Panel A.*

FIG. 5-E-16

Clinical Histories:

CASE 5-14

A 70-year-old woman is seen who had two screening mammograms 1 year apart (Fig. 5-E-14A is the first mammogram, and the one obtained a year later is Fig. 5-E-14B).

CASE 5-15

A 66-year-old woman has this screening mammogram after a previously normal mammogram (Fig. 5-E-15A).

CASE 5-16

A 55-year-old woman presents who had a normal mammogram the previous year (Fig. 5-E-16).

Questions:

5-14. Which of the following statements is false?
   A. The abnormal finding is a spiculated mass.
   B. The rate of change is too slow for a breast cancer.
   C. A malpractice claim should not be encouraged.
   D. The lesion is probably palpable.
   E. This change warrants biopsy.

5-15. With respect to the calcifications, which statement is false?
   A. They may be described as pleomorphic.
   B. The coarse nature of some of the calcifications suggests this is a benign process.
   C. They signal an aggressive malignancy.
   D. They are most likely due to necrosis in duct walls.
   E. Magnification should be performed to assess the extent of disease.

5-16. With respect to the calcifications, which statement is true?
   A. They may be described as granular.
   B. The regional distribution makes them highly suspicious.
   C. Follow-up alone would be inadequate.
   D. The new onset indicates a high probability of malignancy.
   E. They have a less than 20 percent chance of being malignant.

Radiologic Findings:

5-14. This case shows back-to-back craniocaudal views of the right breast obtained 1 year apart. In the interval, a small spiculated mass has appeared (*arrow*).

5-15. The mammogram of the patient in this case shows a cluster of microcalcifications posteriorly in the lateral aspect of the breast. Previous mammograms have been normal.

5-16. Magnification view of a portion of the breast of the patient in this case shows coarse calcifications, some of which are rounded or ringlike.

Discussion:

Case 5-14 illustrates the concept of developing density. A *developing density* is any opacity that increases in size or density over time. All such opacities should be evaluated critically, because they can be signs of carcinoma. This concept is based on the natural behavior of breast cancer, which generally grows slowly. With periodic screening, the early tumor will be imaged but unrecognized on early images and may not be detected until 1, 2, 3, or more years later. Tumors 5 mm or smaller are very difficult to differentiate from normal breast tissue, but masses larger than 1 cm are more easily detected. The typical breast cancer has been present for several years by the time it is 1 cm in size. Therefore, breast cancers are routinely visible in retrospect on previous mammograms if the patient has had frequent screening. This does not mean, however, that malpractice has occurred. If the cancer is still small, no harm has been done and more harm could potentially be done by biopsying all such tiny densities, because most of them would be normal breast (statement *C* is true). Being suspicious but judicious with any developing density, therefore, is necessary to detect breast cancer early without unnecessary biopsy.

This patient has a small (about 1 cm) spiculated mass in the central part of the breast (statement *A* is true). It has increased slightly in size over 1 year, with a growth rate typical for breast carcinoma (statement *B* is false and is the correct answer to Question 5-14). Being so small in a medium-sized breast, it is unlikely to be palpable (statement *D* is true) and, therefore, would require imaging guidance for any biopsy. The spiculated margins, the rate of growth, and the patient's age group all make this a very suspicious lesion, and biopsy is warranted (statement *E* is true). This lesion was an infiltrating ductal carcinoma.

Case 5-15 illustrates a new finding after a previous normal screening. There is a cluster of microcalcifications in the upper outer quadrant. Note that the calcifications are small and irregular, but we do not see their configuration exquisitely, nor can we be confident of the extent of disease, since there may be other smaller calcifications that we do not see. The patient, therefore, requires recall for magnification mammography (Fig. 5-E-15*B*) (statement *E* is true). On magnification, we can appreciate that the calcifications are of many different sizes and shapes (i.e., pleomorphic) (statement *A* is true). Malignant microcalcifications are usually less than 0.5 mm in size, and the very coarse calcifications are classically benign. However, there is significant overlap, and configuration is generally a more helpful sign. Malignant calcifications are usually either granular or linear and branching.

These linear and branching calcifications are typical of intraductal carcinoma. The aggressive type of intraductal carcinoma, comedo or high-nuclear-grade carcinoma, causes necrosis in the cancerous mammary duct walls. Calcifications form in areas of necrosis, forming a "cast" of the duct. This process results in the linear and branching forms of calcification (statements *C* and *D* are true). Pathologic analysis of this tissue showed intraductal carcinoma of the comedo type.

Lesser degrees of necrosis result in smaller, more granular calcifications, whereas extensive necrosis yields rather large, rod-shaped or branched calcifications. Option *B* is false because, although large calcifications alone are usually benign, the mixture of tiny irregular calcifications with the coarse casting calcifications remains very suspicious for malignancy (statement *B* is false and is the correct answer to Question 5-15).

In Case 5-16, the mammogram detail shows typical benign calcifications. Benign calcifications take many forms, but if we see rings with lucent centers, as in this case, we can rest assured that they are benign. These rings are calcifying microcystic areas of fat necrosis. This is a very common benign finding. Punctate, or dotlike, calcifications are also usually benign if uniform and smooth. Granular calcifications are more angular, like broken needle tips, and would be more suspicious (statement *A* is false).

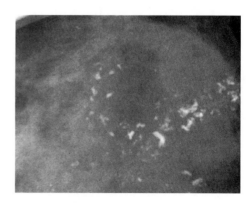

FIG. 5-E-15 (*Panel B*) Magnification view of microcalcifications seen on a screening mammogram of the patient in Case 5-15. Note the pleomorphism of the microcalcifications. The size varies from very fine to coarse, and shapes are bizarre. This appearance is typical of comedocarcinoma.

Benign calcifying processes such as fibroadenoma, sclerosing adenosis, and fat necrosis can all be unifocal, or regional, as well as multifocal or diffuse; therefore, distribution alone does not make calcifications suspicious (statement *B* is false).

Benign processes of many types do present in adulthood and therefore may appear de novo after a previously normal screening examination. Again, the configuration of calcifications is more helpful (statement *D* is false).

For obviously benign calcifications such as these, routine follow-up alone is adequate (statement *C* is false). Some calcifications are obviously malignant, as in Case 5-15. A third group of calcifications is classified as indeterminate, and these require further evaluation, either close mammographic follow-up or some type of biopsy. Taken as a group, biopsied microcalcifications historically have had a rate of malignancy of only 20 percent. Therefore, option *E* is true, since these ringlike calcifications have a better-than-average chance of being benign (statement *E* is true and is the correct answer to Question 5-16).

SUMMARY

In summary, mammography is an exciting subspecialty of radiology that is interesting, challenging, and personally rewarding because it is the best technique we have today to diagnose early breast cancer. Hopefully, the results of screening mammography with detection of cancer at earlier stages will have the positive effect of further reducing mortality from this relatively common disease.

BIBLIOGRAPHY

Homer MJ: *Mammographic Interpretation.* New York, McGraw-Hill, 1991.
Kopans DB: *Breast Imaging.* Philadelphia, Lippincott, 1989.
Love SM: *Dr. Susan Love's Breast Book.* Reading, Mass., Addison-Wesley, 1990.
Svane G et al: *Screening Mammography.* St Louis, Mosby, 1993.
Tabár L, Dean PB: *Teaching Atlas of Mammography.* Stuttgart, Thieme-Verlag, 1985.

PART 3

BONES AND JOINTS

6

MUSCULOSKELETAL IMAGING

Tamara Miner Haygood
Sam T. Auringer
Johnny U. V. Monu

TECHNIQUES
>   **Conventional Radiography**
>   **Mammographic Techniques**
>   **Fluoroscopy**
>   **Conventional Tomography**
>   **Computed Tomography**
>   **Magnetic Resonance Imaging**
>   **Nuclear Medicine**
>   **Biopsy**

TECHNIQUE SELECTION
>   **Trauma**
>   **Bone or Soft-Tissue Tumors**
>   **Metastatic Tumors**
>   **Osteomyelitis**

EXERCISES
>   **6-1: Trauma**
>   **6-2: Local Disease**
>   **6-3: Systemic Disease**

When Wilhelm Conrad Röntgen discovered the x-ray in November 1895, he investigated it thoroughly, testing its ability to penetrate various inanimate objects and observing its effects on fluorescent screens and photographic film. He gazed in amazement at the image of the bones of his own hand as he allowed the new rays to penetrate his flesh. He made a photographic x-ray image of a hand (reportedly his wife's) and sent prints of it together with his paper describing the new phenomenon to a carefully selected list of scientific colleagues.

By mid-February 1896, Röntgen's paper had not only been published but also reprinted in other scientific journals, including the American journal *Science*. Scientists everywhere repeated Röntgen's simple experiments and confirmed the truth of his discovery. Within a year, x-rays were in widespread use for medical purposes—chiefly for imaging of the skeleton.

Since Röntgen's time, many new imaging techniques have been developed that allow radiologists to see the muscles and other soft tissues of the musculoskeletal system as well as the bones. These techniques make skeletal imaging a very exciting area of radiology and one that can enhance patients' quality of life. They also can be very expensive, however. This chapter is intended to introduce you to musculoskeletal imaging techniques and to suggest efficient

ways to use them that will help you not only to make correct diagnoses but also to do so without excessive cost. Naturally, the suggestions made in these pages must be tailored to the needs of individual patients.

TECHNIQUES

Conventional Radiography

Conventional radiographs, or *plain films,* as they are often called, are the most frequently obtained of all imaging studies. They are chiefly useful for evaluation of the bones, but useful information also may be obtained concerning the adjacent soft tissues. Gas may be seen within the soft tissues and may be a clue to an open wound, ulcer, or infection with a gas-producing organism. Calcifications within the soft tissues can indicate a tumor, myositis ossificans, or systemic disorders such as scleroderma or hyperparathyroidism.

To get the most information possible from conventional radiographs, you should carefully choose the study to be ordered. At most hospitals and clinics, standardized sets of views have been developed that are obtained routinely together for evaluation of specific body areas in certain clinical settings. It is useful to know what will be obtained routinely when a certain set of films is ordered. Radiographs of the ankle, for example, usually include a straight frontal view of the ankle, a frontal view obtained with approximately 15 degrees of internal rotation of the ankle (the mortise view), and a lateral view.

There will be some variation among institutions, however. The films used to evaluate the cervical spine of accident victims, for example, vary tremendously. Radiologists at some institutions are satisfied with the lateral, frontal, and odontoid views. Others add one or more of several other views: oblique views, an angled frontal view (the pil-

lar view), or flexion and extension views. In addition to the standard projections obtained as part of these routine sets, many other specialized projections are obtained infrequently but are quite useful in the correct setting.

At a minimum, two views at right angles to each other should be obtained when a fracture or dislocation is suspected, since such injuries are notorious for being very subtle or even invisible in one projection, even when they are glaringly obvious in another view (Fig. 6-1). Another useful principle is that radiographs should be focused on the anatomic area being evaluated, as free as possible of

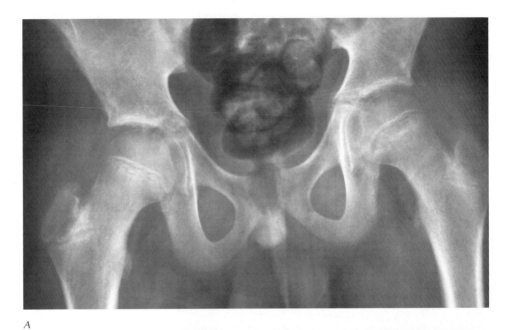

A

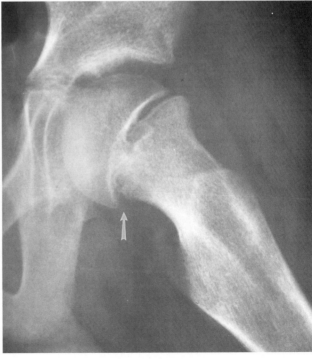

FIG. 6-1 Slipped capital femoral epiphysis. (*A*) Anteroposterior (AP) radiograph of the pelvis. There are signs of a fracture through the physis of the left proximal femur: That femoral epiphysis is less well mineralized than the one on the right, the lucent line demarcating the physis is slightly widened, and the alignment of the edges of the epiphysis and metaphysis is abnormal. These signs are relatively subtle and could easily be missed. (*B*) Frog-leg lateral view of the left hip. This view, a lateral of the proximal femur, is much more obviously abnormal. Along the posterior edge of the femur, the cortices of the epiphysis and metaphysis should be flush but are instead offset by approximately 5 mm (*arrow*).

B

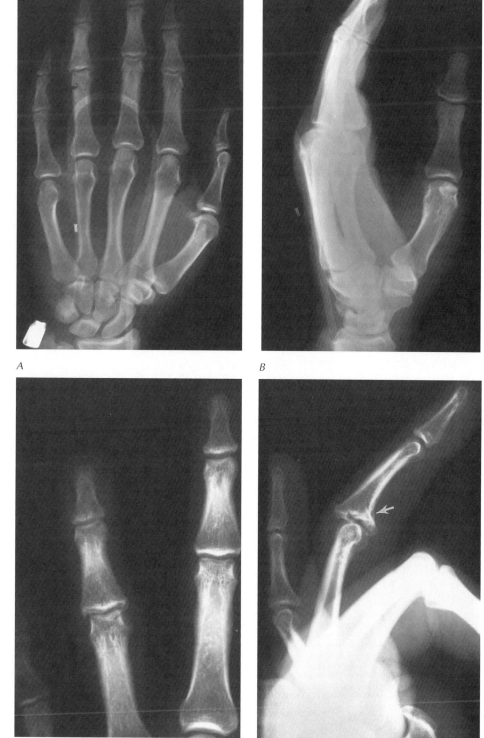

FIG. 6-2 Phalangeal fracture. (*A,B*) AP and lateral radiographs of the hand. This young man was first evaluated for trauma to the ring finger with frontal and lateral views of the whole hand. On the lateral view, all fingers other than the thumb are overlapped. No fracture was found. (*C,D*) AP and lateral radiographs of the finger. The patient returned 2 1/2 months later, complaining that his finger still hurt. This time radiographs were coned more closely to the finger, and care was taken on the lateral view to image the ring finger separately from the others. In that view, the intraarticular fracture of the proximal aspect of the middle phalanx is quite obvious (*arrow*). It is far more subtle on the frontal view.

overlapping, extraneous anatomy (Fig. 6-2). If the knee is the site of trouble, do not order views of the entire tibia and fibula; you will be disappointed with the visualization of the knee. This principle must be abandoned more or less in young children and mentally impaired individuals who may not be able to localize their symptoms well and also in trauma victims with so many injuries that the relatively minor ones may be overlooked.

In addition, when the radiographs will be studied by a consulting radiologist, it is helpful to provide a succinct yet accurate history pinpointing your clinical concerns. Simply indicating the site of injury will improve the likelihood that a subtle fracture will be discovered.

A conventional radiograph of a normal bone will show a smooth, homogeneous cortex surrounding the medullary space. The cortex will be thicker along the shaft (diaphysis) of long bones and thinner in small, irregular bones such as the carpal and tarsal bones and at the ends of long bones (Fig. 6-3). Exceptions are the normal roughening of the cortex at tendon and ligament insertion sites and the normal interruption of the cortex at the site of the nutrient arteries. Naturally, these occur at predictable places that differ from bone to bone. Within the medullary space of a normal bone are trabeculae. These are visible in radiographs as thin, crisp white lines that are arranged not randomly but in predictable patterns that enhance the stress-bearing capability of the bone. It is beyond the scope of this chapter to address the appearance of each bone.

When questions arise concerning whether a particular appearance is normal or abnormal, several solutions are possible. Two books, Keats' *Normal Variants* and Kohler's *Borderlands* (see "Bibliography"), are very useful in helping to distinguish the normal from the abnormal. Correlation with the results of the history and physical examination also may be helpful, as suggested above. Finally, comparison with the patient's prior plain radiographs or with a radiograph of the opposite extremity also may help (Fig. 6-4). Comparison views of the opposite extremity are especially helpful in children, in whom the open physes and accessory centers of ossification may vary a surprising amount from individual to individual.

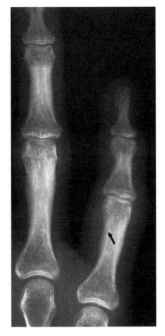 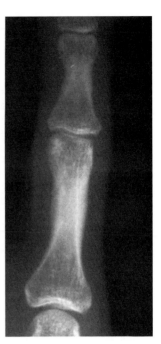

A   *B*

FIG. 6-4   Nutrient canal. PA radiographs of the small finger. (*A*) The smooth white cortex of the radial side of the proximal phalanx of the small finger is interrupted by a thin, obliquely oriented dark line (*arrow*). The soft tissues are swollen, and there is tenderness in this area. How can you distinguish this nutrient canal from a fracture? The appearance of this lucency is more suggestive of a normal nutrient canal than of a fracture. It is in a typical location for a nutrient canal. Its borders are smooth and sclerotic, not jagged. For definitive proof, delve into the patient's film folder. (*B*) The same lucency was present 2 1/2 years earlier. In this case, the soft-tissue swelling was due to cellulitis after a cat bite.

Mammographic Techniques

In mammography, very low energy x-rays emanating from a small focal spot are used to create images of the soft tissues (usually, of course, the breast) characterized by sharp spatial resolution and high contrast between objects of different densities. This technique is seldom used for structures other than the breast, but any soft-tissue area that can be pulled away from the skeleton successfully and placed between the compression paddle and the film may be imaged in this way. In extremity imaging, mammographic technique is occasionally used to search for small calcifications or foreign bodies in the soft tissues.

Fluoroscopy

In fluoroscopy, x-rays are sent through the patient, strike a fluorescent screen, and create an image that is made brighter by an image intensifier and may then be observed on a television screen. Conventional radiographs produce a tangible piece of film on which is permanently recorded the radiographic appearance of a patient as he or she ap-

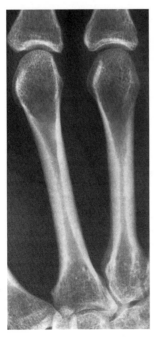

FIG. 6-3   Normal metacarpals. Posteroanterior (PA) radiograph of the second and third metacarpals of a 36-year-old woman. The cortex is thick and homogeneously white in the midshaft of the metacarpal. It becomes progressively thinner as it approaches the ends of the bones. At the articular surfaces the cortex has been reduced to a thin, yet distinct, white line.

peared for a few milliseconds. Radiographs are degraded by patient motion. Fluoroscopy, by contrast, is a dynamic technique. It allows visualization of the skeleton in motion, but unless the images are taped or still radiographs are taken in conjunction with the fluoroscopic examination, it leaves no permanent record. Fluoroscopy plays an important role in evaluation of joint motion and is indispensable in arthrography and joint aspirations.

In areas of skeletal radiology other than joint imaging, fluoroscopy is often used by orthopedic surgeons to monitor placement of hardware. It also may be of assistance in positioning patients for unusual conventional radiographic views.

Conventional Tomography

Tomography is a technique for obtaining images of a cross-sectional "slice" of the body, relatively isolated from adjacent structures in other planes. Because of their frequent use in many hospitals, computed axial tomography (CT) and magnetic resonance (MR) imaging, both of which provide cross-sectional images, may be more familiar than conventional tomography. In conventional tomography, x-rays are projected through the patient onto x-ray film. The tomographic effect is achieved by motion of the x-ray tube, the film, or both. The motion causes the structures above and below the desired plane to be blurry, whereas those at the level of interest are more sharply defined.

There are two types of conventional tomography—planar and complex motion. Complex motion tomography, in which the tube typically moves in a spiral or helical path, is most often advocated for skeletal tomography. The advent of CT, however, has greatly decreased the demand for complex motion tomography. As a result, many radiology departments are eliminating their complex motion tomographic units in order to use the floor space for other equipment and to save money on upkeep.

If complex motion tomographic equipment is not available, acceptable images may be acquired with planar equipment. In fact, if metallic orthopedic implants are present, planar tomography may give superior images if the patient can be positioned so that the direction of tube travel is parallel to the metal. Planar tomographic equipment often will be available, even when complex motion equipment is not, because it is frequently used in genitourinary radiography, where it is very useful for intravenous pyelograms.

Conventional tomography is used chiefly in skeletal imaging for the diagnosis and evaluation of fractures when conventional radiographs have either failed to demonstrate a fracture that is strongly suspected clinically or have demonstrated a fracture but have not displayed it with sufficient clarity to determine the position of the fracture fragments. It is particularly good for demonstrating fracture lines that run in the axial plane and, therefore, may be missed by CT. In the same way, it may provide superior illustration of the alignment of fracture fragments across a flat surface running in the axial plane, such as the tibial plateau or the end plate of a vertebra (Fig. 6-5). This is particularly true if the patient cannot be positioned with the surface of interest almost perpendicular to the gantry of the CT scanner. Conventional tomography is also less expensive than CT at most institutions.

Computed Tomography

CT has two major uses in skeletal imaging. The first is that it is the main alternative to conventional tomography for evaluation of fracture fragment position. It is particularly useful for fractures that run in the coronal or sagittal planes or for evaluation of structures roughly perpendicular to the axial plane. Thus fractures of the medial acetabulum, scapula, and calcaneus are particularly well suited to CT (Fig. 6-6). When multiplanar reconstruction is available, or when a cooperative patient can be appropriately positioned, CT becomes a worthy rival to conventional tomography for evaluation of structures in the axial plane. Because CT is expensive and does expose the patient to more radiation, the decision to use it or not should be based on whether the study will change treatment or will be of sufficient help in operative planning to justify the additional radiation and expense. Scapular fractures, for example, are often treated conservatively, but orthopedic surgeons differ on the treatment of fractures that extend into the glenoid or involve the scapular spine. Some believe these benefit from internal fixation; others do not. CT to evaluate these structures will be more useful to a surgeon who would use internal fixation selectively than to one who would use conservative therapy on all scapular fractures.

Three-dimensional reconstruction is available with many CT scanners. It requires extra technologist time to perform the scan and more films as well, so there is usually an extra charge. This may be justified if it helps the orthopedic surgeon to plan operative intervention and thus decrease the time required for surgery. Three-dimensional images are also useful for teaching purposes, since they can often be understood by less experienced individuals. They do not, however, contain information beyond that available in tomographic images.

The second major use of CT is in evaluation of bone tumors or tumor-like diseases. For this purpose, MR imaging is the principal competing technique. CT is more sensitive than MR imaging in demonstrating small amounts of calcium and can show early periosteal new bone formation or small amounts of matrix calcification before they may be seen with conventional radiography. This finding can be helpful in narrowing the differential diagnosis of a tumor. Before MR imaging was developed, CT also was used widely for determining the extent of bone and soft-tissue tumors. MR imaging, however, is now more often used for staging. Its superior contrast resolution greatly eases the

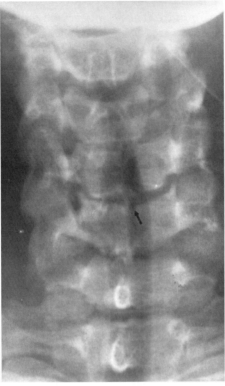
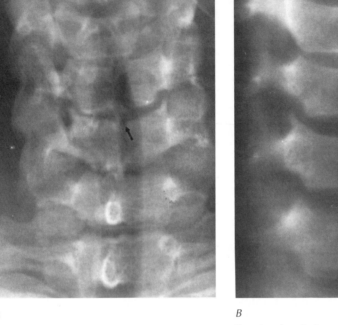

A   *B*

FIG. 6-5 Vertebral fracture. (*A*) AP radiograph of the cervical spine. The vertebral bodies of C5 and C6 are too wide compared with the width of C4, and there is a subtle incongruity of the end plates, most noticeable at the superior end plate of C6 (*arrow*). The edge of the left lateral mass of C4 is also too far from the lateral margin of the C4 vertebral body. (*B*) Coronal tomogram of the cervical spine. A conventional tomogram obtained with poly-directional technique and centered at the level of the middle to posterior vertebral bodies demonstrates the fractures clearly. The amount and direction of displacement of the surfaces of the end plates can be assessed accurately. A distinct lucency through the left lateral mass of C4 indicates a fracture there as well as through the C5 and C6 vertebral bodies. CT is more often used for evaluation of cervical spine injuries. (*Courtesy of José F. Garcia, M.D.*)

task of determining tumor extent within bone marrow and muscle or other soft tissues (Fig. 6-7).

In addition to these two uses, CT may be obtained to assist the orthopedic surgeon in operative planning. It is particularly useful when surgical intervention is needed in a patient with altered anatomy such as a previous joint replacement or a history of developmental dysplasia of the hip.

Magnetic Resonance Imaging

MR imaging uses radio waves, rather than x-rays, to produce tomographic images. Unlike CT and conventional tomography, which are restricted as to the planes that may be chosen, MR images can be obtained at practically any angle without the loss of information that occurs when CT images are postprocessed or reconstructed into planes other than the one in which the images were originally acquired. As stated previously, the exquisite contrast seen with MR imaging makes it ideal for evaluation of soft tissues. Its most frequent use in skeletal imaging, therefore, is

for diagnosis of injuries to muscles, tendons, or ligaments about joints.

This superb contrast resolution of MR imaging also makes it very useful for evaluating disorders of the bone marrow, including neoplasms, marrow-packing diseases such as Gaucher's disease, osteomyelitis, fractures that are occult on conventional radiographs, and avascular necrosis. Unfortunately, although MR imaging is very sensitive to these abnormalities, it is also very nonspecific. Many diseases of marrow cause similar signal alterations. One must then narrow the differential diagnosis based on the distribution of the abnormalities together with the clinical history.

Nuclear Medicine

Several nuclear medicine studies are used for skeletal disease. The two most common are the technetium bone scan and the technetium- or indium-labeled white blood cell scan. One of several phosphate compounds of technetium-99m is selected for use in a bone scan. Methylene diphos-

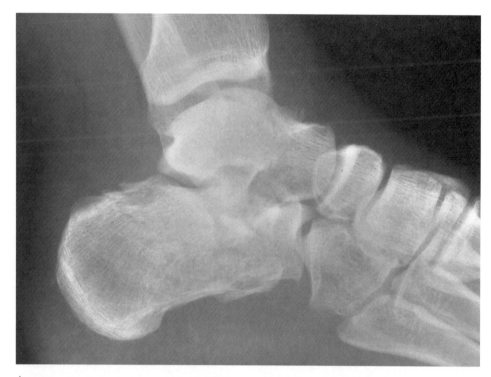

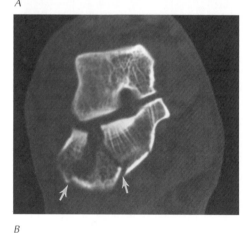

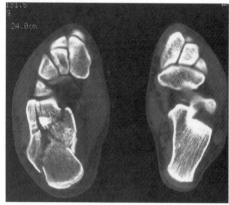

FIG. 6-6 Calcaneal fracture. (*A*) Lateral radiograph of the foot. The calcaneus of this 27-year-old man has a comminuted fracture that can easily be diagnosed with this conventional radiograph, but the degree of involvement of the articular surfaces is difficult to appreciate. (*B*) Direct coronal CT image through the posterior and middle subtalar joints demonstrates obliquely oriented fracture lines entering the posterior facet (*arrows*). There is a gap of approximately 8 mm between the fracture margins, and the lateral fragment has been rotated outward. (*C*) Axial CT image demonstrates a comminuted fracture of the inferior aspect of the calcaneocuboid joint.

phonate is probably used most frequently. If there is a specific anatomic area of interest, images may be acquired over that area at the time the radionuclide is injected, as well as 3 to 4 h later. The immediate images reflect the amount of blood flow to the area; the delayed images reflect the amount of bone remodeling occurring there.

Bone scintigraphy is a sensitive but nonspecific technique. Most osseous abnormalities of clinical significance will cause an increase in radiolabeling. Exceptions are destructive lesions that incite little reparative reaction in the host bone or that destroy bone so quickly that it cannot remodel.

Because of their sensitivity, and because they provide physiologic rather than anatomic information, bone scans can be used to find abnormalities before they are detectable by conventional radiography. In particular, they are often used for screening for bone metastases in patients with known malignancy. Both multiple myeloma in adults and Langerhans cell histiocytosis in children, however, are notorious for causing no increased accumulation on bone scans. Therefore, in these diseases conventional radiographs or skeletal surveys are better than bone scans for screening for osseous involvement.

Early detection of avascular necrosis, historically an indication for bone scanning, has largely been usurped by MR imaging because it is more sensitive and provides greater anatomic detail. Legg-Calvé-Perthes disease (spontaneous avascular necrosis of the capital femoral epiphysis) in children is an exception, however, since bone scans may be more sensitive than MR imaging in this diagnosis. MR imaging also may prove to be better than bone scans for the detection of occult fractures.

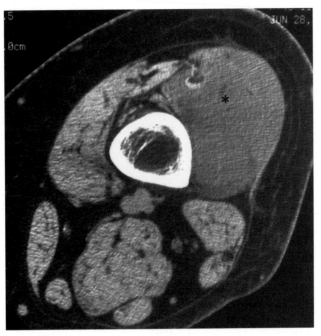

A

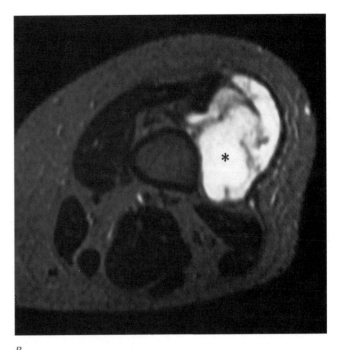

B

FIG. 6-7 (*A*) Axial CT image of the distal thigh. This 49-year-old woman complained of a palpable mass in her thigh. It had been present for a year and was painless. The internal architecture of the vastus lateralis muscle (*) is disrupted. The interdigitated fat and muscle tissue evident in the patient's other muscles has been replaced with a more homogeneous mass of decreased attenuation. There is no apparent associated calcification. The mass closely approximates the femur but is not causing osseous de-struction. (*B*) T2-weighted (2500/80) MR image of the thigh at approximately the same level. While this tumor (*) could be seen on the CT scan, on the MR image it is far more obvious and more easily distinguished from normal tissue. The superiority of MR imaging in detecting soft-tissue neoplasms makes it excellent for determining the extent of primary soft-tissue tumors such as this myxoid liposarcoma, as well as for evaluating the spread of primary bone tumors into adjacent soft tissues.

White blood cell scans are performed by labeling a sample of the patient's leukocytes with indium or technetium and reinjecting them. Scanning is then done 3 to 4 h later if technetium is used and 24 to 48 h later if indium is used. The study has but one use in skeletal imaging; it vies with MR images and bone scans as a method of detecting osteomyelitis. Which technique or combination of techniques is best is far from certain. Some studies have favored nuclear medicine; others have favored MR imaging. Both bone scans and MR imaging are sensitive but lack specificity. White blood cell scans are relatively specific for infection but often cannot distinguish cellulitis from osteomyelitis with certainty. All three techniques are expensive.

Biopsy

When tumor or infection is suspected, it is often useful to obtain a tissue sample for cytologic or histologic analysis or for culture. This may be accomplished by means of an "open" procedure in the operating room or a percutaneous needle puncture of the lesion to obtain a cellular aspirate or slender core of tissue. Needle biopsies of palpable lesions need no radiologic intervention. When the lesion is not pal-pable, however, biopsy may be accomplished under fluoroscopic or CT guidance.

When a skeletal lesion should be biopsied and by whom are important questions that can have a tremendous impact on the patient's outcome. For example, sarcomas have been reported to grow along the surgical or needle tracks after diagnostic biopsies. Therefore, when planning biopsies of suspected musculoskeletal sarcomas, great care must be taken to approach the lesion through a track that can be resected en bloc with the tumor at the time of ultimate excision. These biopsies should be carried out in close consultation with the surgeon who will be performing the definitive surgery.

When systemic disease such as metastatic carcinoma is the primary consideration, percutaneous needle biopsy is the most efficacious means of making a diagnosis if the lesion is amenable to this procedure. In this setting, the yield of needle biopsy is very good (90 percent or more of such biopsies yield a positive diagnosis when tumor is truly present), and a negative result is less likely to lead to open biopsy than it would in some suspected primary tumors. Nonetheless, biopsy should still be performed in consultation with the oncologist or other physician giving overall care.

TECHNIQUE SELECTION

In general, as in most other organ systems, the plain radiograph is the initial imaging test after history and physical examination. The selection of subsequent (often more expensive) imaging tests depends not only on medical need but also on a variety of other factors, including availability, expense, and the preferences of the radiologist, clinician, and patient.

Trauma

Rely primarily on conventional radiography. When a strongly suspected fracture is not identified, you may choose among repetition of conventional radiographs in 7 to 10 days, nuclear medicine bone scanning, and MR imaging. If a fracture is noticed and more information is needed concerning the location of fragments, either conventional tomography or CT is useful.

Bone or Soft-Tissue Tumors

Conventional radiography is the technique of choice for generating a differential diagnosis of primary bone tumors.

For local staging of both bone and soft-tissue neoplasms, MR imaging is the best technique. When a bone tumor is suspected but is not discovered with conventional radiographs, MR imaging is a useful secondary screening tool.

Metastatic Tumors

Symptomatic sites suspected of being involved by metastatic neoplasm are best evaluated initially with plain radiographs. An overall survey for osseous metastases may be performed by nuclear medicine bone scan. Conventional radiography is then used to evaluate sites of possible tumor involvement. Suspected soft-tissue metastases are best evaluated by MR imaging.

Osteomyelitis

Conventional radiographs should be obtained first. If these are normal or inconclusive, MR imaging, nuclear medicine bone scan, or white blood cell scanning may be helpful.

EXERCISE 6-1: TRAUMA

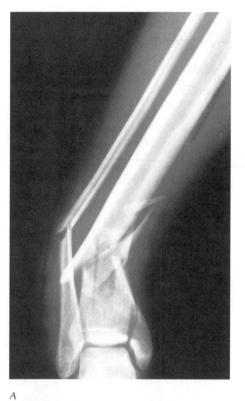
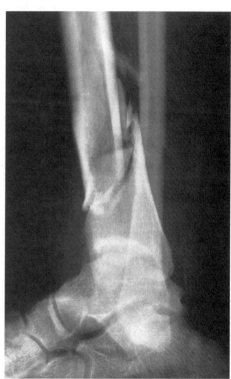

FIG. 6-E-1 (*Panels A and B*) AP and lateral views of the distal tibia and fibula.

A   B

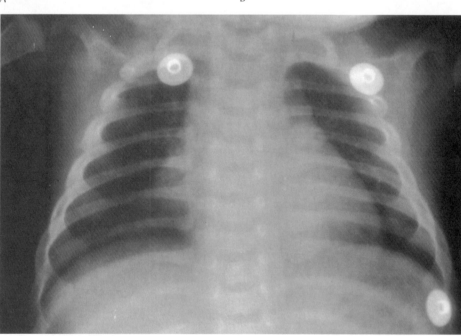

FIG. 6-E-2 (*Panel A*) Frontal view of the chest.

Clinical Histories:

CASE 6-1

On the first day of your medical school rotation in orthopedic surgery, the resident and attending physician send you to the emergency room to see a 26-year-old man with a broken leg (Fig. 6-E-1*A,B*).

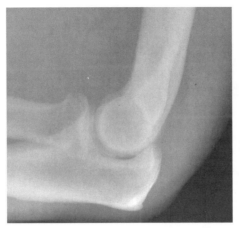

FIG. 6-E-3 (*Panel A*) Lateral view of the elbow.

FIG. 6-E-4 (*Panel A*) AP view of the ankle.

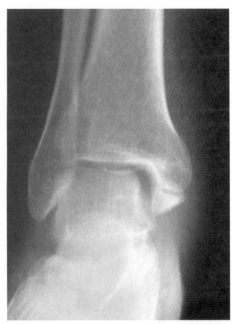

FIG. 6-E-5 (*Panels A and B*) AP and lateral views of the ankle.

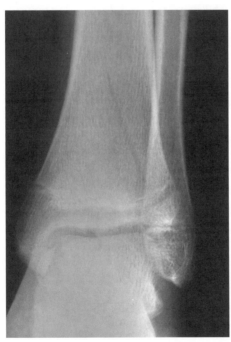

A

B

CASE 6-2

Infant with low-grade fever. You obtain a chest radiograph to "rule out pneumonia" (Fig. 6-E-2A).

CASE 6-3

While moonlighting in the emergency department of a small community hospital, you examine a 25-year-old man who fell on an outstretched hand and now complains of elbow pain. You obtain frontal and lateral views of his elbow (Fig. 6-E-3A).

CASE 6-4
A week later you are once again moonlighting in the same small emergency department when a 29-year-old man is carried in complaining of ankle pain after a twisting injury. His ankle is swollen and ecchymotic, and he is tender to palpation along the medial malleolus. He has no other complaints. You order frontal, lateral, and oblique views of the ankle (Fig. 6-E-4A).

CASE 6-5
A 15-year-old boy complains of ankle pain after a fall (Fig. 6-E-5A,B).

Questions:

6-1. You are supposed to look at the radiographs and call your colleagues in the operating room to describe the fracture. Which of the following statements concerning the fracture would you not wish to make?
  A. The distal tibial fragment is displaced 1 cm posteriorly.
  B. There is comminution of the metaphyseal component of the tibial fracture.
  C. There is slight valgus angulation of the distal tibial fragment.
  D. A tibial fracture line extends to the articular surface.
  E. This is an open fracture.

6-2. 1. You interpret the chest radiograph and render the following diagnosis:
    A. Normal chest radiograph.
    B. Round pneumonia.
    C. Viral pneumonia.
    D. Multiple healing rib fractures.
    E. Pneumothorax.

  2. What should you do next?
    A. Prescribe antibacterials and discharge the patient.
    B. Perform a workup for sepsis.
    C. Reassure the parents "it's just a cold."
    D. Reexamine the child and obtain a skeletal survey.
    E. Obtain a radiology consult.

6-3. 1. You first examine the lateral view of the elbow. You find:
    A. A lytic lesion in the distal humerus.
    B. A fracture through the proximal ulna.
    C. Displacement of the anterior and posterior fat pads of the elbow.
    D. Dislocation of the elbow.

  You do not see any abnormalities on the other film.

  2. What should you do next?
    A. Send him home with instructions to use ice packs and acetaminophen to treat his soft-tissue contusion.
    B. Treat him for a presumed radial head fracture.
    C. Biopsy the lytic lesion in the humerus.
    D. Perform arthrocentesis to see if he has a joint effusion.
    E. Order MR imaging of the elbow.

6-4. You examine the radiographs. Only the anteroposterior (AP) view is shown here. You tell the patient he has broken his ankle, but you want to get one more study:
  A. Contralateral ankle, for comparison purposes.
  B. Ipsilateral foot, to exclude a fracture of the fifth metatarsal.
  C. Remainder of the ipsilateral tibia and fibula, to exclude more proximal fractures.
  D. CT, for more precise evaluation of the alignment of the fracture.

6-5. 1. What is the abnormality?
A. Triplane fracture of the distal tibia
B. Fracture of the distal fibula
C. Stress fracture of the talus
D. Ankle sprain
E. Avascular necrosis of the talus

2. What imaging study would be most useful?
A. Nuclear medicine bone scan
B. Repeat radiographic examination in 10 days
C. CT
D. MR imaging

Radiologic Findings:

6-1. There are comminuted fractures of the distal tibia and fibula with intraarticular extension of the tibial fracture. Gas dissects through the soft tissues and indicates communication between the fracture and the skin.

6-2. A row of rounded opacities in the left chest represents posterior healing rib fractures.

6-3. This patient's anterior fat pad is pushed away from the bone, creating a small triangular "sail." The posterior fat pad is visible when it should not normally be visible at all. There is no visible fracture or dislocation.

6-4. Transverse fracture of the distal medial malleolus with widening of the medial aspect of the ankle joint.

6-5. There are abnormal lucencies running vertically through the epiphysis on the frontal view and obliquely through the metaphysis on both the frontal and the lateral views. The lateral aspect of the distal tibial physis or growth plate is widened.

Discussion:

6-1. Your mission is to describe accurately and succinctly the features of this fracture that will affect treatment and outcome. All the features mentioned under "Radiologic Findings" should be included.

You also should discuss the alignment of the largest tibial and fibular fragments. You should address both displacement and angulation. Displacement is always described in terms of the position of the distal fragment relative to that of the proximal fragment. There is obvious displacement in the lateral view, since the distal tibial fragment is displaced 1 cm posteriorly.

On the frontal view there is obvious angulation. Angulation may be described either in terms of the direction of shift of the distal fragment or in terms of the direction in which the apex of the angle points. In either case, it is better to give a measurement than to use subjective modifiers such as *slight* or *moderate*. This angulation may correctly be described as "30 degrees of varus angulation of the distal fragment" or "30-degree lateral apical angulation" (Fig. 6-E-1*C,D*) (*C* is the incorrect statement and the correct answer to this question).

6-2. Rib fractures in a young child suggest child abuse (the correct answer to Question 1 is *D*). Since most rib fractures in infants are caused by nonaccidental injury, you should reexamine the child for other stigmata of child abuse, such as bruises, welts, burns, or retinal hemorrhages, notify protective services, and obtain a skeletal survey (the correct answer to Question 2 is *D*). If you were unsure of your diagnosis or desired confirmation of the radiographic findings, you should have obtained a radiology consult, since discharging the patient could place the child in serious danger.

Figure 6-E-2*B* from the skeletal survey reveals the classic metaphyseal "corner" (*large arrows*) and "bucket-handle" (*small arrows*) fractures virtually pathognomonic of infant abuse. The astute observer also will note a healing fracture of the superior pubic ramus. In summary, radiologic findings with moderate to high specificity for infant

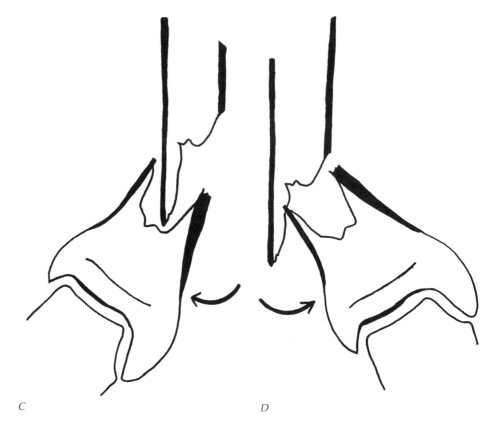

FIG. 6-E-1 Varus and valgus angulation. (*Panel C*) The distal tibial fragment has shifted laterally with respect to the proximal tibia. This is valgus angulation. (*Panel D*) The distal tibial fragment has shifted medially with respect to the proximal fragment. This is varus angulation.

C

D

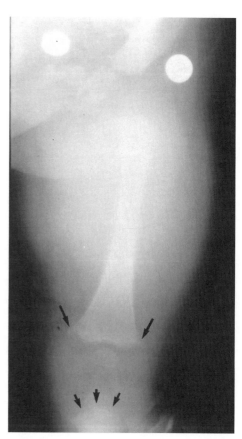

FIG. 6-E-2 (*Panel B*) AP view of the femur. There are metaphyseal fractures of both the femur (*arrows*) and the tibia (*small arrows*).

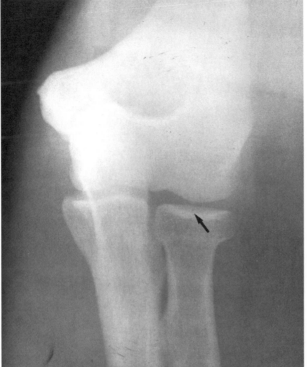

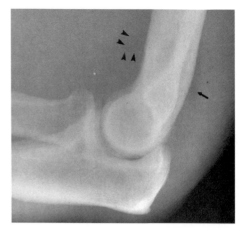

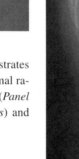

B

FIG. 6-E-3 (*Panel B*) Frontal view of the elbow demonstrates a tiny linear lucency on the articular surface of the proximal radius (*arrow*). This is a nondisplaced radial head fracture. (*Panel C*) Lateral view of the elbow with anterior (*arrowheads*) and posterior (*arrow*) fat pad signs.

FIG. 6-E-4 (*Panel B*) AP view of the knee. The proximal fibula is fractured.

abuse include posterior rib fractures, metaphyseal fractures, multiple fractures, and fractures at differing stages of healing.

6-3. When examining a radiograph for a suspected fracture, it is important to evaluate not only the bones themselves but also the adjacent soft tissues. In a number of areas of the body there are normal deposits of fat, termed *fat pads,* that may be displaced by accumulation of blood or fluid in the underlying tissues. The fat pads of the elbow are particularly helpful (*C* is the correct answer to Question 1).

Displacement of the elbow fat pad is a nonspecific sign that indicates distension of the joint. Effusions due to rheumatoid arthritis, an infected joint, or hemorrhage, especially in a patient with a bleeding disorder, could all cause the "fat pad sign" seen in this patient. In an otherwise healthy person who has suffered trauma, however, a radial head fracture should be suspected, since it is the most common elbow fracture in an adult (*B* is the correct answer to Question 2). This patient's frontal view (Fig. 6-E-3*B,C*) did actually demonstrate a small lucent fracture line in the radial head. Even without that, however, the most prudent course is to treat the patient as though he had a radial head fracture and also arrange for follow-up care with a physician accustomed to caring for fractures.

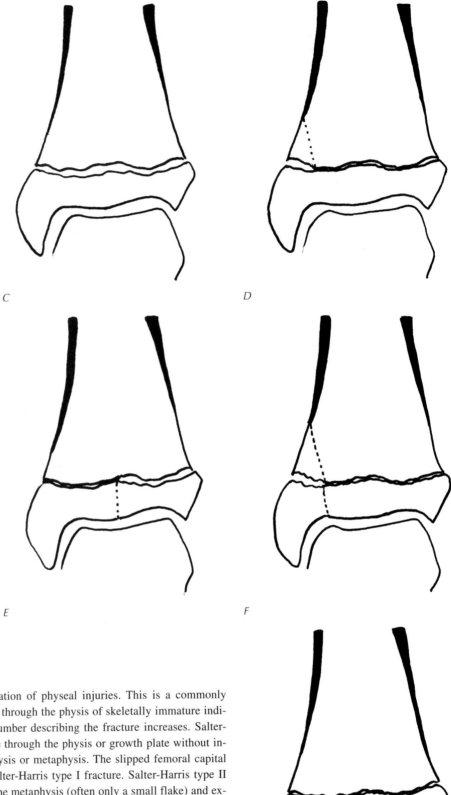

FIG. 6-E-5 Salter-Harris classification of physeal injuries. This is a commonly used method of describing fractures through the physis of skeletally immature individuals. Outcome worsens as the number describing the fracture increases. Salter-Harris type I fractures (*Panel C*) are through the physis or growth plate without involvement of the bone of the epiphysis or metaphysis. The slipped femoral capital epiphysis shown in Fig. 6-1 is a Salter-Harris type I fracture. Salter-Harris type II fractures (*Panel D*) involve part of the metaphysis (often only a small flake) and extend to the physis. Salter-Harris type III fractures (*Panel E*) involve the epiphysis and extend to the physis. The Salter-Harris type III fracture illustrated here is similar to the epiphyseal and physeal components of the triplane fracture (*Panel A*) without extension to the metaphysis. It also is a fairly common injury pattern. The Salter-Harris type IV fracture (*Panel F*) involves both the metaphysis and epiphysis. The Salter-Harris type V injury (*Panel G*) involves only the physis and is a compressive injury secondary to axial loading forces.

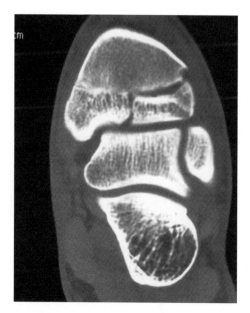

FIG. 6-E-5 (*Panel H*) Coronal CT scan of the ankle. This image was obtained with direct coronal technique. The patient was positioned with his feet on the CT table and knees bent. Images were then obtained about 15 degrees from a true coronal through the tibiotalar joint. Had the image been reconstructed from data acquired during axial imaging, it would not have been as sharp and detailed. Putting together the information on multiple such images allows more precise evaluation of fracture fragment position than is possible with conventional radiographs. This image demonstrates widening of the physis laterally and the sagittal split through the epiphysis.

6-4. The correct answer to this question is *C*. Transverse medial malleolar fracture usually accompanies eversion of the ankle and is often associated with a fibular fracture. The fibular injury may occur at any level from the ankle to the knee. When there is no apparent distal fibular fracture, the remainder of the bone should be imaged. In this case, there is indeed a fracture of the proximal fibula (Fig. 6-E-4*B*). This fracture indicates rupture of the interosseous membrane all along its course from the ankle to the fibular fracture, so this is an unstable injury that many orthopedic surgeons will treat with open reduction and internal fixation of the malleolar component and of the syndesmosis.

Fractures of the proximal fifth metatarsal may accompany ankle inversion and may be difficult to distinguish clinically from other ankle injuries; therefore, that part of the foot should always be included on at least one view of the ankle. If it is not, then it is prudent, when possible, to obtain one more view, but this should not ordinarily be considered a separate study or incur an additional charge. CT is not necessary in this case and would be money ill-spent.

6-5. This adolescent patient has suffered a relatively common growth-plate injury with a typical but somewhat complex fracture pattern. It is called a *triplane fracture* because it has components that run, more or less, in all three primary planes of section. It travels in the sagittal plane through the epiphysis, in the axial plane through the unfused portion of the physis or growth plate, and in the coronal plane through the metaphysis (*A* is the correct answer to Question 1). It is a Salter-Harris type IV fracture (Fig. 6-E-5*C* to *G*). It can be diagnosed easily on the conventional radiographs. Overlapping of several bones in the ankle region, together with the inferiorly concave shape of the articular surface of the distal tibia, the tibial plafond, complicates evaluation of fracture fragment position, and so a CT scan was obtained (Fig. 6-E-5*H*) (*C* is the correct answer to Question 2).

EXERCISE 6-2: LOCAL DISEASE

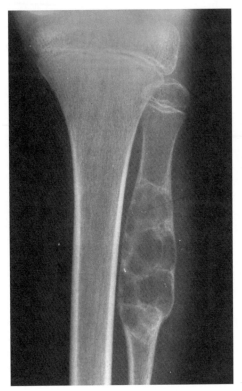 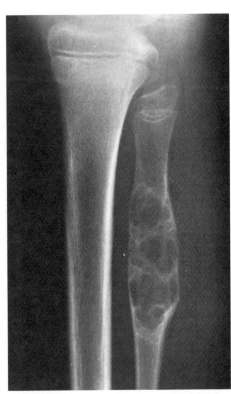

FIG. 6-E-6 (*Panels A and B*) AP and lateral views of the proximal tibia and fibula.

A　　　　*B*

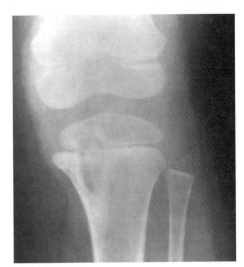

FIG. 6-E-7 (*Panel A*) AP view of the knee. (*Courtesy of Murray K. Dalinka, M.D.*)

Clinical Histories:

CASE 6-6
A 12-year-old girl comes to your pediatrics office complaining of 2 weeks of knee pain. There is no history of trauma. She is slightly swollen, tender, and erythematous over the proximal fibula. You obtain frontal and lateral views of the tibia and fibula (Fig. 6-E-6A,B).

CASE 6-7
This 5-year-old girl has been limping off and on for 2 months. Her knee is warm and swollen (Fig. 6-E-7A).

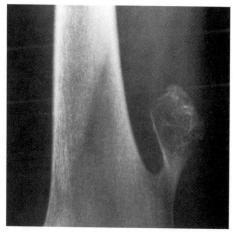

FIG. 6-E-9 (*Panel A*) AP view of the distal femur.

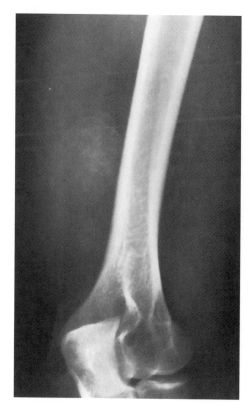

FIG. 6-E-8 AP view of the arm.

CASE 6-8

A 35-year-old man complains of a lump in the soft tissues of the right arm. He first noticed the lump 6 months ago after hurting his arm in a fall from a bicycle (Fig. 6-E-8).

CASE 6-9

A 10-year-old girl complains of a lump on the inside of her thigh near the knee. It has been there as long as she can remember but has been annoying her since she recently took up horseback riding (Fig. 6-E-9A).

Questions:

6-6. 1. Based on the history, physical examination, and radiographs, which of the following choices is the best working diagnosis?
   A. A bone tumor, most likely benign
   B. A bone tumor, most likely malignant
   C. Osteomyelitis
   D. A stress fracture of the proximal fibula

2. What should you do next?
   A. Refer the patient to an orthopedic surgeon who specializes in treatment of tumors.
   B. Obtain a bone scan, MR imaging study, and CT scan to narrow the differential diagnosis and evaluate the local extent of this disease.
   C. Order a percutaneous needle biopsy of the lesion in the fibula.
   D. Try a 2-week course of antibiotics.

6-7. What is the most likely diagnosis?
   A. Osteomyelitis
   B. A bone tumor, most likely malignant
   C. A Salter-Harris type IV fracture
   D. Langerhans cell histiocytosis (eosinophilic granuloma)

6-8. What should you do about the calcified lump in this patient's arm?
  A. Needle biopsy
  B. Open excisional biopsy
  C. Reassure the patient
  D. Bone scan

6-9. What is this lump?
  A. An osteosarcoma
  B. An osteochondroma
  C. A normal variant
  D. A soft-tissue sarcoma

Radiologic Findings: 6-6. Focal lytic lesion in the proximal fibular metadiaphysis with an intact shell of new cortex and a well-defined, short zone of transition between itself and adjacent normal bone.

6-7. There is a well-defined lytic lesion in the proximal tibia. Its edges are slightly sclerotic. It extends across the physis to involve portions of both the metaphysis and epiphysis.

6-8. A well-defined ossified mass projects in the musculature of the posterolateral arm. It has a thin but distinct cortex surrounding trabeculae.

6-9. Arising from the medial cortex of the femur is an ossified mass topped by a cauliflower-like thin shell of cortex. The cortex of the remainder of the femur is continuous with the cortex of the tumor, and the trabecular bone of the femoral metaphysis blends imperceptibly with that of the mass. The mass has grown away from its metaphyseal place of origin and points toward the diaphysis and away from the joint.

Discussion: 6-6. The radiographs demonstrate a focal lytic lesion in the proximal fibular metadiaphysis. The cortex appears intact around the lesion, and the bone is widened. Cortex is not pliable; it will not stretch to accommodate a growing lesion. Instead, it will slowly remodel by resorption of endosteal bone and deposition of periosteal new bone. The intact cortex implies a slow growth rate for this lesion. Another indication of a slow growth rate is the sharp demarcation or short zone of transition between the lesion and adjacent normal bone.

In general, osteomyelitis will not cause apparent expansion of bone the way this lesion has. Stress fractures are usually linear lesions. Stress fractures may be lucent, if a gap in cortical bone is their primary manifestation, or sclerotic, due either to compression of trabeculae with resultant overlap or to healing. The periosteal reaction that they engender may cause them to be mistaken for bone tumors, but they will not look like this particular lesion (Fig. 6-E-6*C*).

Of the choices given in the first question, the remaining ones are benign and malignant bone tumor. For the most part, malignant bone tumors in children have a rapid growth rate. This will cause them to have poorly defined borders with adjacent normal bone. In addition, where they destroy cortex, the periosteum will be unable to contain them with solidly mineralized new bone, as has occurred here. There may be gaps in the cortex where tumor has broken through (Fig. 6-E-6*D*). The periosteal new bone may mineralize at 90-degree angles to the diaphysis or may be lamellated (like onion skin) or incomplete. The intact shell of periosteal new bone seen in this patient and the short zone of transition are more typical of a benign than a malignant tumor (*A* is the correct answer to the first question).

A primary bone tumor, no matter how benign its appearance, is most appropriately handled by an orthopedic surgeon experienced with tumor patients. Since you have been stipulated to be a pediatrician, the best answer to Question 2 is *A,* and the patient should be sent to an orthopedic surgeon who specializes in treatment of tumors.

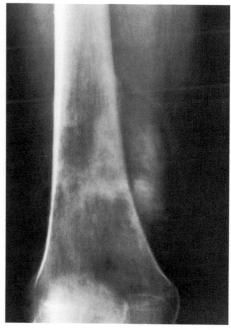

D

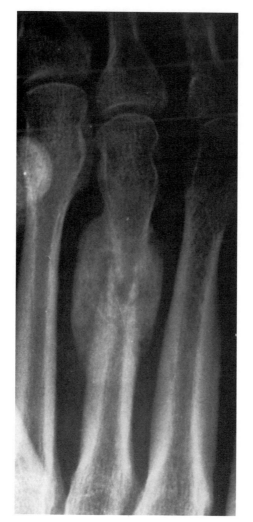

C

FIG. 6-E-6 (*Panel C*) Stress fracture. Oblique view of the third metatarsal. This typical healing stress fracture demonstrates both a transverse, linear lucency and abundant callus formation. (*Panel D*) AP view of the distal femur. Many of the radiographic features of this osteosarcoma mark it as a malignant tumor. The abnormal area of mottled lucent and sclerotic tumor in the metaphysis fades gradually into the shadows of surrounding normal bone. It is difficult to see where the tumor begins and ends. There is a large soft-tissue mass adjacent to the bone. The periosteum has been unable to maintain a shell of mineralized new bone around this mass. The sclerotic areas within the bone and the mineralized portions of the soft-tissue mass both have a relatively amorphous, smudged appearance that is seen with calcified osteoid matrix.

Performing a percutaneous needle biopsy (option *C*) has the potential to cause great harm if a poorly chosen route is taken. For example, if the needle passed close to the common peroneal nerve and then the lesion proved unexpectedly to be malignant, the nerve might have to be sacrificed in order to obtain a curative resection.

Obtaining additional imaging studies to evaluate this lesion further is not a bad idea. It is better, however, to allow the orthopedic surgeon to whom the patient will be referred (in consultation with the radiologist) to decide which imaging tests are most appropriate to evaluate the lesion more thoroughly before ordering additional tests.

6-7. The edges of malignant tumors are usually not as well defined as those of this lesion. Malignant tumors may extend across the growth plate, but it is uncommon for them to do so while they are still as small as this lesion.

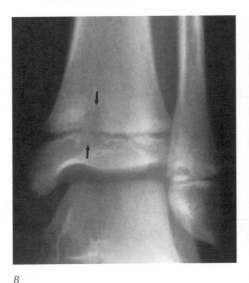

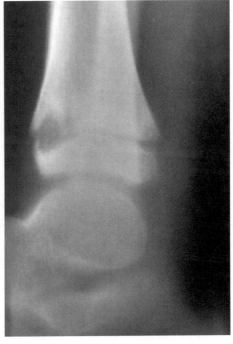

FIG. 6-E-7 AP view (*Panel B*) and sagittal tomogram (*Panel C*) of the ankle. This focus of osteomyelitis (arrows), occurring in a 5-year-old boy, also crosses the growth plate. It is radiographically indistinguishable from the case of tuberculous osteomyelitis, yet it was due to *Staphylococcus*. The distinction between pyogenic and tuberculous osteomyelitis must be made on clinical grounds and proven by biopsy.

Osteomyelitis, on the other hand, often breaches the growth plate (*A* is the correct answer). The most common organisms to cause osteomyelitis are species of *Staphylococcus* and *Streptococcus* (Fig. 6-E-7*B,C*). The relatively long history of limping, however, should suggest a more indolent organism. This case was due to *Mycobacterium tuberculosis*. Skeletal tuberculosis is uncommon and thus often is overlooked as a diagnostic possibility. Because it is curable yet responds to very different drugs than would be used for pyogenic osteomyelitis, it is important to keep it in mind. It may occur at any site, but it is most common in the spine. In the extremities it most often occurs in or near the hip and knee.

Langerhans cell histiocytosis (eosinophilic granuloma) is much less common than osteomyelitis and is thus not as likely a diagnosis. When it does occur, its favorite location is the skull.

6-8. This ossified mass represents myositis ossificans, also known as *heterotopic new bone formation*. Though often associated with trauma, it also may be seen in patients without a distinct history of trauma. When it resembles mature bone as closely as in this patient, it is not a diagnostic dilemma, and you may reassure the patient that there is a benign cause for his lump (*C* is the correct answer).

Occasionally, myositis ossificans warrants excision on the basis of mechanical interference with the use of a muscle or joint. Recurrence is less likely if excision is performed after the lesion has matured. A bone scan may help to distinguish between mature and immature lesions. An immature lesion that is still undergoing ossification will exhibit marked radionuclide uptake. Once ossification is complete, radionuclide accumulation will resemble that of other bones.

Myositis ossificans may be diagnosed more confidently with radiography than with histology. An immature lesion will be full of immature, rapidly proliferating cells that may be mistaken for a sarcoma by the pathologist. Radiologically, however, there is a

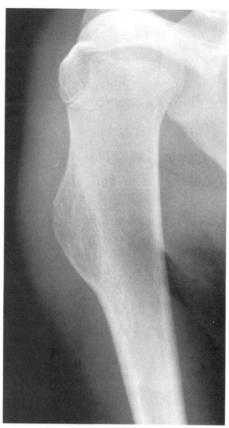

FIG. 6-E-9 (*Panel B*) AP view of the proximal humerus. There is a sessile osteochondroma on the lateral aspect of this child's humerus. Proton-density (*Panel C*) and T2-weighted (*Panel D*) coronal MR images of the knee. On the former, a very tiny osteochondroma arises from the lateral metaphysis of the distal femur (*arrow*). Notice that the signal intensity (shade of gray) inside this diminutive tumor is the same as that of the adjoining marrow space. The bright area (*arrow*) over the osteochondroma in *Panel D* represents a small, fluid-filled bursa. This patient complained of a snapping sensation that most likely was due to movement of the iliotibial band back and forth over the osteochondroma.

B

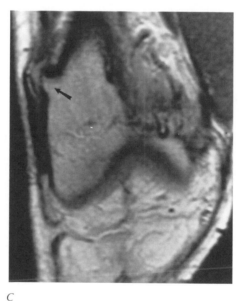

C

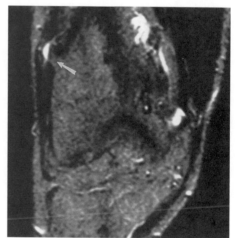

D

distinct difference between the two. Myositis ossificans ossifies from the outside in. Sarcomas ossify from the inside out. (Look back at Fig. 6-E-6D and notice that the central portion of the soft-tissue mass of the osteosarcoma is ossified, whereas the outer portion is not.) If it is not entirely clear from conventional radiographs where and how the ossification is occurring, a CT scan is the test of choice because of its sensitivity to calcium.

6-9. This mass has the characteristic appearance of an osteochondroma, the most common of all benign cartilaginous neoplasms. Osteochondromas may be very large or very small, pedunculated or sessile (Fig. 6-E-9B). They grow as the child grows and should cease growth by adulthood. Often asymptomatic, they may be an incidental finding. They may, however, cause a wide range of symptoms. The most common complaint is that they interfere with activities or with wearing certain clothes, such as tight blue jeans. They may be painful as a result of irritation of an overlying bursa, and they are subject to fracture. An uncommon (1 percent or less) but feared complication is malignant transformation, usually resulting in a chondrosarcoma. Signs of such transformation include enlargement of the osteochondroma in an adult, thickening of the cartilaginous cap that covers the tumor, development of a soft-tissue mass, and destruction of bone.

When further radiologic studies are needed, MR imaging is probably the most useful modality. It can demonstrate the cartilage cap and any associated soft-tissue mass. When the diagnosis is not as obvious as in this case by conventional radiography, MR imaging can assist in confirming the identity of the tumor by demonstrating continuity between the cortices and medullary spaces of the tumor and the host bone (Fig. 6-E-9C,D).

EXERCISE 6-3: SYSTEMIC DISEASE

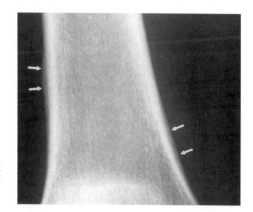

FIG. 6-E-11 (*Panel A*) AP view of the right distal femur. Arrows indicate the periosteal new bone formation.

FIG. 6-E-12 (*Panels A and B*) PA and lateral views of the chest.

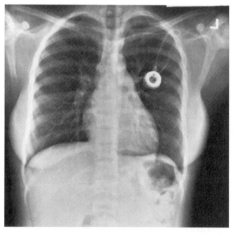

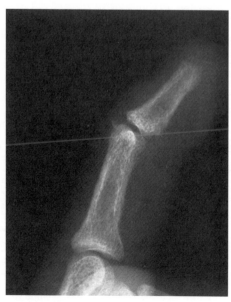

A

B

FIG. 6-E-13 (*Panel A*) AP views of the index, middle, and ring fingers. (*Panel B*) Lateral view of the index finger.

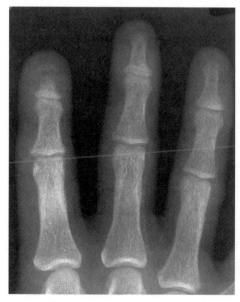

A

B

Clinical Histories:

CASE 6-10
As a medical student on the oncology team you see in clinic a 45-year-old woman with a history of breast cancer diagnosed 5 years previously. She underwent surgery and since that time has been free of disease. She has come for her routine follow-up appointment and complains only of vague, aching discomfort in her left hip.

CASE 6-11
A 40-year-old man complains of knee pain and swelling of 3 weeks' duration. He has no other known disease. You order conventional radiographs of the knees. You notice some periosteal elevation on both femurs and tibiae (Fig. 6-E-11A).

CASE 6-12
This chest radiograph was obtained to exclude pneumonia in a chronically ill 26-year-old woman (Fig. 6-E-12A,B).

CASE 6-13
In a 50-year-old man with diabetes, radiographs of the hand were obtained to exclude fracture after a fall (Fig. 6-E-13A,B).

Questions:

6-10. Which of the following studies do you not want to order today?
A. Chest radiograph
B. Conventional radiographs of the left hip and pelvis
C. Bone scan
D. Skeletal survey
E. Mammography

6-11. What is the next study you should order?
A. Bone scan
B. MR imaging of the knees
C. Hand films
D. Chest radiograph

6-12. There is no evidence of pneumonia, but there are several abnormalities that are clues to the nature of this patient's chronic illness. Which finding listed below is not such a clue?
A. Surgical clips in the gallbladder bed
B. Enlargement of the pulmonary artery segment of the mediastinum
C. Depressions in the end plates of numerous vertebrae
D. Irregular sclerosis of both humeral heads

6-13. Which of the following statements is most likely to be correct?
A. The patient has not suffered a fracture.
B. A metastatic tumor is destroying the distal phalanx of the index finger.
C. The bones are normally mineralized.
D. Renal failure has developed.

Radiologic Findings:

6-11. A thin rim of calcium added to the bony contour of both sides of the right femoral metaphysis (arrows) is due to periosteal elevation. Similar findings were present on the left femur and both tibiae. This helped to distinguish this small amount of periosteal new bone from the normal irregularity of the cortex at muscle attachment sites.

6-12. There are surgical clips in the right upper quadrant. The humeral heads have an abnormal, mottled, sclerotic appearance. Many vertebral bodies, as best appreciated in the lateral view, are shaped like the letter H lying on its side.

6-13. The distal interphalangeal joint of the middle finger is held in slight flexion. A small triangular chip of bone projects in the soft tissues dorsally and a few millimeters proximally to the proximal aspect of the distal phalanx. The tufts of all the fingers are abnormal. This patient's phalanges are too short and too narrow at their tips. The cortex has been resorbed in many places. It is difficult to decide exactly where the edge of the bone is. Besides resorption of the most distal portion of the tuft of the index finger, there is also irregular resorption or destruction of the central portion of the distal phalanx.

Discussion:

6-10. Options *A*, a chest radiograph, and *E*, mammography, are both reasonable screening examinations often obtained yearly in asymptomatic cancer patients. These would be good tests to order for this patient even without new symptoms. Indeed, mammography should be obtained in any woman of 45 years every year or two for screening purposes, irrespective of her history. Bone scans are also often ordered as screens for metastatic disease in asymptomatic breast cancer patients, particularly for the first 2 to 3 years after diagnosis. Because this patient is complaining of skeletal pain, both a bone scan (Fig. 6-E-10*A*) and conventional radiographs of the affected area (Fig. 6-E-10*B*) are indicated. A skeletal survey is not appropriate (*D* is the correct answer to this question).

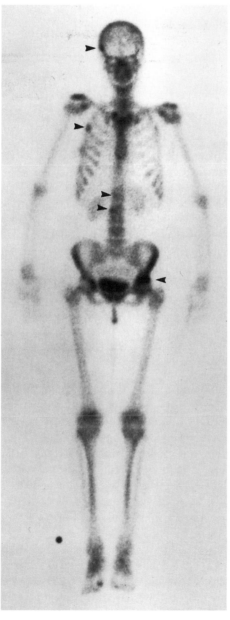

A

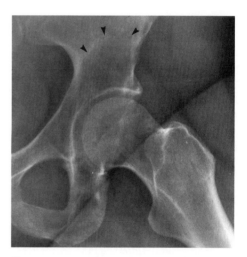

B

FIG. 6-E-10 (*Panel A*) Anterior view from a ⁹⁹ᵐTc-MDP whole-body bone scan. In several areas more radionuclide has accumulated than in the remainder of the skeleton, and these areas appear darker: left acetabulum, two upper lumbar vertebrae, the lateral aspect of the right third rib, and the right side of the skull (*arrowheads*). Numerous foci of increased radioactivity, sprinkled somewhat haphazardly about the body but mostly involving the axial skeleton, are very typical of the appearance of metastatic cancer. (*Panel B*) Frog-leg lateral view of the left hip. The ilium just above the acetabulum is too lucent, and a thin, irregular white line (*arrowheads*) appears to demarcate the edge of the lucency. On a frontal view of the pelvis (not shown), this area also seemed slightly too lucent in comparison with the other side.

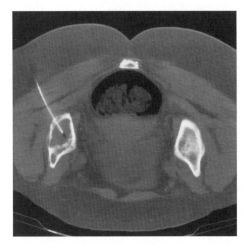

C

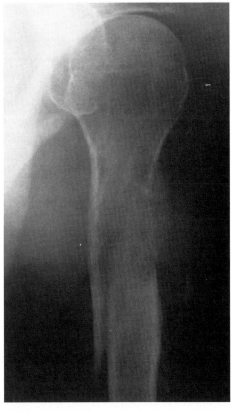

D

FIG. 6-E-10   (*Panel C*) Axial CT scan obtained with the patient in prone position. The trabecular bone of the left ilium has been replaced by material of approximately the same density as the muscle. Using a percutaneous approach through the left buttock, a needle has been placed into the center of the lesion. Aspiration of cells yielded a diagnosis of metastatic breast carcinoma. The needle appears to be wholly embedded within the patient because it has traveled an oblique course. The rest of it would be apparent on scans taken cranially or caudally to this one. (*Panel D*) AP view of the proximal left humerus of a different patient. An acute fracture has occurred through an area of bone destruction caused by metastatic carcinoma. (The same radiographic appearance could be seen in a healing fracture through previously normal bone.) Conventional radiographs are used to identify bony metastases that have destroyed enough bone to make a pathologic fracture likely.

In general, a skeletal survey is utilized in oncology only for screening for multiple myeloma and Langerhans cell histiocytosis.

In this patient's case, a bone scan revealed multiple areas of abnormally increased accumulation of radionuclide, including the left acetabulum (Fig. 6-E-10*A*). The multiplicity of lesions, together with the history of breast cancer (which often metastasizes to bone and may do so after a disease-free interval of many years), is very suggestive of metastatic disease. Some oncologists would choose to treat the patient for presumed metastatic disease on the basis of the bone scan, history, and current symptoms. Others would prefer a biopsy before proceeding to further treatment. This patient underwent a CT-guided needle aspiration of the acetabular lesion, which revealed metastatic tumor (Fig. 6-E-10*C*). To evaluate for possible impending pathologic fracture (Fig. 6-E-10*D*), most oncologists also would request conventional radiographs of areas demonstrating increased activity on the bone scan.

6-11. Periosteal elevation is a nonspecific finding that occurs with local disorders such as fracture, bone tumors, and osteomyelitis, as well as with systemic or multifocal disorders such as bone infarction (Fig. 6-E-11*B*), venous stasis, and secondary hypertrophic osteoarthropathy. Because this finding is bilateral, it is more likely due to a systemic or multifocal disorder than to a local one.

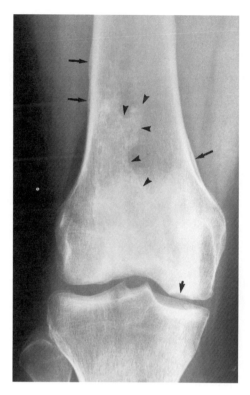

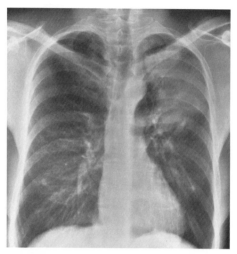

FIG. 6-E-11 (*Panel B*) AP view of the knee. This is an example of periosteal new bone formation (*arrows*) associated with bone infarction. The infarction is marked by an irregular sclerotic area in the metaphysis (*arrowheads*), as well as a small, rounded lucent defect in the articular surface of the medial femoral condyle (*short arrow*).

FIG. 6-E-11 (*Panel C*) PA view of the chest. A large mass in the left upper lobe represents a primary lung carcinoma.

Of all the systemic disorders that may be associated with periosteal new bone formation, secondary hypertrophic osteoarthropathy is the most important to exclude. At one time it was called *hypertrophic pulmonary osteoarthropathy* because it is usually caused by pulmonary disease. The designation *secondary hypertrophic osteoarthropathy* reflects current understanding that this disorder also may be due to nonpulmonary diseases such as inflammatory bowel disease or congenital cardiac anomalies. Nonetheless, pulmonary disease, specifically lung cancer, remains the most common cause (*D* is the correct answer). This patient, in fact, had lung cancer (Fig. 6-E-11*C*).

A bone scan could be useful if you did not notice the periosteal new bone or were not sure of its presence. Hand films could demonstrate clubbing, which may be seen with some of the same disorders that cause hypertrophic osteoarthropathy, but simple physical inspection of the patient's hands would accomplish the same thing. MR imaging of the knees will not be helpful in this case.

6-12. This patient has sickle cell disease. The surgical clips in the right upper quadrant of the abdomen are from a prior cholecystectomy. People with sickle cell disease are prone to early development of cholelithiasis.

The peculiar shape of multiple vertebral bodies is very characteristic of sickle cell anemia, though it may occasionally be seen in other diseases affecting the marrow cavity, particularly Gaucher's disease. It may be caused by infarction of bone beneath the end plates, with remodeling of the cortex to produce the H shape.

When red blood cells sickle, they clump together and may block blood vessels. In bone this leads to avascular necrosis, which may be widespread, involving many bones simultaneously. The mottled appearance of the humeral heads is due to avascular necrosis and is a common finding in patients with sickle cell anemia.

Modest enlargement of the pulmonary artery, as seen in this patient, is so common in young women that it is considered normal in that population (*B* is the correct answer).

Though it was not included among the possible answers to the question, another finding of interest on this examination involves the appearance of the left upper quadrant. The gas-filled splenic flexure of the colon occupies too much of the left upper quadrant on the frontal view. There is no room for a spleen of normal size. In sickle cell pa-

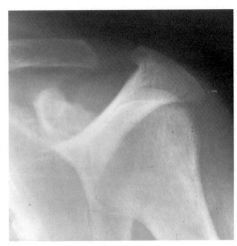

D

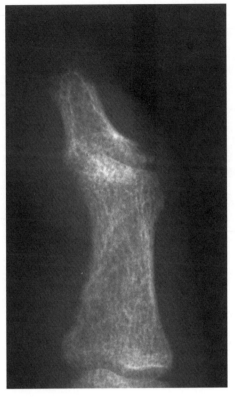

C

FIG. 6-E-13   (*Panel C*) Oblique view of the middle finger. Note the many tiny erosions of the cortex of the radial side of the middle phalanx. (*Panel D*) Oblique view of the acromioclavicular joint. The clavicle is too short by approximately 1 cm, and the cortex of the distal end of this bone is fuzzy and ill-defined.

tients the spleen is often infarcted so that by the time they reach adulthood it has shrunk to a small fraction of normal size.

6-13. This patient has many findings of hyperparathyroidism. Primary hyperparathyroidism usually results from a hyperfunctioning parathyroid adenoma, which is usually detected and removed before the osseous findings of hyperparathyroidism develop. Secondary hyperparathyroidism is most often associated with chronic renal failure, a common complication of diabetes mellitus (*D* is the correct answer).

Parathyroid hormone stimulates the action of osteoclasts and thus causes resorption of bone. Acroosteolysis (resorption of the tufts of the fingers) is one manifestation of hyperparathyroidism. Two other places where such resorption often occurs are also seen in this patient's hands. One is intracortical, where resorption is causing longitudinal striation in the cortex. The other is subperiosteal. Notice that the cortex of the lateral or radial side of each of the middle phalanges is finely serrated (Fig. 6-E-13*C*). This is caused by resorption of bone in the troughs, and the peaks are areas where the cortex has maintained a more normal thickness. Subperiosteal resorption in this location is often the earliest radiographic sign of hyperparathyroidism. It is also nearly pathognomonic of this disorder. For this reason, hand films may be obtained to monitor patients with renal failure for early evidence of hyperparathyroidism. Another common site of bone resorption in hyperparathyroidism is the distal clavicle (Fig. 6-E-13*D*).

Resorption of the central portion of the distal phalanx of the index finger also may be due to the hyperparathyroidism, but other causes such as osteomyelitis or tumor also should be considered. Of the two, osteomyelitis is more common and may occur in the fingers as a result of direct implantation of organisms from a puncture wound. Metastasis may occur in any bone but favors the axial skeleton and is uncommon in the hands.

Finally, the chip of bone at the distal interphalangeal joint of the middle finger is likely to represent an avulsion fracture of the attachment site of the extensor tendon.

BIBLIOGRAPHY

Edeiken J et al: Edeiken's Roentgen Diagnosis of Diseases of Bone, 4th ed. Baltimore, Williams & Wilkins, 1990.

Keats TE: Atlas of Normal Roentgen Variants That May Simulate Disease, 4th ed. Chicago, Year Book Medical Publishers, 1988.

Köhler A, Zimmer E-A: Borderlands of Normal and Early Pathologic Findings in Skeletal Radiology, 4th ed. New York, Thieme Medical Publishers, 1993.

Schultz RJ: The Language of Fractures, 2d ed. Baltimore, Williams & Wilkins, 1990.

7

IMAGING OF JOINTS

Johnny U. V. Monu
Thomas L. Pope, Jr.

Conventional plain-film radiography remains the foundation of joint evaluation, although other imaging methods or specialized techniques can be used to obtain direct or indirect information about a joint. Some of these other techniques and modalities include plain-film tomography, ultrasonography, computed tomography (CT), magnetic resonance (MR) imaging, radionuclide imaging, and arthrography.

TECHNIQUES AND NORMAL ANATOMY

Plain Film

The plain-film examination uses x-rays, which are a form of ionizing radiation. Plain films provide a panoramic view of the joint and yield information that allows identification of the joint (knee joint, shoulder joint, etc.). They also give gross information about the status of a joint. Ionizing radiation is a disadvantage, however, because that method cannot be used very frequently, especially in pediatric patients or pregnant women.

Conventional Tomography

This technique is a variation on the plain film and requires specialized equipment. Images made with this modality show only a defined layer or tissue plane in focus, and other structures outside this selected imaging plane are blurred. This test is used to acquire very specific information, e.g., the presence of a radiopaque intraarticular fragment, and is useful when overlying opaque material impedes adequate evaluation. Its major disadvantages are a high radiation dose to the patient, relatively poor image resolution, and the fact that images can be obtained in only one plane (Fig. 7-1).

Arthrography

Prior to the advent of MR imaging, arthrography was the only method by which articular structures could be evaluated. In this technique, the joint was imaged indirectly by the intraarticular injection of contrast material followed by radiographs, CT, or both. The radiographic contrast material may be either air or an iodine-containing water-soluble compound used either singly or in combination (Figs. 7-2 and 7-3). MR arthrography is preferred in some centers but

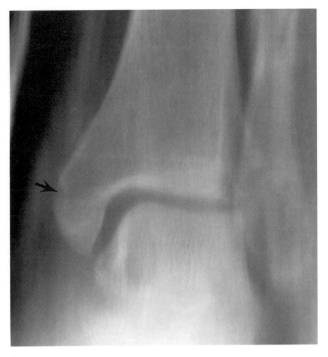

A

FIG. 7-1 (*A*) Anteroposterior (AP) tomogram of left ankle after trauma showing a nondisplaced fracture (*arrow*) of the medial malleolus not seen on the routine plain-film examination. (*B*) Lateral view of the traumatized ankle showing a fracture through the posterior aspect (posterior malleolus) of the distal tibia (*arrow*). The tomogram was obtained to assess the offset between the articular surfaces of the fragments of the fracture.

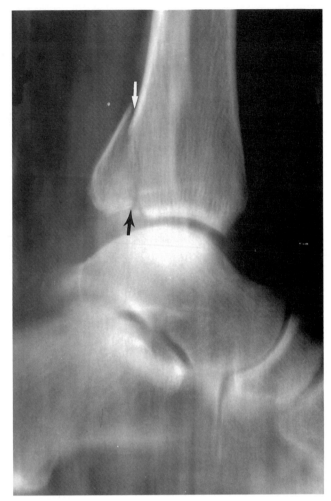

B

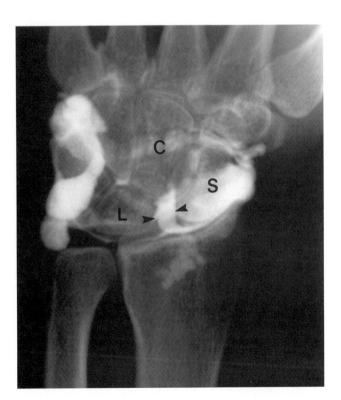

has not yet gained wide acceptance. Arthrography may be useful when MR imaging is contraindicated or when the patient has had previous surgery, such as reevaluating the shoulder in a patient who has had prior rotator cuff repair.

Computed Tomography

Computed tomography (CT) also uses ionizing x-rays to generate images. Because older CT units acquired images only in axial planes, joints with axial orientation were not optimally imaged. Newer CT units, such as spiral or helical CT scanners, acquire images in a way that allows easy reconstruction of the data so that the images can be displayed in other planes. The spatial resolution of CT images is sig-

FIG. 7-2 Contrast arthrogram with plain films. AP wrist arthrogram view obtained after injection of contrast material into the radiocarpal joint shows contrast material passing through the scaphoid (*S*)–lunate (*L*) space from the radiocarpal joint into the midcarpal joint (*arrowheads*). This indicates a tear in the scapholunate ligament (*C*, capitate bone).

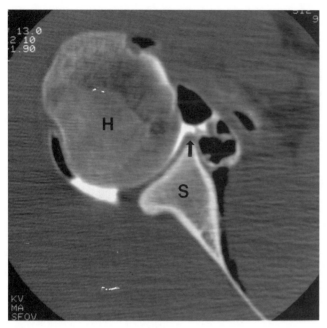

FIG. 7-3 Air-contrast arthrogram with CT. Axial (transverse) CT image of the shoulder of a patient after injection of air and contrast material into the joint. This so-called double-contrast study shows the anterior glenoid labrum surrounded by contrast (*black arrow*). Radiographic contrast material and air can be seen outlining the rest of the joint (*H,* humeral head; *S,* the glenoid process of scapula).

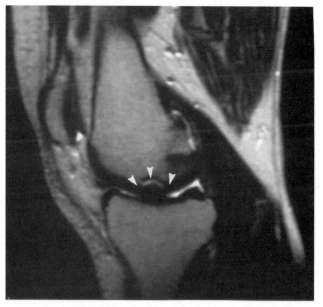

FIG. 7-4 MR imaging of avascular changes in bone. Sagittal MR image of the knee shows an area of bone infarct in the femur just below the cortex (*arrowheads*). This abnormality was not seen on the plain radiograph. MR imaging also can show these changes in the femoral head long before the plain film shows any abnormality.

nificantly better than that of plain films, and the radiation dose is lower than that delivered by plain-film tomography. In most instances, CT is preferable to plain-film tomography for imaging of joints. Exceptions include cases in which overlying or adjacent structures or artifacts will introduce significant and unacceptable image degradation. Because of its excellent spatial resolution, CT depicts the fine details about the constituents of a joint (see Fig. 7-3).

MR Imaging

MR imaging has tremendous advantages over other imaging modalities in the evaluation of joints because of its excellent soft-tissue contrast, high resolution, and ability to image in every plane. MR imaging may show pathophysiologic events even before these alterations are visible on plain x-ray films, such as showing the very early changes of avascular necrosis of bone (Fig. 7-4). When there is a possibility of soft-tissue injury in relation to a joint abnormality, MR imaging should be the next study performed after the plain-film examination. Unfortunately, some patients have contraindications to undergoing MR imaging. The most common exclusions are patients with cardiac pacemakers and those with electronic implants and ferromagnetic implants. MR imaging is also an expensive technique that should be used appropriately.

Ultrasonography

Ultrasonography is a technique in which ultrahigh-frequency sound waves are transmitted into joints, and computer processing is then used to generate images. It is a good technique for children, since it does not involve ionizing radiation. Ultrasound equipment is also relatively inexpensive, and the units can be transported to the patient's bedside. Bone absorbs all the sound at the frequencies that are used commonly in ultrasound, and therefore, diagnostic images of bone cannot be produced with this technique. However, nonosseous intraarticular structures, particularly cartilage and ligaments, can be imaged, and this feature makes ultrasonography an excellent test for evaluating some clinical problems such as suspected neonatal hip dysplasia and rotator cuff disease of the shoulder. The major drawbacks of ultrasonography are that it is operator-dependent and requires specialized skill to interpret the images (Fig. 7-5).

Radionuclide Imaging

In this technique, radioactive tracers, most commonly technetium-99 methylene diphosphonate, are injected into the patient, and images are acquired a few hours later by computer equipment that measures radioactivity. The radiotracers accumulate in areas with hyperemia or high metabolic activity such as inflamed joints. Radionuclide studies are not used routinely for investigation of joint abnormalities.

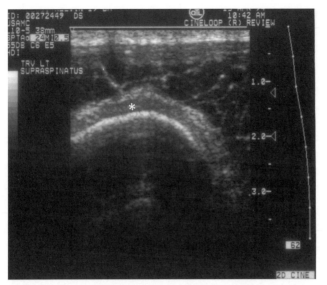

FIG. 7-5 Ultrasonography of the shoulder. An axial (transverse) ultrasonographic image of the shoulder shows an intact supraspinatus tendon (*), seen as a zone of hypoechogenicity (low-signal echoes) on the scan. This technique is very operator dependent.

Normal Anatomy: The Typical Joint

A typical joint is the synovial joint and consists of at least two articulating bones enclosed in a synovium-lined joint capsule. The apposing bony surfaces are covered by smooth articular hyaline cartilage. On plain-film radiographs, every joint has a lucent interval or articular space between the adjacent bones representing the region occupied by the hyaline or articular cartilage, meniscus, and joint fluid, depending on which joint is imaged. These structures are not normally depicted on plain radiographs because of the limited soft-tissue contrast of plain films (Fig. 7-6).

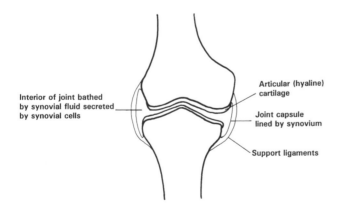

Interior of joint bathed by synovial fluid secreted by synovial cells

Articular (hyaline) cartilage

Joint capsule lined by synovium

Support ligaments

FIG. 7-6 Schematic drawing of normal knee joint. Note the arrangement of the various components.

Signs of Joint Disease

Joint disease is manifested clinically by abnormal function such as reduced mobility, hypermobility, and pain. Altered function may be due to pain, discomfort, apprehension, or instability. The wide range of imaging features of joint disease is summarized below. Most of these processes are shown or discussed in the exercises. Any of these signs may occur singly or in combination with any others.

Radiographically, joint disease is seen as

1. Incongruity of the articulating bone, as is seen with dislocations (e.g., traumatic dislocation or dislocations caused by arthropathy, as in lupus arthritis).
2. Irregularity of articulating bone ends and margins, as in erosions (e.g., in psoriasis or gout).
3. Increased density or sclerosis of articulating bone ends (also described as *eburnation*), as in osteoarthritis.
4. Bony outgrowth at bone ends, known as *osteophytes*.
5. Diffuse reduced density of bone ends, described as juxtaarticular or periarticular osteopenia (e.g., rheumatoid arthritis, tuberculous arthritis).
6. Focal areas of loss of medullary bone substance beneath the articular cortex, known as *subchondral cysts* or *geodes* (e.g., osteoarthritis, rheumatoid arthritis).
7. Loss of joint space because of destruction of articular cartilage (e.g., septic arthritis, osteoarthritis).
8. Joint effusion. Excess joint fluid is a common manifestation of joint disorders. The fluid may be synovial fluid, blood, or even pus, depending on the etiology of the joint disease.
9. Calcification of articular (hyaline) cartilage or fibrocartilage or intraarticular soft-tissue calcification, such as that seen in chondrocalcinosis or scleroderma.
10. Synovial proliferation or abnormal increase in the synovial lining, such as that seen with pigmented villonodular synovitis (PVNS).

TECHNIQUE SELECTION

Plain radiography should always be the initial imaging test to evaluate the joints and should only be obtained after the patient has had a thorough history and physical examination. In obtaining the radiograph of the specified joint, various projections may be used depending on the clinical indication or the situation. Often plain radiographs alone will suffice for confirming a clinical diagnosis or suggesting an entirely different one. Often, however, it may be necessary to obtain more expensive radiographic techniques to clarify the findings on the plain film or to evaluate significant clinical symptoms and signs or laboratory abnormalities if the plain-film results are normal. The following paragraphs discuss selection of imaging techniques in certain clinical situations.

Congenital Diseases

If the clinical question concerns a suspected congenital or pediatric joint abnormality, or if a limp is present in a child, a plain film of the joint should be obtained first. Because the joint structures are not well mineralized in the neonate, further evaluation of the joint with ultrasonography or MR imaging often will be required to make a definitive preoperative diagnosis because they are the best techniques to visualize nonmineralized structures. If MR imaging facilities are not available, the congenital abnormality may be investigated with a combination of plain-film radiography, contrast arthrography, CT with or without intraarticular contrast enhancement, and ultrasonography.

Acute Trauma

In acute trauma, the first line of radiologic investigation is the plain film. If fractures are identified, further imaging will depend on the needs of the clinician or subspecialist physician as dictated by the clinical situation. Generally, fractures that extend into the joint surface (intraarticular fractures) should be treated most aggressively with the aim of reestablishing the integrity of the joint. Intraarticular fractures are often treated with intraoperative reduction and internal fixation if the fracture fragments are severely displaced. CT examination of the involved limb and joints is often also performed preoperatively for surgical planning and then postoperatively to assess the results of surgery. The advantages of CT are that it enables precise assessment of joint reconstitution and also confirms or excludes the presence of any intraarticular fragments that may interfere with proper reduction and healing.

Subacute and Remote Trauma

If the trauma is subacute or remote, the investigation also should begin with the plain film. If the joint is normal and there is a strong clinical suspicion of injury, the patient may benefit from radionuclide bone studies or MR imaging. As already mentioned, MR imaging has the advantage of superior tissue contrast and resolution. It is therefore particularly well suited for investigation of the soft-tissue intraarticular and periarticular structures, such as tendons and ligaments, that maintain the integrity of a joint.

Nontraumatic Cases

After an initial plain-film examination, MR imaging is the modality of choice if the plain film is normal. If the joint is abnormal, it may be cost-effective to aspirate the joint, especially if there is evidence of effusion. The joint aspirate is then analyzed for cell types and chemical composition.

EXERCISE 7-1: CONGENITAL JOINT DISORDERS

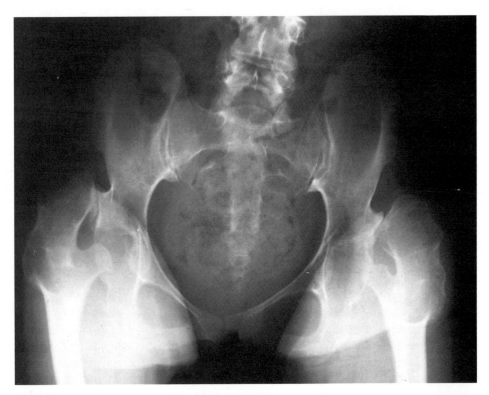

FIG. 7-E-1

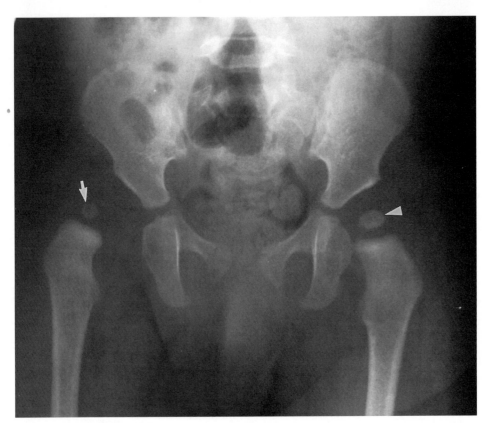

FIG. 7-E-2

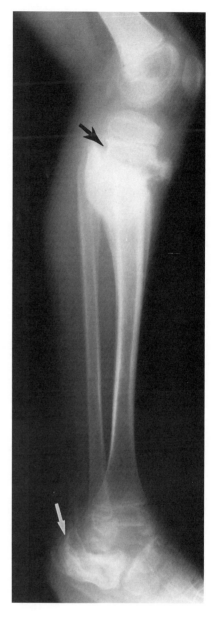

FIG. 7-E-3

Clinical Histories:

CASE 7-1
A 25-year-old woman presents with hip pain that is gradually becoming unbearable. She always walked abnormally and had some discomfort as long as she could remember. Her pelvic radiograph is shown in Fig. 7-E-1.

CASE 7-2
A child is seen who was examined by a pediatrician because of developmental delay. He has not tried to walk and is still crawling at 2 years of age. Several radiographs were ordered. Figure 7-E-2 is a radiograph of the pelvis.

CASE 7-3
A young boy presents who was examined by a pediatrician because "he walks funny," according to his mother. He denies any pain, especially in the ankle. A film of the tibia and fibula is shown in Fig. 7-E-3.

Questions:

7-1. The most likely diagnosis in Fig. 7-E-1 is
- A. bilateral congenital dysplasia of the hips (CDH).
- B. Legg-Calvé-Perthes disease.
- C. proximal focal femoral deficiency syndrome (PFFDS).
- D. neuropathic joint disease.

7-2. In Case 7-2, the next best imaging test would be
- A. plain-film tomography of both hips.
- B. MR imaging of the pelvis.
- C. radionuclide bone scans of the pelvis.
- D. CT of the hips.

7-3. The patient in Case 7-3 has congenital insensitivity to pain (asymbolia), which may accompany neuropathic joint disease. The signs of a neuropathic joint disease include
- A. multiple fractures.
- B. soft-tissue swelling.
- C. joint disorganization.
- D. all of the above.

Radiologic Findings:

7-1. Both hip joints in the patient in this case (Fig. 7-E-1) are abnormal. The femoral heads and necks are malformed and dislocated superiorly from the acetabular fossae, which are also malformed, being more vertically oriented than normal. The patient had congenital dislocation of the hips that had been ignored by her parents (*A* is the correct answer to Question 7-1). The diagnosis should have been made at birth or shortly thereafter to avoid this complication.

7-2. In this case (Fig. 7-E-2), the capital femoral epiphysis on the right (*arrow*) is laterally displaced and smaller than its counterpart on the left (*arrowhead*). The acetabular fossa on the right side is also malformed and more vertical than the one on the left. Normal development of the acetabulum depends on a normally located femoral head, and this is the explanation for this abnormality. These findings are the classic imaging features of CDH.

7-3. In this case (Fig. 7-E-3), the calcaneus is deformed (*white arrow*). The talus is poorly visualized because of its complete dislocation from its normal position below the tibia, and there are subluxations at the tibiotalar, talocalcaneal, and talonavicular joints. There is overall frank disorganization of this ankle joint, and clinically, there was diffuse soft-tissue swelling around the ankle (not appreciated on this lateral film). There is also a metaphyseal fracture of the proximal tibia with exuberant periosteal/callus formation (*black arrow*). All these findings in this patient are caused by congenital insensitivity to pain with chronic respective trauma (*D* is the correct answer to Question 7-3).

Discussion:

Congenital joint disorders are uncommon, but they should be diagnosed as early as possible after birth because delayed diagnosis complicates management. Some of the more common congenital joint disorders include

1. Congenital dislocation of the hips (a bone dysplasia manifesting as a joint disorder)
2. Arthrogryposis multiplex or hypermobile joints
3. Congenital insensitivity to pain (asymbolia)

Congenital hip dislocation is actually a bone dysplasia. The femoral head is dysplastic and does not provide adequate stimulation for proper development of the acetabulum. Usually the femoral head is displaced laterally out of an unusually shallow (i.e., more vertically oriented) acetabulum (Fig. 7-E-2). Diagnosis should be made and treatment of CDH should begin at birth or in the perinatal period to avoid complications.

Historically, hip arthrograms have been used to document the location of the femoral head, which at birth is a cartilaginous structure and therefore radiolucent on plain radiographs. Ultrasonography is an excellent test to assist in the diagnosis in the neonatal period because it requires no ionizing radiation. However, interpretation of the ultrasound is variable and depends on the expertise and experience of the imager. MR imaging can show the soft-tissue structures surrounding the hip well, and it is at present the modality of choice in the evaluation of CDH (*B* is the correct answer to Question 7-2). If patients are not treated or are poorly treated, they will eventually develop secondary osteoarthritic changes. However, MR imaging is of no diagnostic value at this stage because the advanced nature of the disease can be ascertained just as well from plain films.

Proximal focal femoral deficiency is a disease of uncertain etiology that is characterized by congenital absence of a segment or all of the proximal third of the femur. The incidence is higher in children born to diabetic mothers, and it is associated with congenital hip dysplasia in a large number of cases. MR imaging is also the imaging modality of choice in evaluating such children.

A neuropathic joint is one that is chronically damaged by trauma from the impairment of sensation. Such joints are characterized by soft-tissue swelling or effusion, fragmentation of the bony structures, and general disorganization of the joint. The most common causes of neuropathic joints in the lower extremities include tabes dorsalis (neurosyphilis) and diabetes mellitus. Asymbolia, or congenital insensitivity to pain, as exhibited in Case 7-3 (Fig. 7-E-3), is a group of uncommon congenital disorders in which there is a variable degree of loss of pain sensation, and this is an unusual cause of neuropathic joint. Patients with asymbolia almost always acquire deformities of the extremities after repeated trauma. This diagnosis should be considered in the young patient with multiple healing fractures and no signs of child abuse syndrome.

EXERCISE 7-2: JOINT TRAUMA

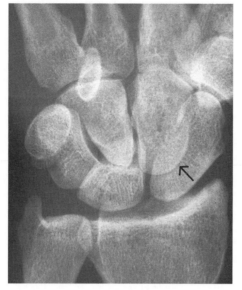

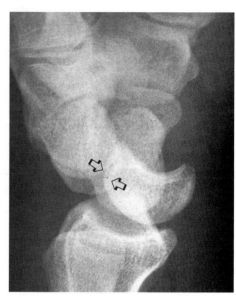

FIG. 7-E-4   (*Panels A and B*)

A

B

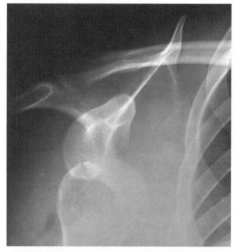

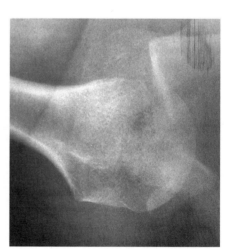

FIG. 7-E-5   (*Panels A, B, and C*)

A

B

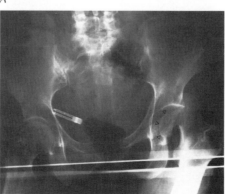

C

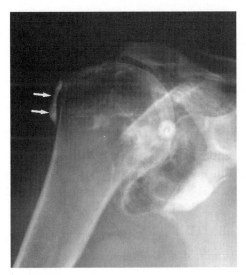

FIG. 7-E-6

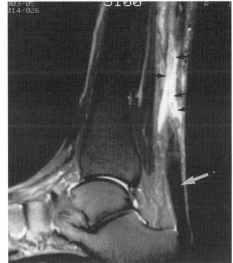

FIG. 7-E-7

Clinical Histories:

CASE 7-4

A 25-year-old man presents who fell on his hands while running. Figure 7-E-4A is an anteroposterior (AP) view of the wrist, and Fig. 7-E-4B is a lateral plain radiograph of the wrist.

CASE 7-5

You are shown plain-film radiographs of an elderly couple, Bill and Lori, who had been drinking and were involved in a head-on collision with another car. You are shown AP (Fig. 7-E-5A) and axillary (Fig. 7-E-5B) radiographs of Bill's shoulder and a pelvic film of his wife, Lori (Fig. 7-E-5C).

CASE 7-6

A 57-year-old man had sudden onset of pain in the right shoulder. He described the pain as somewhat different from the shoulder pain he had just before his recent coronary artery bypass surgery. His plain radiographs were normal, and because of persistent pain, his physician requested MR imaging of his shoulder. The radiologist, after talking to the patient, canceled the MR imaging study and performed shoulder arthrography instead. You are shown a selected film from the arthrogram (Fig. 7-E-6).

CASE 7-7

A 36-year-old man who was already the vice-president of his company agreed to participate in a fund-raiser basketball tournament. He had not engaged in any sporting activity since he left college, so he decided to practice before the tournament. On his first day on the court, as he jumped to block a pass, he felt a "pop" and a sudden snap. There was immediate diffuse ankle swelling, and he had to be helped off the court because of his severe pain. What might you do to best evaluate this problem if you initially saw this man in the emergency department? You are shown one film from the MR imaging study of the ankle (Fig. 7-E-7).

Questions:

7-4. Study the radiographs of Case 7-4 (Fig. 7-E-4A,B), and indicate the most likely diagnosis.

A. Lunate dislocation

B. Perilunate dislocation

C. Transcaphoid fracture-dislocation

D. None of the above

7-5.   In Fig. 7-E-5*A,B,* the most likely diagnosis is
   A.   subglenoid anterior dislocation of the shoulder.
   B.   intertubercular sulcus on the humeral head.
   C.   posterior dislocation of the humerus.
   D.   none of the above.

7-6.   What is the correct diagnosis of Fig. 7-E-5*C?*
   A.   Fracture of the right iliac wing
   B.   Rupture of the sacrotuberous ligament
   C.   Posterior dislocation of the right hip
   D.   Diastasis of the symphysis pubis
   E.   Fracture or dislocation of the head of the left femur

7-7.   The most likely diagnosis in Fig. 7-E-6 is
   A.   dislocation of the right shoulder.
   B.   tear of the anterior glenoid labrum.
   C.   dislocation of the biceps tendon.
   D.   tear of the rotator cuff of the shoulder.

7-8.   The reason for performing shoulder arthrography instead of an MR imaging study
   in this patient is
   A.   a history of recent repair of the rotator cuff tendon(s).
   B.   recent surgery to vital organs with possible presence of ferromagnetic clips.
   C.   the presence of a cardiac pacemaker.
   D.   a history of repeated shoulder dislocation.

7-9.   The most likely diagnosis in Case 7-7 (Fig. 7-E-7) is
   A.   complete rupture of the Achilles tendon.
   B.   partial tear of the peroneus longus tendon.
   C.   changes of osteochondritis dissecans of the talar dome.
   D.   none of the above.

Radiologic Findings:

7-4. In the frontal projection (Fig. 7-E-4*A*), there is disorganization of the carpal arcs. The capitate is no longer articulating with the lunate and partly overlaps the scaphoid (*arrow*). The scaphoid is elongated on this view but not fractured. On the lateral projection (Fig. 7-E-4*B*), the lunate is still in line with the distal radius, but the capitate has been dislocated dorsally (*open arrows*). Therefore, the patient has a dorsal perilunate dislocation (*B* is the correct answer to Question 7-4).

7-5. In Fig. 7-E-5*A,* the humeral head is displaced inferiorly and medially to the glenoid process. On the axillary view (Fig. 7-E-5*B*), the humeral head is displaced inferiorly and anteriorly to the glenoid. Therefore, the patient has an anterior dislocation of the humeral head (*A* is the correct answer to Question 7-5). The intertubercular sulcus or bicipital groove is not normally seen on the axillary view of the shoulder. In Fig. 7-E-5*C,* the femoral head is displaced superiorly and laterally to the acetabulum. The arrowheads show a semilunar piece of bone (part of the femoral head) still within the acetabulum that was sheared off during the posterior dislocation (*C* is the correct answer to Question 7-6).

7-6. Figure 7-E-6 is an image from a right shoulder arthrogram. Contrast material (*white arrows*) is seen lateral to the humerus and beyond its anatomic neck. This contrast material resides in the subdeltoid bursa, which is normally separated from the joint by the rotator cuff muscles. The patient has a large complete tear of the supraspinatus muscle (rotator cuff tear) that allowed contrast material injected within the joint to spill into the bursa (*D* is the correct answer to Question 7-7). The patient in this case recently had cardiac surgery. A chest radiograph showed metallic clips, a potential contraindication for MR imaging. The radiologist could not determine whether the clips were ferromagnetic; therefore, the patient was scheduled for arthrography instead (*B* is the correct answer to Question 7-8).

  7-7. The patient in this case underwent an MR imaging examination as soon as possible. The MR imaging study (Fig. 7-E-7) is a sagittal T2-weighted MR image of the ankle showing complete disruption of the Achilles tendon with high-signal-intensity hemorrhage and edema (*short arrows*) interposed between the tendon fragments (*A* is the correct answer to Question 7-9). The white arrow points out the distal Achilles tendon.

Discussion:

Dislocation or subluxation. The terms *subluxation* and *dislocation* are often used interchangeably. However, *subluxation* denotes partial and *dislocation* complete loss of congruity between articulating bone ends or surfaces. Disruption or loss of integrity of the restraining ligaments around the joint leads to instability and thus permits dislocation to occur. Traumatic dislocations are often caused by severe hyperflexion or hyperextension forces, often with associated fractures.

CARPAL DISLOCATION

The normal carpal arrangement as seen on the AP view of the wrist (Fig. 7-E-4*C*) shows three smooth, parallel arcs to the proximal and midcarpal rows. The lateral view of the wrist (Fig. 7-E-4*D*) shows that the radius, lunate, and capitate are in an almost straight line. There are two major types of carpal dislocation in the wrist: perilunate and lunate dislocations. In a perilunate dislocation, the lunate maintains its normal articulation with the radius, and the capitate is displaced dorsally. In a lunate dislocation, the lunate is displaced volarly from its normal articulation, and the radius and capitate maintain their normal relationship. Wrist dislocations are usually produced by a fall on the outstretched hand and are more common in young adults. The diagnosis is usually made by plain-film examination, although CT or plain-film tomography may be used after reduction to evaluate the wrist for joint congruity and for the presence of loose bodies (intraarticular fracture fragments).

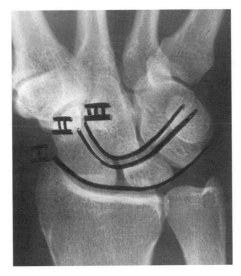

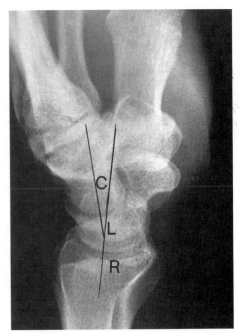

FIG. 7-E-4 (*Panel C*) AP view of the normal wrist showing the three parallel arcs of the radiocarpal joint (I) and the midcarpal joint (II and III). (*From Poehling G et al: Arthroscopy of the Wrist and Elbow. New York, Raven Press, 1994; used with permission.*) (*Panel D*) Lateral view of the normal wrist showing the almost linear arrangement (*straight lines*) of the distal radius (*R*), lunate (*L*), and capitate (*C*).

C   D

SHOULDER DISLOCATION

The two main types of shoulder dislocation are anterior and posterior dislocations. Anterior dislocation, usually caused by falls, is most common and is seen in about 95 percent of cases. In an anterior dislocation, the humeral head is displaced anteriorly and inferiorly to the scapular glenoid fossa. There are three subtypes of anterior dislocations: subglenoid, subcoracoid, and medial. These subtypes are based on the location of the humeral head relative to the glenoid fossa and coracoid process.

Posterior dislocation is relatively uncommon. It is produced by severe contraction of the muscles of the shoulder girdle, which occurs in electric shock or convulsions. A diagnosis of posterior dislocation in one shoulder should prompt investigation of the other shoulder, since the injury is often bilateral.

After an initial dislocation, if the postreduction plain radiographs appear normal, there is no need for another imaging study in the acute setting. However, if there is a recurrence of dislocation, or if the patient remains chronically symptomatic, MR imaging or CT arthrography of the shoulder should be obtained to clarify the causes of these symptoms.

CT arthrography and MR imaging are used to investigate the shoulder for cartilage and soft-tissue injuries resulting from shoulder dislocation. After an anterior dislocation, there is frequently associated injury to the anterior glenoid labrum that is produced by the impacted posterolateral aspect of the humeral head beneath the glenoid process. There also may be an accompanying compression fracture of the humeral head, referred to as the *Hill-Sachs deformity.*

HIP DISLOCATION

The hip is a relatively stable joint because of the surrounding strong muscles and joint capsule, and significant trauma is required for dislocations to occur. The most common dislocating direction of the femur is posterior, and when this occurs, the femoral head often ends up superior to its native acetabulum. In posterior dislocations, there is almost always an associated fracture of the acetabular rim or the femoral head. Anterior hip dislocation is uncommon and is produced by a blow to the hip when the femur is internally rotated and abducted. Central dislocation of the hip usually occurs with direct lateral forces, and there is an associated fracture of the quadrilateral plate (medial aspect) of the acetabulum.

ACHILLES TENDON RUPTURE

The history of the patient in Case 7-7 is classic for Achilles tendon rupture. The injury occurs most frequently in patients in the fourth and fifth decades of life and, although it can affect anyone, is most common in individuals who do not exercise regularly.

The clinical history and physical findings are enough to make a diagnosis of Achilles tendon rupture. Plain-film stress views should not be performed in the setting of a suspected Achilles tendon rupture because the stress may actually make the tear worse. Any question of whether the tear is partial or complete rupture usually should be resolved, since the treatment for each of these is different. Moreover, the clinician needs to know the level of injury and how far the tendon fragments are separated. MR imaging is currently the imaging technique of choice to evaluate the Achilles tendon for abnormalities, since the whole length of the tendon, including its origin on the calcaneus, and any associated injury to it can be shown in great detail. In cases of complete rupture of the tendon, the MR images show separation of the normally low-signal-intensity fibers of the Achilles tendon by high-signal-intensity edema and hemorrhage (Fig. 7-E-7). The frayed ends of each of the separated fragments also may be seen. In partial tears, areas of intermediate or high signal, which represent regions of partial disruption, are seen within the normal low signal intensity, and some of the fibers of the tendon remain intact.

EXERCISE 7-3: JOINT INSTABILITY

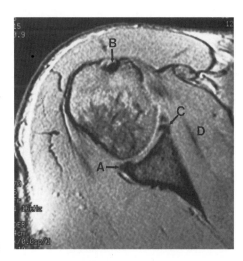

FIG. 7-E-8   *(Panel A)*

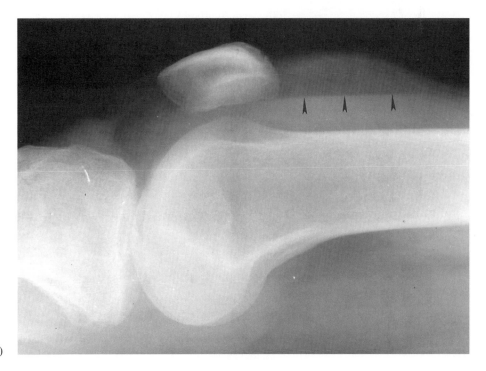

FIG. 7-E-9   *(Panel A)*

Clinical Histories:

CASE 7-8

A 45-year-old former baseball pitcher had recurrent dislocation of the shoulder, pain, and inability to reach around to his back pocket. He also feels a click and catching sensation when he moves his arm. Plain radiographs of his shoulder are normal, and his physician, who prefers not to request MR imaging, requests arthrography with CT to follow (CT arthrogram). The radiologist, after talking with the patient and conferring with the physician, performed MR imaging of the shoulder. A selected MR image is shown to assist you in answering the questions (Fig. 7-E-8*A*).

CASE 7-9

A 20-year-old football player was examined in the emergency department after being tackled particularly hard. A plain radiograph was obtained first (Fig. 7-E-9*A*).

Questions:

7-10. The most likely diagnosis in Fig. 7-E-8*A* is
A.   dislocation of the shoulder.
B.   myositis ossificans.
C.   tear of the anterior glenoid labrum.
D.   none of the above.

7-11. In Fig. 7-E-8*A*, the structure labeled as *B* is the
A.   subscapularis muscle.
B.   tendon of the long head of the biceps tendon.
C.   supraspinatus muscle.
D.   glenoid labrum.

7-12. Regarding Fig. 7-E-9*A*, the arrowheads indicate
A.   fracture of the patella.
B.   lipohemarthrosis.
C.   tear of the anterior cruciate ligament.
D.   all of the above.
E.   none of the above.

7-13. The football player had an MR imaging study to further characterize the plain-film finding. Selected images from this study are shown (Figs. 7-E-9*B,C*). Match the label with the structures listed below.

Label

A _____	(1) Medial collateral ligament
B _____	(2) Posterior cruciate ligament
C _____	(3) Quadriceps tendon
D _____	(4) Iliotibial band
E _____	(5) Medial meniscus

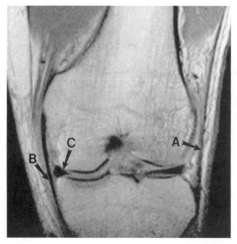 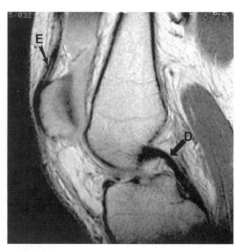

FIG. 7-E-9   (*Panels B and C*)

B   *C*

Radiologic Findings:

7-8. Figure 7-E-8*A* is an axial image from an MR imaging study of the right shoulder showing a tear of the anterior glenoid labrum. Note the high-signal-intensity (white) line running through the triangular anterior glenoid labrum (*arrow* from *C*) (*C* is the correct answer to Question 7-10). In Fig. 7-E-8*A*, *A* is the posterior labrum, *B* is the biceps tendon, *C* is the anterior labrum, and *D* is the subscapularis tendon (*B* is the correct answer to Question 7-11).

7-9. Figure 7-E-9*A* is a lateral plain radiograph of the knee obtained with a horizontal x-ray beam. A large joint effusion with a fat-fluid level (*arrowheads*) can be seen. The presence of a fat-fluid level in the knee in this setting indicates a lipohemarthrosis, and frequently there is a fracture to account for the presence of free fat (from the bone marrow) in the joint (*B* is the correct answer to Question 7-12). Fat-fluid levels also may be seen in patients who have an acute tear of the anterior cruciate ligament.

Discussion:

INSTABILITY DISORDERS

These are functional disorders generally manifested by pain, feeling of insecurity around the joint, or a sensation of the joint giving way and abnormal motion around the joint. There may be no plain-film evidence of joint abnormality, since often only soft-tissue injuries, such as ligamentous or fibrocartilaginous tears, are present. The abnormality may be demonstrated only by stress, plain-film, or MR imaging examinations of the joint in question.

SHOULDER INSTABILITY

The glenohumeral joint is an inherently unstable ball-in-socket joint. The major stability of the shoulder joint is provided by the joint capsule, the rotator cuff muscles, and the ligaments and tendons that surround it. The glenoid labrum, a fibrocartilaginous structure, contributes to shoulder joint stability by deepening the socket (glenoid labral complex) for this ball (humeral head).

A number of soft-tissue injuries are associated with the instability syndrome. A tear of the glenoid labrum is a common cause of persistent shoulder pain in this setting. A less common disorder is medial dislocation of the biceps tendon from chronic repetitive or acute trauma. Ruptures of the tendons of the rotator cuff [supraspinatus, subscapularis, infraspinatus, and teres minor (SITS) muscles] are other common causes of shoulder joint dysfunction and instability. Of these, the supraspinatus is the most commonly torn tendon in the shoulder. Tears most frequently occur about 1 cm proximal to the tendon's insertion on the greater tuberosity of the humerus (Fig. 7-E-8*B*).

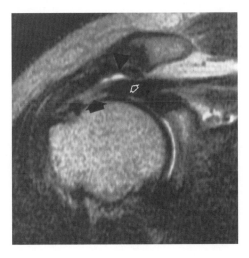

FIG. 7-E-8 (*Panel B*) Coronal T2-weighted MR scan showing a complete tear of the supraspinatus tendon (*black arrow*). The arrowhead represents fluid in the subacromial bursa, and the white open arrow is the retracted supraspinatus tendon.

The shoulder joint is best evaluated with MR imaging if there is a suspicion of tendon or ligamentous abnormality. Shoulder arthrography and CT arthrography, as originally requested by the orthopedic surgeon, are also used as alternative investigational tools in the patient who has undergone repair of the rotator cuff, in the patient who has had recent surgery to vital structures with residual ferromagnetic metallic clips, and in the patient who has aneurysm clips or metallic substances in the eye.

KNEE JOINT INSTABILITY

Stability of the knee joint, which is a hinge joint, is provided partly by the muscles and the ligamentous complexes, including the anterior cruciate ligaments, the posterior cruciate ligament, the lateral collateral ligament complex, and the medial collateral ligament. The muscles that cross the joint include the quadriceps tendon and patella ligament anteriorly, the biceps femoris tendon and tensor fasciae latae and popliteus muscles laterally, the pes anserinus tendons (sartorius, gracilis, and semitendinosus muscles) medially, and the gastrocnemius and plantaris muscles posteriorly. All these structures can be exquisitely demonstrated with MR imaging, which is the best imaging test to evaluate instability in this joint. In Fig. 7-E-9*B,C, A* is the iliotibial band, which is a continuation of the tensor fasciae latae muscle, *B* is the medial collateral ligament, *C* is the medial meniscus, *D* is the posterior cruciate ligament, and *E* is the quadriceps tendon.

Rupture of any of the tendons, ligaments, or muscles compromises stability of the knee joint. Commonly injured structures that are easily evaluated by MR imaging are the anterior cruciate ligament, the medial collateral ligament, and the medial meniscus (Fig. 7-E-9*D*).

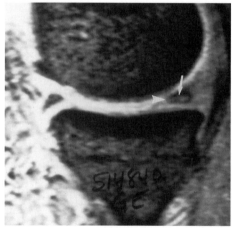

FIG. 7-E-9 (*Panel D*) Sagittal T2-weighted MR image of the knee showing an oblique tear in the posterior horn of the medial meniscus, a common location for meniscal tears (*arrow*). The tear is seen as linear high signal intensity (a *white line* in this image) that extends to the articular surface (*arrowhead*).

EXERCISE 7-4: ARTHRITIDES

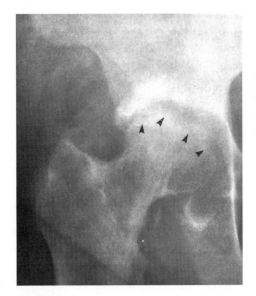

FIG. 7-E-10

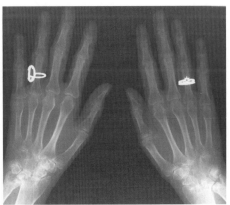

FIG. 7-E-11   (*Panel A*)

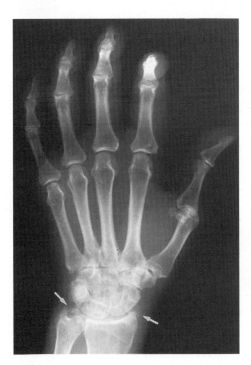

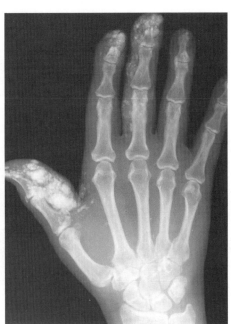

A   *B*

FIG. 7-E-12   (*Panel A*) A 45-year-old man with chronic joint pain. (*Panel B*) A 42-year-old woman complaining of skin dryness and tightness. (*Panel C*) A 33-year-old man with eye and genitourinary complaints. (*Panel D*) A 55-year-old man who was known to "take a few drinks" and who had an elevated serum abnormality. (*Panel E*) A 36-year-old man with low back pain, a "skin rash," limitation of spinal motion, and thickening of his nail beds. (*Panel F*) A 51-year-old man with knee pain laterally. (*Panel G*) Plain radiograph of the right hand in a patient with inflammatory osteoarthritis. There are erosions at the articular surfaces of the bones at the second and third distal interphalangeal joints of the fingers (*white arrows*). There is loss of joint space at the third and fourth proximal interphalangeal joints. Observe the erosions at the first and second carpometacarpal joints (*black arrows*).

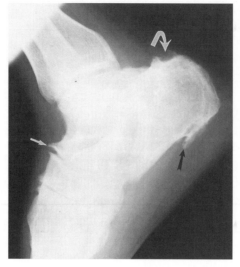

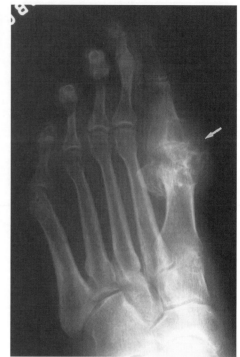

FIG. 7-E-12   (*Continued*)

C

D

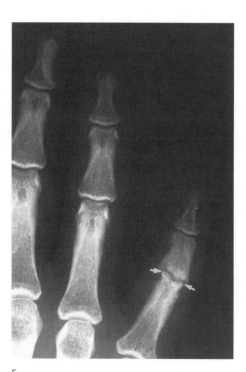

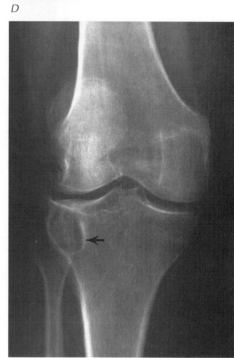

E

F

Clinical Histories:

CASE 7-10

A 59-year-old black woman was examined in the emergency department after a 2-day history of right hip pain. She gave a history of a fall 8 days ago. On examination, she was exquisitely painful and had limited range of motion. She is a long-standing hemodialysis patient. Figure 7-E-10 shows her right hip.

CASE 7-11

A 45-year-old woman with generalized body pain and joint aches of 4 to 6 months' duration presented to a rheumatologist. There were no areas of point tenderness. The patient's erythrocyte sedimentation rate (ESR) was elevated at 70 mm. Figure 7-E-11A shows both hands.

CASE 7-12

Six representative images (Fig. 7-E-12A–F) are shown from different patients who have various types of arthritis. Identify the disease process, and complete Question 7-16.

Questions:

7-14. The radiograph of the right hip in Case 7-10 (Fig. 7-E-10) shows all the following features except
  A. bony erosions.
  B. geode formation.
  C. loss of joint space.
  D. mixture of osteopenia and osteosclerosis.

7-15. Your observations concerning the wrist in case 7-11 include all the following except
  A. diffuse osteopenia in her hands.
  B. symmetrical loss of radiocarpal joint space.
  C. erosions at the metacarpal heads.
  D. periostitis (periosteal new bone formation).

7-16. Regarding the radiographs in Case 7-12, match the image with the correct diagnosis.

Diagnosis	Imaging
(1) Scleroderma	Figure 7-E-12A _____
(2) Osteoarthritis	Figure 7-E-12B _____
(3) CPPD	Figure 7-E-12C _____
(4) Psoriasis	Figure 7-E-12D _____
(5) Gout	Figure 7-E-12E _____
(6) Reiter's disease	Figure 7-E-12F _____

Radiologic Findings:

7-10. The radiograph of the right hip in this case (Fig. 7-E-10) shows irregularity of the femoral head (*arrowheads*) and acetabulum and narrowing of the hip joint. There is also minimal osteopenia and osteosclerosis. No subchondral cysts (geodes) or osteophytes are demonstrated. The findings are classic for septic arthritis of the hip (*B* is the correct answer to Question 7-14).

7-11. Plain-film examination of both hands of the woman in this case (Fig. 7-E-11A) shows moderate osteopenia with loss of radiocarpal joint spaces and radiocarpal erosions best seen in the lunate, both radii, and both ulnas. Erosions are also present in the right third, fourth, and fifth metacarpal heads and in the left second metacarpal head. Minimal erosive changes are present in the left third and fourth proximal interphalangeal joints. These changes show bilateral symmetry, and no periostitis is seen. The characteristics of these changes are typical of rheumatoid arthritis (*D* is the correct answer to Question 7-15).

7-12. Figure 7-E-12A is a radiograph of the hand demonstrating intraarticular calcification in the radiocarpal joint (*arrows*). There are degenerative cysts in the bones of the wrist and at the second and fifth metacarpophalangeal joints. The findings are consistent with calcification in the triangular fibrocartilage in a patient with CPPD (3 is the correct match for Fig. 7-E-12*A* in Question 7-16).

Figure 7-E-12*B* shows a radiograph of the right hand. There are multiple areas of amorphous soft-tissue calcification in all the fingers. Careful examination shows resorption of the tufts of the terminal phalanges of the second and third fingers. There are no erosions, and the bone density is normal. The patient suffers from scleroderma (progressive systemic sclerosis) (1 is the correct match for Fig. 7-E-12*B* in Question 7-16).

Figure 7-E-12*C* shows a lateral radiograph of the hindfoot. The predominant finding is exuberant proliferative changes at the inferior aspect of the calcaneus (*black arrow*) and at the talonavicular and navicular-cuneiform joint (*white arrow*). An erosion is also present at the superior aspect of the calcaneus where the Achilles tendon inserts (*curved arrow*). This patient has typical plain-film findings of Reiter's disease (6 is the correct match for Fig. 7-E-12*C* in Question 7-16). The patient's complaints were urethritis and uveitis.

Figure 7-E-12*D* shows a plain radiograph of the forefoot of a patient with an elevated uric acid level. It depicts soft-tissue swelling over the first metatarsophalangeal joint and joint space narrowing with bony proliferation at the first metatarsophalangeal joint (*arrow*) and the first cuneiform-metatarsal joint. There are cysts in the head of the first metatarsal. The findings are classic for gout, and in this location it is called *podagra* (5 is the correct match for Fig. 7-E-12*D* in Question 7-16).

Figure 7-E-12*E* shows a coned-down view of the third, fourth, and fifth fingers. There is narrowing of the proximal interphalangeal joint of the fifth finger (*white arrows*). There is diffuse erosion of the articular bone ends with minimal telescoping of the proximal phalanx into the base of the middle phalanx. Subtle cortical thickening (due to periostitis) is present. Observe the diffuse cortical thickening (sclerosis at the medial aspect of the terminal phalanx of the middle finger). These findings are common in the arthropathy associated with the seronegative spondyloarthropathies. In this patient, it is psoriasis (4 is the correct match for Fig. 7-E-12*E* in Question 7-16).

Figure 7-E-12*F* shows a plain radiograph of the right knee demonstrating a large subchondral cyst (or geode) in the lateral tibial condyle (*arrow*) with large marginal osteophytes on the lateral aspects of the femur and tibia. These findings of articular space narrowing, subchondral sclerosis, osteophyte formations, and subchondral cysts are typical of osteoarthritis (2 is the correct match for Fig. 7-E-12*F* in Question 7-16).

Discussion:

SEPTIC ARTHRITIS

Septic arthritis is usually blood-borne (hematogenous) and tends to be monarticular (involving only one joint at any time). A common cause of septic arthritis in the adult is *Staphylococcus aureus,* although other infective agents including *Streptococcus, Gonococcus,* and gram-negative organisms are also encountered. *Streptococcus* and gram-negative organisms are particularly important in the pediatric age group.

In this setting, the plain-film examination of the patient in Case 7-10 provides general anatomic information and helps to determine whether further imaging is necessary and what type of further intervention may be appropriate. Her physicians were very worried about septic arthritis in this clinical setting of previous renal transplant, and a hip aspiration was requested. Twenty milliliters of blood-stained turbid fluid was aspirated and was sent to the microbiology laboratory for Gram's stain, culture, and sensitivity studies. The cultures grew *S. aureus,* a common pathogen in septic arthritis.

Septic arthritis is a serious condition and is treated aggressively. The joint should be drained surgically, and the patient should be treated with systemic antibiotics.

Osteoarthritis (OA) is a degenerative disorder of synovial joints most commonly caused by aging. The radiographic findings of OA in the hip can be summarized as loss of articular joint space, osteophyte formation, sclerosis (or eburnation) of contiguous bone ends, and subchondral cyst formation (or geodes). Not all these features are necessary to make the diagnosis of OA, since they represent a continuum. Note that osteopenia

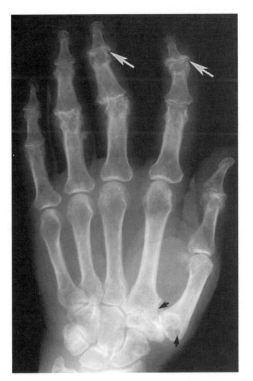

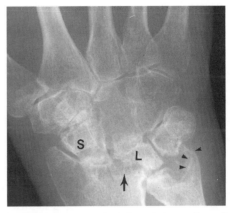

FIG. 7-E-11 (*Panel B*) Coned down view of the wrist in the same patient. Observe the narrowing of the ulna styloid as a result of erosions (*arrowheads*). Also observe erosions in the distal radius (*arrow*). There is marked deformity of the proximal carpal row of bones, especially the lunate (*L*) and the scaphoid (*S*). This patient has advanced changes in her wrist.

G

FIG. 7-E-12 (*Continued*)

and bony erosions are not usual features of OA. Patients with a variant of OA known as *erosive* or *inflammatory osteoarthritis* may have episodic painful bouts of the disease in the hands and may show erosions at the distal interphalangeal joints that may mimic psoriatic arthritis or even rheumatoid arthritis. Another prominent feature of OA is degenerative change at the trapezio–first metacarpal joint (*black arrows* in Fig. 7-E-12*G*).

CONNECTIVE-TISSUE DISEASES

Generally, a history of polyarticular stiffness suggests polyarthritis, and the first line of radiographic investigation is a plain-film survey of the affected joint or joints. This survey is intended to check the most common regions of involvement and usually includes films of the hands, wrists, pelvis, knee, feet, and ankles. The findings on these films, coupled with ESR values, should indicate whether a connective-tissue disorder is the cause of the arthropathy.

Rheumatoid arthritis (RA) is one of the more common connective-tissue diseases. It affects females more often than males, and its exact cause is uncertain. It is thought to be due to a malfunction of the immune system with production of the so-called rheumatoid factor, and the ESR is usually greatly elevated. The peripheral joints are often involved by the disease process in a symmetrical fashion. The pathologic process in RA is primarily a synovitis, with synovial proliferation manifested on the radiograph as periarticular soft-tissue swelling. In the early stages of the disease, there is osteopenia followed by loss of articular cartilage (seen as joint space loss or narrowing) and erosions. Subsequently, the disease may progress to secondary degenerative changes and eventually to ankylosis of the joint (usually fibrous). In the wrist, the carpal bones will show osteopenia carpal crowding or subluxations. In fact, the ulnar styloid is often one of the first sites of erosions and "penciling" (Fig. 7-E-11*B*). Juxtaarticular osteopenia is seen in the bones of the hands and wrists. Symmetrical swelling at the proximal interphalangeal joints of the hand is present, and bone ends show erosions, especially at the metacarpophalangeal and proximal interphalangeal joints.

Systemic lupus erythematosus (SLE) is a connective-tissue disorder that can be seen in conjunction with other connective-tissue diseases (the so-called overlap syndrome). SLE is associated with profound osteopenia, including resorption of the tufts. It also may produce joint instability with multiple subluxations at the wrists and metacarpophalangeal joints. In fact, SLE is the most common cause of a nonerosive subluxing arthropathy. Subluxations also occur in RA, but the subluxations in RA do not occur without erosions.

Scleroderma (progressive systemic sclerosis, or PSS) is a disorder characterized by fibrosis and skin thickening, resulting in calcification of the connective tissue. The major effects of this disease are not on the joints per se but are secondary to the diffuse sclerosis with resultant joint stiffness for which the patient may seek treatment initially. About 10 percent of patients with PSS have synovitis that is indistinguishable from RA at diagnosis, and many of these patients eventually develop Raynaud's phenomenon. The typical imaging findings are periarticular calcification and resorption of the terminal phalangeal tufts. Scleroderma also may be discovered along with other connective-tissue disorders such as RA and SLE.

Psoriasis, one of the seronegative spondyloarthropathies (the others are Reiter's disease, ankylosis spondylitis, and inflammatory bowel disease), is another connective-tissue disorder that primarily affects the skin. However, about 15 percent of patients with psoriasis develop bone and joint changes that may be the initial manifestations of the disease. Plain-film findings of psoriasis include periosteal reaction (periostitis), focal cortical thickening in the digits, or both. Initially, these manifest as juxtaarticular osteopenia that is less profound than in RA. There are erosions at the bone ends (marginal erosions), and these erosions are more common in the distal interphalangeal joints, unlike those in patients with RA, which are predominately in the proximal interphalangeal joints. Patients with psoriasis and other seronegative spondyloarthropathies also develop abnormalities of the spine and sacroiliac joints (hence the term *spondyloarthropathy*).

Reiter's disease is a postinfective disorder of the immune system that is characterized by the triad of nongonococcal urethritis, conjunctivitis/iritis, and arthritis. Seen most frequently in male patients, Reiter's disease was originally thought to be caused by *Chlamydia,* but other organisms, including *Escherichia coli* and *Salmonella* organisms, also have been implicated. The range of imaging findings is almost identical to the findings in psoriatic arthritis except that the feet are more commonly involved than the hands. The bones show periostitis, erosions, and gross enthesopathy. An *enthesis* is an area of attachment of a ligament or tendon to bone by the perforating fibers of Sharpey. An *enthesopathy,* therefore, is an abnormality at this site and is seen on the radiograph as bony excrescences in these areas. An example is the bony excrescence on the inferior aspect of the calcaneus in Fig. 7-E-12C (*black arrow*), which is an enthesopathy at the site of attachment of the plantar fascia and the short flexors in the foot.

CRYSTAL DEPOSITION DISEASES

Gout, a disorder more common in middle-aged men, is an inflammatory arthritis caused by abnormal deposition of urates (called *tophi*) in the soft tissues and cartilage, which causes episodic joint inflammation. In the earlier stages of the disease, radiographs of the bone and joints are normal. A classic initial presentation of gout is podagra, an acute inflammation of the first metatarsal-phalangeal joint (Fig. 7-E-12D). The patient has severe joint pain, and the overlying soft tissue is swollen and red. With repeated attacks, bony erosions with overhanging edges (or overhanging margins) develop adjacent to the joint but not within the joint. When the patient is severely incapacitated by pain, osteopenia, the result of disease, can be seen on radiographs. Occasionally, osteopenia may be due to intraosseous deposition of tophaceous material. The typical areas to screen for gout changes include the first metatarsal-phalangeal joint, the heel, the back of the elbow joint, and the hands and wrists. Joint aspiration is probably the best way to confirm the clinical suspicion of gout and will show birefringent uric acid crystals in the synovial fluid.

Calcium pyrophosphate dihydrate crystal deposition (CPPD) disease is the proto-type of the crystal deposition joint disorders. In CPPD disease there is calcification in the fibrocartilage and hyaline articular cartilage (called *chondrocalcinosis*). The most common predisposing factor for chondrocalcinosis is aging. The presence of calcification alone is not diagnostic of CPPD, however. The clinical syndrome of pain from the presence of abnormal cartilage calcification is referred to as the *CPPD syndrome*. Symptoms may be provoked by various stresses (e.g., surgical procedures). Differential diagnosis of chondrocalcinosis includes pseudogout (CPPD disease), gout, ochronosis, and hemochromatosis.

EXERCISE 7-5: MISCELLANEOUS JOINT DISORDERS

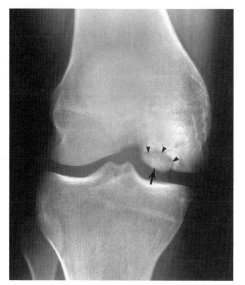

FIG. 7-E-13

FIG. 7-E-14

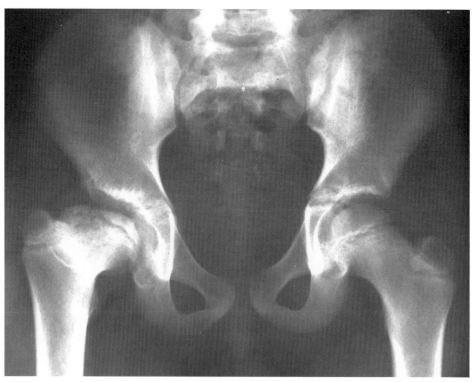

FIG. 7-E-15

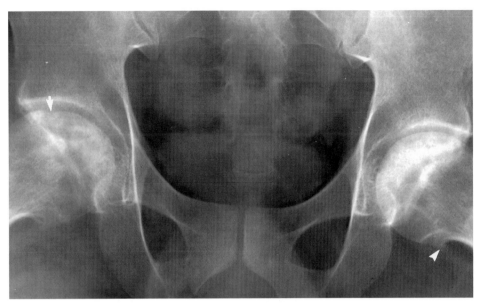

FIG. 7-E-16   *(Panel A)*

Clinical Histories:

CASE 7-13

A 24-year-old male medical student, an avid tennis player, had intermittent joint swelling and minimal knee pain. Lately the pain had worsened and was interfering with his tennis game. Nonsteroidal anti-inflammatory agents were not working well, and an orthopedic resident requested he get a knee x-ray (Fig. 7-E-13). After looking at the radiograph, the resident scheduled an appointment for the student with an attending surgeon.

CASE 7-14

A 20-year-old man presents complaining of a feeling of fullness and gritty sensations in his right shoulder. He has never had a shoulder dislocation, although on several occasions he has been unable to raise the shoulder and has felt a painful "catch" at times. A plain radiograph of his right shoulder was obtained (Fig. 7-E-14).

CASE 7-15

A 10-year-old boy was referred to an orthopedic surgeon for investigation of a limp. There was no reliable history of trauma. A plain radiograph of the pelvis is shown and is abnormal (Fig. 7-E-15).

CASE 7-16

A 35-year-old man with episodic right hip pain that began 4 to 6 months ago presents with a dull aching pain now in both hips. A plain radiograph of both hips was obtained (Fig. 7-E-16*A*).

Questions:

7-17. In the radiograph of the knee for Case 7-13 (Fig. 7-E-13), the most likely diagnosis is

  A. synovial osteochondromatosis.
  B. pigmented villonodular synovitis.
  C. avascular necrosis of the femoral condyle.
  D. osteochondritis dissecans (OCD) of the femoral condyle.

7-18. Concerning Fig. 7-E-14, the most likely diagnosis is
    A. hemochromatosis.
    B. synovial osteochondromatosis.
    C. pigmented villonodular synovitis.
    D. calcified Heberden's nodes.

7-19. The most likely diagnosis of the patient in Fig. 7-E-15 is
    A. chronic changes of transient synovitis of the right hip.
    B. chronic changes of slipped capital femoral epiphysis (epiphysiolysis).
    C. chronic changes of Legge-Calvé-Perthes disease of the right hip.
    D. none of the above.

7-20. Concerning Fig. 7-E-16*A*, the observations include all the following except
    A. osteophytes in both femoral heads.
    B. irregularity and loss of sphericity of the right femoral head.
    C. depression/subchondral fracture of right femoral head.
    D. bilateral acetabular sclerosis.

Radiologic Findings:

7-13. The AP view of the right knee in this case (Fig. 7-E-13) shows only an ovoid bony fragment on the inner aspect of the medial femoral condyle (*arrow*) separated from the native femur by a lucency (*arrowheads*). This appearance is diagnostic of osteochondritis dissecans (OCD) of the knee (*D* is the correct answer to Question 7-17).

7-14. The plain radiograph of the right shoulder in this case (Fig. 7-E-14) shows multiple rounded calcific bodies overlying the proximal humerus and glenoid process of the scapula. The distribution of these is within the joint and axillary recess (*arrows*). The appearance is classic for synovial osteochondromatosis (SOC) (*B* is the correct answer to Question 7-18).

7-15. The radiograph of the pelvis in this case (Fig. 7-E-15) shows collapse of the right capital femoral epiphysis, which is broad and short and forms an acute angle with the shaft of the femur. The femoral head is displaced laterally and is not completely covered by the mildly deformed acetabulum. The left hip is normal. The findings are characteristic of late changes in Legg-Calvé-Perthes disease (*C* is the correct answer to Question 7-19).

7-16. The radiograph of both hips in this case (Fig. 7-E-16*A*) demonstrates that the right femoral head is no longer smooth and spherical (loss of sphericity), and this is due to the presence of subchondral collapse in the superolateral aspect (*arrow*). The left femoral head is still spherical but shows sclerosis. Also note the marginal osteophytes arising from the inferior and medial aspects of the left femoral head (*arrowhead*). The acetabuli are normal (*D* is the correct answer to Question 7-20).

Discussion:

Osteochondritis dissecans (OCD) is a bone disorder that produces joint symptoms because of the intraarticular location of the abnormality. OCD, as classically demonstrated in Fig. 7-E-13, is seen on radiograph as a semicircular focus of bone and overlying cartilage separated from the convex articular surface of the native bone by a lucency. The etiology is uncertain, but current opinion favors repetitive microtrauma and vascular causes as predisposing factors. Most joints are affected, but the knee (distal femur), ankle (dome of the talus), and elbow (capitellum) joints are the more commonly involved sites. The disease is slightly more common in active young men, but it is developing more frequently in young women because they are more actively involved in athletics today. In the knee, OCD typically involves the medial aspect of the lateral femoral condyle. Reformatted images from the CT scan will be necessary to evaluate the lesion properly, and reformatted images do not have the high resolution of the original images. Knee arthrography has the dual disadvantages of being an invasive procedure and using ionizing radiation. Today, MR imaging is the best test to stage the lesion, predict whether the fragment may become separated entirely, and plan definitive treatment. Therefore, MR imaging is currently the investigation of choice for OCD. Historically, plain films, arthrograms, and bone scans have been used to stage the lesion prior to treatment.

Synovial osteochondromatosis (SOC) is a joint abnormality characterized by the presence of cartilaginous and osseous loose bodies within the synovial cavity in the joint. The exact cause is not known, but the primary type is thought to occur secondary to synovial metaplasia, and the secondary type is assumed to be due to fractures of osteophytes or articular cartilage that shed into the joint cavity. A plain radiograph may show only a joint effusion if the fragments are not ossified but will show multiple intraarticular bodies if they have been ossified (Fig. 7-E-14, *arrows*). MR imaging is an excellent preoperative test to show both ossified and nonossified intraarticular fragments and to evaluate the other soft-tissue structures around the joint.

Pigmented villonodular synovitis (PVNS) is a condition of unknown etiology characterized by hyperplasia or excessive villous proliferation of the synovium. The condition may occur in localized or diffuse patterns and is characterized by repeated hemorrhage within the joint. The hemosiderin-laden macrophages give the synovium a pigmented appearance best appreciated on gross examination. On plain films there is often a joint effusion with preservation of the joint space and bone mineral density. The later stages of the disease produce erosions on both sides of the joint. Joint aspiration yields dark brown (chocolate-colored) fluid caused by the hemosiderin-laden macrophages. MR imaging is an excellent preoperative test to evaluate PVNS because the pigmented material (hemosiderin) shows low signal intensity on both the T1-weighted and T2-weighted MR images, and this is a very specific appearance of the disease.

Osteonecrosis can occur in any bone and is associated with a variety of disorders, including sickle cell hemoglobinopathy, Gaucher's disease, SLE, pancreatitis, alcoholism, steroid treatment, and barotrauma. When the process occurs at a bone end, it is known as *avascular necrosis;* when it occurs in the diaphysis of the bone, it is commonly referred to as a *bone infarct.* Eponyms have been used to designate osteonecrosis in a particular site. For example, *Perthes' disease* (*Legg-Calvé-Perthes disease*) is idiopathic osteonecrosis of the femoral head occurring in a child, as shown in Case 7-15 (Fig. 7-E-15); *Freiberg's infraction* involves the head of the second or third metatarsal; *Köhler's disease* involves the tarsal navicular; *Panner's disease* involves the capitellum of the humerus; whereas *Kienböck's disease* involves the lunate.

The exact mechanism of the development of osteonecrosis is unknown, although bone marrow edema after thrombosis and occlusion of the osseous capillaries and end arterioles are believed to be primarily responsible.

Plain films are rather insensitive diagnostic tools for evaluating the early manifestations of osteonecrosis. On plain films, osteonecrosis causes zones of increased and decreased density in the affected bone (Fig. 7-E-16A). If the disease is not diagnosed and treated early, the affected bone may go through a phase of subchondral collapse and become deformed. Subsequently, secondary osteoarthrosis will develop in the affected joint as a complication of neglected or poorly treated disease. Traditionally, nuclear medicine bone scanning has been used in this setting, but today MR imaging is the most sensitive available modality for the early diagnosis of this disease. A coronal T1-weighted image of the pelvis of a patient with osteonecrosis of both hips is shown in Fig. 7-E-16B. Note the focal areas of abnormally low signal intensity in both femoral heads superiorly (*arrowheads*). The low signal (dark) areas are separated from the normal bone by linear high signal (bright). The MR imaging features are classic of bilateral avascular necrosis of the femoral heads.

Hemochromatosis is a rare disorder of iron metabolism in which iron is deposited in the skin, parenchymal organs, and articular cartilage leading to degenerative disease of the joint. In the joint there is loss of joint space and formation of peculiar hooked osteophytes, especially at the metacarpal heads. Heberden's nodes are a disfigurement of the interphalangeal joints as a result of severe osteoarthritis. Initially, they are due to soft-tis-

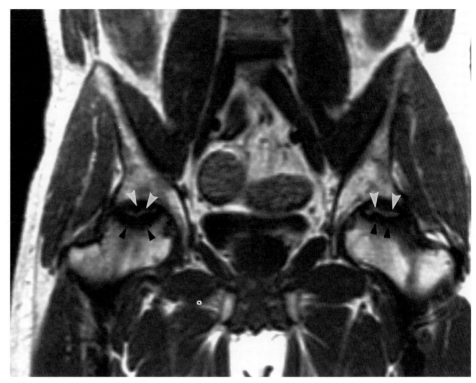

FIG. 7-E-16   (*Panel B*) Coronal T1-weighted image of the pelvis in a patient who takes steroids and has bilateral hip pain.

sue inflammatory changes and subsequently are due to bony changes at the distal interphalangeal joints. Heberden's nodes are seen more commonly in female patients.

BIBLIOGRAPHY

Bassett LW et al: *Musculoskeletal Disease: Test and Syllabus.* Reston, Va, American College of Radiology, 1994.

Brower AC: *Arthritis in Black and White.* Philadelphia, Saunders, 1988.

Forrester DM, Brown JC: *The Radiology of Joint Disease.* Philadelphia, Saunders, 1987.

Renton P: *Orthopaedic Radiology.* London, Martin Dunitz, 1990.

Weissman BNW, Sledge CB: *Orthopedic Radiology.* Philadelphia, Saunders, 1986.

PART IV

ABDOMEN

8

PLAIN FILM
OF THE ABDOMEN

Michael Y. M. Chen

In recent years, new techniques such as ultrasonography and computed tomography (CT) have been used widely and have altered the use of plain films of the abdomen in the evaluation of abdominal diseases. Plain films of the abdomen are still used primarily to assess calcifications and intestinal perforation or obstruction. They may be used as a preliminary study for other procedures, such as CT, barium enema, and oral cholecystography. In addition, plain abdominal radiography is employed routinely before intravenous urography because some faint stones in the urinary tract can be obscured by iodinated contrast material but may be shown on plain abdominal radiographs. The yield of plain film is higher in patients with moderate or severe abdominal symptoms and signs than in those with minor symptoms.

TECHNIQUE AND NORMAL IMAGING

Technique

The most common plain film of the abdomen is an anteroposterior (AP) view with the patient in the supine position. The AP view of the abdomen is also called by the acronym *KUB film* because it includes the kidneys, ureters, and bladder. When acute abdominal disease is suspected clinically, an erect film of the abdomen and a posteroanterior (PA) view of the chest are also required.

Normal Imaging

SOFT TISSUE
The abdomen is composed primarily of soft tissue. The density of soft tissue is similar to the density of water, and the difference in density between solid and liquid is not distinguishable on plain film. The liver is a homogeneous structure located in the right upper quadrant; the hepatic angle delineates the lower margin of the posterior position of the liver (Fig. 8-1). In the left upper quadrant a similar angular structure, the splenic angle, can be identified by the fat shadow around the spleen (see Fig. 8-1).

Organ enlargement can be recognized by the effect of displacement on nearby bowel loops or by obliteration of the adjacent normal fat or gas pattern. Hepatomegaly may compress the proximal transverse colon below the right kidney. Splenomegaly may push the splenic flexure of the colon downward. A large fused renal shadow across the psoas muscle and lumbar spine suggests a horseshoe kidney.

FAT SHADOW
Fat density, which is between that of soft tissue and that of gas, outlines the contour of solid organs or muscles. In obese patients, fat may not be distinguishable from ascitic fluid on plain abdominal film. The flank stripe, also called the *properitoneal fat stripe,* is a line of fat next to the muscle of the lateral abdominal wall (see Fig. 8-1). The flank

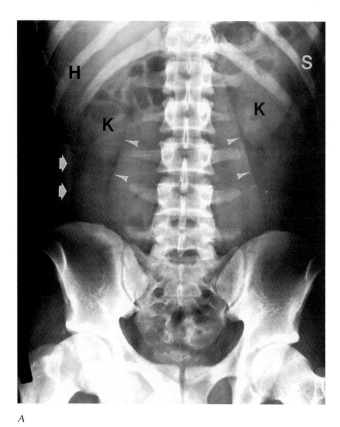

A

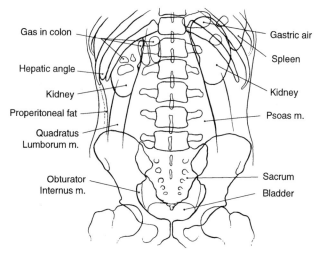

B

FIG. 8-1 (*A*) Normal plain film of the abdomen. The lower margins of the posterior portion of the liver, the hepatic angle (H), and the lower part of the spleen (S) are delineated by a fat shadow. Both kidneys (K) and the psoas muscle shadows (*arrowheads*) are outlined by a fat shadow. The properitoneal fat stripe is also shown bilaterally (*arrows*). (*B*) Diagram of normal abdominal plain film.

stripes are symmetrically concave or slightly convex in obese people, located along the side of the abdominal wall. The normal properitoneal fat stripe is in close proximity to the gas pattern in the ascending or descending colon.

Widening of the distance between the properitoneal fat stripe and the ascending or descending colon suggests fluid, such as abscess, ascitic fluid, or blood within the paracolic gutter.

Fat is present in the retroperitoneal space adjacent to the psoas muscle (see Fig. 8-1). The psoas muscle shadow may be absent unilaterally or bilaterally as a normal variant or as a result of inflammation, hemorrhage, or neoplasms of the retroperitoneum. Unilateral convexity of the psoas muscle contour suggests an intramuscular mass or abscess. The quadratus lumborum muscles may be delineated by fat located lateral to the psoas shadow (see Fig. 8-1). In the pelvis, the fatty envelope of the obturator internus muscle is seen on the inner aspect of the pelvic inlet (see Fig. 8-1). The dome of the urinary bladder may be delineated by fat.

GAS PATTERN

Gas has the lowest density (radiolucency) in the abdomen. It is seen in the stomach and colon, but it is rarely seen in the normal small bowel because the air rapidly traverses the organ. Presence of more than a minimal amount of gas in the small bowel should be considered abnormal and is indicative of a functional ileus or mechanical obstruction. Identification of the differences between the gas shadows of the jejunum, ileum, or colon helps to assess the location of bowel obstruction (Fig. 8-2). A gas pattern in distended intestinal loops is usually limited above the point of mechanical obstruction, but functional ileus has a more diffuse distribution in both the small intestine and the colon. If the gas shadow in the intestine is displaced to an unusual location, a soft-tissue mass, either inflammatory or neoplastic, may be suspected. The presence of air-fluid levels in a distended small intestine on upright films suggests either functional ileus or mechanical obstruction. Fluid levels within the stomach or colon are ordinarily of no pathologic importance, because fluid may be introduced by oral agents or by cleansing enemas. The presence of solid material with a mottled appearance and small bubbles of gas surrounded by the colonic contour suggests feces in the colon.

A large amount of gas seen in the peritoneal cavity indicates postoperative status or bowel perforation. Air bubbles in the peritoneal cavity mean that there is a perforated viscus, abscess, or necrotic tumor. In the right upper quadrant, air that is seen in the biliary tree or around the gallbladder suggests cholecystoenteric fistula or emphysematous cholecystitis. A finely arborizing gas pattern over the right upper quadrant that extends peripherally to the edge of the liver is characteristic of hepatic portal vein gas. In the bowel wall, multiple air bubbles may indicate pneumatosis cystoides intestinalis. Extraluminal gas also may appear within the retroperitoneal structures, including the lesser omental bursa, a subhepatic site, the paraduodenal fossae, and the pericecal or periappendiceal areas. A gas pattern seen below the bony pelvis indicates an inguinal or femoral hernia.

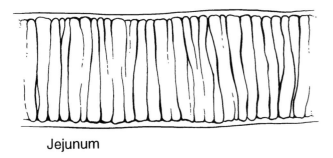

Jejunum

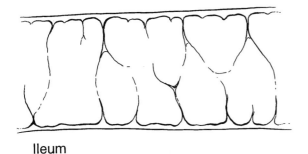

Ileum

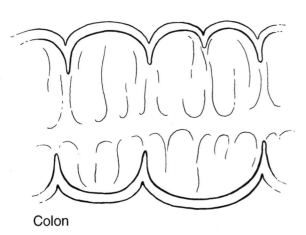

Colon

FIG. 8-2 Schematic illustration of portions of bowel. The jejunum shows numerous mucosal folds, and the ileum has fewer folds. Both serosa of the jejunum and the ileum are smooth. The colon has serosa indented by haustra, and mucosal folds do not cross the lumen.

BONY STRUCTURE OR CALCIFICATION

Bony structures or calcifications have the highest density (radiopacity) that is seen on the plain film. Bony structures comprise the ribs superiorly, the lumbar spine, and the pelvis. Calcifications in the abdomen include calcified arteries, calculi in the urinary or biliary tract, prostatic cal-

culi, pancreatic calcifications (which are usually indicative of chronic pancreatitis, with or without carcinoma), appendicolith, or ectopic gallstone in the small bowel associated with mechanical obstruction from gallstone ileus. Some foreign bodies, including ingested foreign bodies, bullets, or surgical clips, may be seen in the abdomen. Other rare structures, such as parasitic, metastatic, or heterotopic bone formations, also may be seen in the abdomen.

Suspicion of urinary calculi or gallstones is a common indication for abdominal radiography. About 15 percent of gallstones are radiopaque and are seen on abdominal plain film. Ultrasound or oral cholecystography will demonstrate radiolucent gallstones. On the other hand, 85 to 90 percent of calculi in the urinary tract are opaque and can be detected on plain abdominal films; the remaining 10 to 15 percent are radiolucent and are not seen on plain film.

TECHNIQUE SELECTION

The routine abdominal films consist of supine and upright views. If the patient cannot stand for an erect abdominal film and a PA view of the chest, the cross-table lateral projection with the right side elevated may be used to assess pneumoperitoneum and air-fluid levels. As little as 1 to 2 mL of free air in the peritoneal space may be identified if the films are appropriately obtained. The PA view of the chest is usually obtained as part of an acute abdominal series because an abnormality in the chest may have symptoms referred to the abdomen.

Inspiratory and expiratory films are used to assess the mobility of the kidneys. The normal kidney moves approximately 5 cm between inspiration and expiration or in the change from the erect to the supine position. Decreased mobility or fixation of the kidney occurs if it is affected by an adjacent neoplastic or inflammatory process.

Oblique views and conventional tomography of the abdomen are obtained, especially in examination of the urinary tract, where full delineation of the ureters and depiction of the renal collecting system are desirable. Likewise, oblique studies of the urinary bladder are helpful in delineating abnormalities of that organ.

Plain abdominal radiography is less sensitive in evaluating solid organs or metastases. In recent years, increased use of cross-sectional techniques, such as ultrasonography and CT, has shown them to be more sensitive in assessing disorders of the abdominal solid organs and metastatic disease. Acute cholecystitis is better assessed by ultrasound or nuclear medicine studies.

EXERCISE 8-1: UPPER ABDOMINAL CALCIFICATIONS

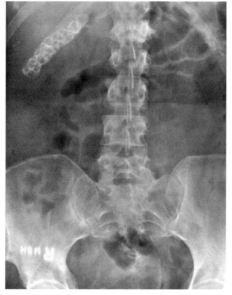

FIG. 8-E-1

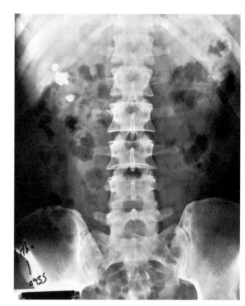

FIG. 8-E-2

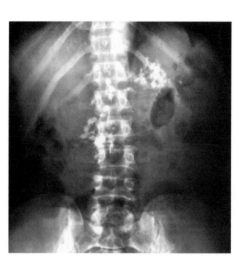

FIG. 8-E-3

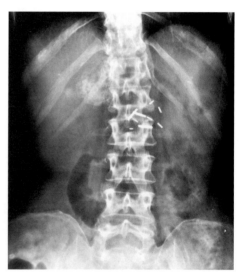

FIG. 8-E-4

Clinical Histories:

CASE 8-1
A 44-year-old woman presents with right upper quadrant pain (Fig. 8-E-1).

CASE 8-2
A 36-year-old woman presents with flank pain (Fig. 8-E-2).

CASE 8-3
A 48-year-old man presents with epigastric pain (Fig. 8-E-3).

CASE 8-4
A 59-year-old woman is seen who underwent colectomy surgery for colon cancer 10 years ago (Fig. 8-E-4).

Questions:

8-1. The most likely diagnosis in Cases 8-1 and 8-2 is
  A. calcified gallstones and acute pancreatitis.
  B. calcified gallstones and chronic pancreatitis.
  C. calcified gallstones and staghorn calculi in the kidney.
  D. kidney stones and adrenal calcification.
  E. kidney stones and calcified gallstone.

8-2. Are the following statements true or false?
  A. About 15 percent of gallstones are radiopaque on plain abdominal film.
  B. Most gallstones are composed of pure cholesterol.
  C. About 85 percent of renal calculi are radiopaque.
  D. Staghorn calculi are uncommonly related to urinary tract infection.
  E. Adrenal calcifications should be triangular in shape.

8-3. The most likely diagnoses in Cases 8-3 and 8-4, respectively, are
  A. primary calcified mucoproducing adenocarcinoma in the colon and adrenal calcification.
  B. adrenal calcification and pancreatic calcification.
  C. pancreatic calcification and gallstone calcification.
  D. pancreatic calcification and calcified hepatic metastases.
  E. pancreatic calcification and adrenal calcification.

8-4. Are the following statements true or false?
  A. Alcoholism is the most common cause of chronic pancreatitis and pancreatic calcification.
  B. Cholelithiasis is a cause of acute pancreatitis.
  C. Cholelithiasis frequently causes calcific pancreatitis.
  D. Hepatic tumor may cause calcification in the liver.
  E. Hepatic calcified granulomas from tuberculosis and histoplasmosis are common.

Radiologic Findings:

8-1. This case demonstrates multiple faceted calcifications in the right upper quadrant which are characteristic for gallstones.

8-2. This case shows three separate deposits of calcific density confined to the right renal shadow. The largest one measures 2 cm in greatest diameter (*C* is the correct answer to Question 8-1).

8-3. This case shows multiple stippled calcifications in the upper abdomen adjacent to the lumbar spine. In a patient with a history of alcoholism, pancreatic calcification from chronic pancreatitis would be the most likely diagnosis.

8-4. This case shows stippled and discrete calcifications overlying the right twelfth rib, just above the renal outline. When calcification in the lung base, skin, retroperitoneum, pancreas, kidney, and adrenal glands is excluded, hepatic calcification should be considered in a patient with a history of colon cancer (*D* is the correct answer to Question 8-3).

Discussion:

About 15 to 20 percent of gallstones are calcified sufficiently to be seen on plain abdominal film (Statement 8-2*A* is true). Most gallstones comprise mixed components, including cholesterol, bile salts, and biliary pigments. Pure cholesterol and pure pigment stones are uncommon (Statement 8-2*B* is false).

Most renal calculi (85 percent) contain calcium salts that are radiographically opaque (Statement 8-2*C* is true). Renal calculi are usually small and lie within the pelvicalyceal system. They may remain and increase in size, or they may pass distally. When calcifications are seen projecting over the renal shadows on routine films of the abdomen, an oblique view or conventional tomography is often needed to localize the densities in relation to the kidneys. A staghorn calculus contains magnesium ammonium phosphate (struvite) and forms in alkaline-infected urine (Statement 8-2D is false).

The adrenal gland is located at the superomedial part of the adjacent kidney. The right gland is lower than the left. Normally, the adrenal gland measures less than 2.5 × 3 cm. Stippled, mottled, discrete, or homogeneous calcifications may appear as a portion of the adrenal gland or may occupy the entire organ, forming a triangular clump in the adrenal glands (Statement 8-2E is false). Most adrenal calcifications are incidental findings in normal-sized glands. They are caused by neonatal adrenal hemorrhage, prolonged hypoxia, severe neonatal infection, or birth trauma. Less than one-fourth of patients with Addison's disease have adrenal calcifications.

In the United States, 85 to 90 percent of patients with pancreatic lithiasis are alcoholics (Statement 8-4A is true). Conversely, less than half of patients with chronic pancreatitis ever develop pancreatic calcifications visible on plain film. Although gallstones passing through the biliary tract can cause acute pancreatitis (Statement 8-4B is true), chronic pancreatitis or pancreatic calcification is rarely caused by cholelithiasis (Statement 8-4C is false).

Primary hepatic tumors, both benign and malignant, may have calcifications. Colonic carcinoma is the most frequent primary tumor causing calcified metastases in the liver. Other primary neoplasms in the thyroid gland, lung, pancreas, adrenal gland, stomach, kidney, ovary, and breast may cause calcified hepatic metastases (Statement 8-4D is true). Inflammatory calcified granulomas related to tuberculosis or histoplasmosis are common in miliary calcifications (Statement 8-4E is true). Calcified cystic lesions, such as *Echinococcus* disease in the liver, are commonly seen in areas of the world where the causative organism is endemic.

EXERCISE 8-2: PELVIC CALCIFICATIONS

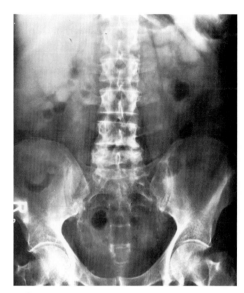

FIG. 8-E-5

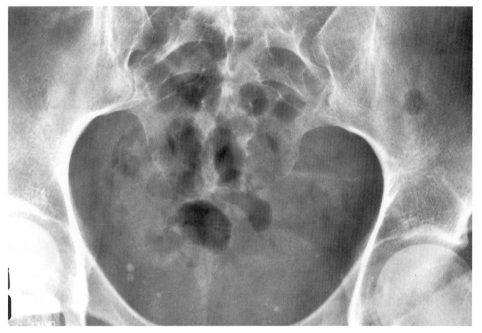

FIG. 8-E-6

Clinical Histories:

CASE 8-5
A 15-year-old boy presents with right lower quadrant pain and fever (Fig. 8-E-5).

CASE 8-6
A 50-year-old woman presents with back pain (Fig. 8-E-6).

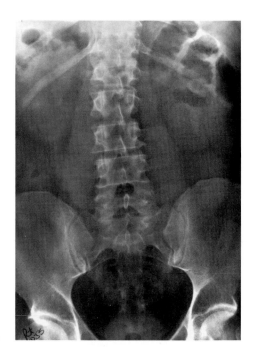

FIG. 8-E-7 *Panel A.*

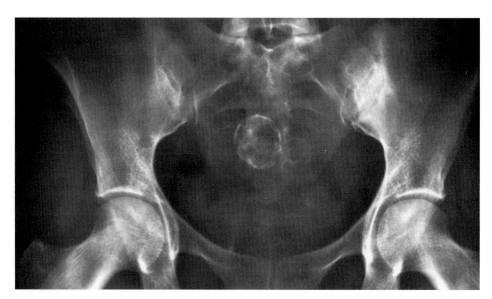

FIG. 8-E-8

CASE 8-7
A 47-year-old man presents with hematuria (Fig. 8-E-7*A*).

CASE 8-8
A 48-year-old woman presents with lower abdominal fullness (Fig. 8-E-8).

Questions:

8-5. What would be the most likely diagnosis in Case 8-5?
   A. Calcified abscess
   B. Ectopic gallstone
   C. Right ureteral calculus
   D. Pelvic phlebolith
   E. Appendicolith

8-6. In Case 8-6, what is the most likely origin of the multiple pelvic calcifications?
A. Multiple ureteral calculi
B. Multiple phleboliths
C. Multiple bladder calculi
D. Calcified carcinoma in the colon
E. Uterine fibroid calcification

8-7. In Case 8-7, what is the most likely diagnosis?
A. Renal tuberculosis
B. Right ureteral calculus
C. Left ureteral calculus
D. Bladder calculus
E. Appendicolith

8-8. In Case 8-8, what would be the most likely diagnosis?
A. Dermoid cyst of the ovary
B. Chondrosarcoma of the sacrum
C. Bladder calculus
D. Cystadenoma of the ovary
E. Uterine fibroid calcification

Radiologic Findings:

8-5. This case is that of a boy with acute appendicitis (*E* is the correct answer to Question 8-5). An oval calcification measuring 0.8 cm in diameter projects over the iliac bone and laterally to the right sacroiliac joint with a distended appendiceal lumen filled with gas. At surgery, gangrenous appendicitis with perforation and an obstructing appendicolith were found.

8-6. This case demonstrates multiple pelvic calcifications projecting below the level of the ischial spines bilaterally. Most of these calcifications are round or oval, and some have radiolucent centers. In the absence of specific urinary tract symptoms, multiple phleboliths would be the first consideration (*B* is the correct answer to Question 8-6). The patient's back pain is not related to phleboliths.

8-7. In this case, one small density 5 mm in diameter projected over the left transverse process of L4 (Fig. 8-E-7*B*). With the patient's history of hematuria, the most likely choice would be left ureteral calculus (*C* is the correct answer to Question 8-7). A subsequent intravenous urogram shows left hydronephrosis with columnization of the proximal ureter superiorly to the calculus (Fig. 8-E-7*C*).

8-8. In this case, large, 2-cm-diameter, mottled and curvilinear calcifications are seen in the midpelvis. These calcifications overlie the sacrum and are consistent with calcification in uterine fibroids (*E* is the correct answer to Question 8-8).

Discussion:

Calcified appendiceal stones are present in only about 10 percent of patients with appendicitis; however, in a symptomatic child, an appendicolith indicates at least a 90 percent chance of acute appendicitis. Prophylactic appendectomy has been recommended in the child with an incidentally discovered appendicolith because of a high incidence of gangrene and perforation.

Phleboliths are thrombi within the pelvic veins, and this location accounts for their circular shape. Calcification within these thrombi starts peripherally with a typical radiolucent center that is seen radiographically. Phleboliths have little clinical significance except that they can be confused with other pelvic densities, particularly distal ureteral calculi. In general, ureteral stones lie above and medially to the ischial spines, and they lack a radiolucent center.

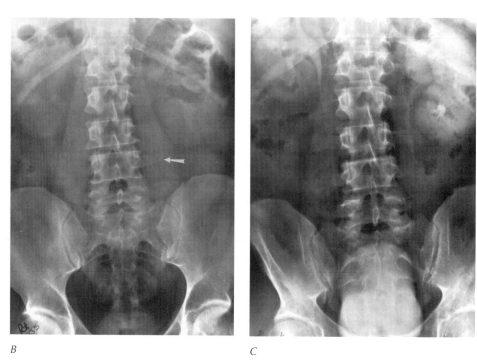

B   *C*

FIG. 8-E-7   Plain film (*Panel B*) and intravenous pyelography (*Panel C*) of the patient. A left ureteral calculus overlaps the transverse process of the L-4 vertebra is seen on plain film (*arrow*) but is obscured by contrast density on intravenous pyelography. Left hydronephrosis and dilatation of the proximal ureter above the ureteral calculus are seen.

Ureteral calculi are always a consideration in patients with hematuria. Since 80 to 90 percent of urinary calculi are radiographically opaque, the plain abdominal film is important as the initial examination. Close scrutiny of the abdominal film is crucial because ureteral calculi may be elusive when they project over the lumbar transverse processes or the sacroiliac region. To confirm a ureteral calculus, intravenous urography is often needed to localize the density to the ureter.

Most uterine leiomyoma calcifications appear as multiple mottled or speckled calcifications or as dense, smooth, curvilinear calcifications around the mass. The real soft-tissue mass is often larger than the area of calcification. Other calcifications in the pelvis include calcified dermoid cysts, bladder calculi, foreign material, lymph nodes, lithopedion, prostatic calculi, or calcified vas deferens.

EXERCISE 8-3: INCREASED ABDOMINAL DENSITY OR MASSES

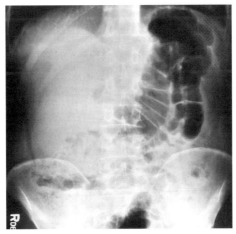

FIG. 8-E-9   *Panel A.*

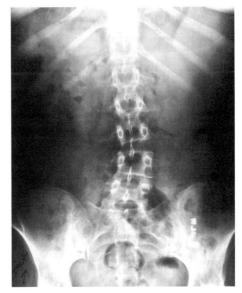

FIG. 8-E-10   *Panel A.*

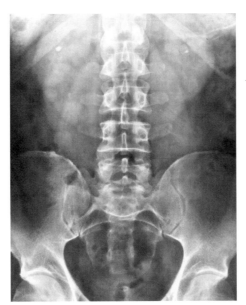

FIG. 8-E-11   *Panel A.*

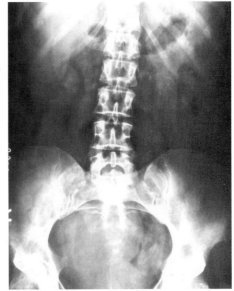

FIG. 8-E-12

Clinical Histories:

CASE 8-9
A 57-year-old man presents with history of hepatitis (Fig. 8-E-9*A*).

CASE 8-10
A 35-year-old woman presents with fever and anemia (Fig. 8-E-10*A*).

CASE 8-11
A 40-year-old man presents with back pain (Fig. 8-E-11*A*).

CASE 8-12
A 45-year-old woman presents with lower abdominal fullness (Fig. 8-E-12).

Questions:

8-9. In Case 8-9, what would be the most likely consideration?
- A. Hepatomegaly
- B. Splenomegaly
- C. Cirrhosis
- D. Nephromegaly
- E. Ascites

8-10. In Case 8-10, the inferior displacement of the gas pattern in the splenic flexure of the colon is most likely due to
- A. gastric outlet obstruction.
- B. adrenal carcinoma.
- C. renal cell carcinoma.
- D. hepatomegaly.
- E. splenomegaly.

8-11. In Case 8-11, what would be the most likely diagnosis?
- A. Gastric outlet obstruction
- B. Gastric carcinoma
- C. Horseshoe kidney
- D. A pseudotumor sign of small bowel obstruction
- E. Hepatomegaly

8-12. In Case 8-12, what would be the most likely consideration?
- A. Pelvic abscess
- B. Ovarian cyst
- C. Pelvic lymphoma
- D. Pelvic hematoma
- E. Ectopic pregnancy

Radiologic Findings:

8-9. In this case, the right side of the abdomen shows increased density and is relatively free of gas. Displacement of the gas pattern in the duodenum and jejunum to the left side is indicative of hepatomegaly (Fig. 8-E-9*B*) (*A* is the correct answer to Question 8-9). A radionuclide liver scan showed hepatic metastases from lung cancer.

8-10. In this case, a soft-tissue mass in the left upper quadrant displaces the gas in the splenic flexure of the colon downward (Fig. 8-E-10*B*). Left adrenal or renal cell carcinoma rarely presents as a large mass to the left of the midline. The most likely diagnosis is splenomegaly (*E* is the correct answer to Question 8-10).

8-11. In this case, a mass in the midabdomen delineates the lower poles of both kidneys, which are fused at the midline, consistent with horseshoe kidney (*C* is the correct answer to Question 8-11). Small renal calculi are present bilaterally (Fig. 8-E-11*B*).

8-12. In this case, there is a soft-tissue mass in the pelvis. In a middle-aged woman, an ovarian or uterine mass would be the most likely considerations. Ultrasound of the pelvis showed a large, fluid-filled mass, confirmed surgically as an ovarian cyst (*B* is the correct answer to Question 8-12).

Discussion:

Although abdominal plain films are useful in detecting splenomegaly, they are of little use in diagnosing hepatic disease, particularly if hepatomegaly is not present. Other imaging modalities, such as ultrasound, CT, and radionuclide liver scans, are more sensitive and accurate for evaluating hepatic primary diseases or metastases. In addition, barium studies of the gastrointestinal tract and intravenous urograms may be helpful in excluding gastric outlet obstruction, carcinoma, or renal cell carcinoma.

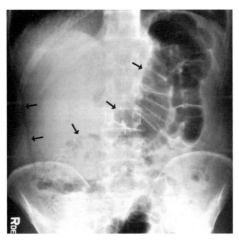

FIG. 8-E-9 (*Panel B*) Hepatomegaly is shown as a soft-tissue density (*arrows*) at the right upper quadrant, displacing the air-filled transverse colon.

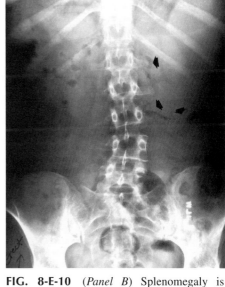

FIG. 8-E-10 (*Panel B*) Splenomegaly is demonstrated as a soft-tissue mass (*arrows*) in the left upper quadrant, displacing the splenic flexure of the colon downward.

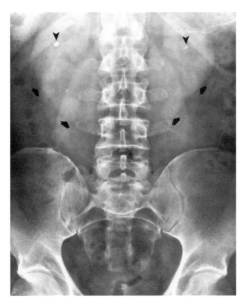

FIG. 8-E-11 (*Panel B*) Horseshoe kidney appears as a soft-tissue mass at midabdomen (*arrows*), and two renal calculi (*arrowheads*) are shown on plain film.

Fusion of the kidneys may occur in the embryologic stage during the second month of gestation. Most (95 percent) of these fusions occur at the lower poles of the kidneys. Intravenous urography shows the kidney to be vertical or even in the reverse oblique direction and its position to be lower than normal. Horseshoe kidney may be associated with other congenital anomalies, as well as a high incidence of urinary tract obstruction, infection, or stone formation. A horseshoe kidney also may deviate the upper ureters laterally.

When the plain film suggests the presence of a pelvic mass, a specific diagnosis often is not possible. Intravenous urography and barium enema are useful in excluding a mass arising from the lower urinary tract or colon and in showing extrinsic involvement of these structures. On the other hand, pelvic ultrasound or CT better demonstrates the pelvic organs and their interrelationship and will differentiate between solid or fluid content in the mass.

EXERCISE 8-4: INTESTINAL DISTENSION

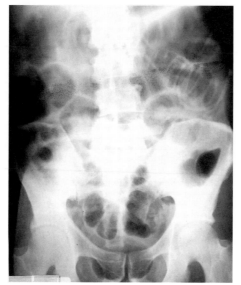

FIG. 8-E-13   *Panel A.*

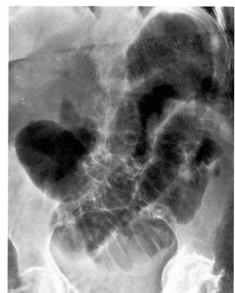

FIG. 8-E-14   *Panel A.*

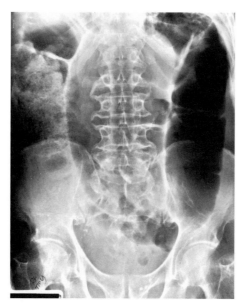

FIG. 8-E-15   *Panel A.*

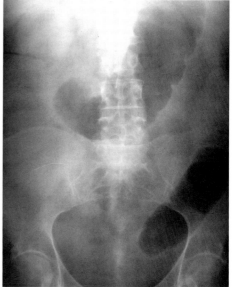

FIG. 8-E-16   *Panel A.*

Clinical Histories:

CASE 8-13
A 66-year-old man presents with fever, chills, and abdominal pain (Fig. 8-E-13A).

CASE 8-14
A 65-year-old woman presents with abdominal distension and a history of abdominal surgery (Fig. 8-E-14A).

CASE 8-15
A 70-year-old man presents with abdominal distension (Fig. 8-E-15A).

CASE 8-16
A 66-year-old woman presents with abdominal distension and constipation for 3 days (Fig. 8-E-16*A*).

Questions:

8-13. In Case 8-13, the most likely diagnosis would be
   A. functional ileus of the bowel.
   B. mechanical obstruction of the small bowel.
   C. mechanical obstruction of the colon.
   D. pneumoperitoneum.
   E. air in the retroperitoneum.

8-14. In Case 8-14, the most likely diagnosis is
   A. gastric outlet obstruction.
   B. functional ileus of the bowel.
   C. mechanical obstruction of the duodenum.
   D. mechanical obstruction of the small intestine.
   E. pneumoperitoneum.

8-15. In Case 8-15, the most likely conclusion would be
   A. functional ileus of the bowel.
   B. pneumoperitoneum.
   C. sigmoid volvulus.
   D. cecal volvulus.
   E. small-bowel volvulus.

8-16. In Case 8-16, the most likely diagnosis is
   A. mechanical obstruction at the small bowel.
   B. mechanical obstruction at the colon.
   C. functional ileus of the bowel.
   D. ascites.
   E. sigmoid volvulus.

Radiologic Findings:

8-13. In this case, a diffuse abnormal gas pattern in the patient's small bowel, colon, and rectum suggests functional ileus. Two days later the patient underwent laparotomy, and enteric ischemia was found during surgery (Fig. 8-E-13*B*) (*A* is the correct answer to Question 8-13).

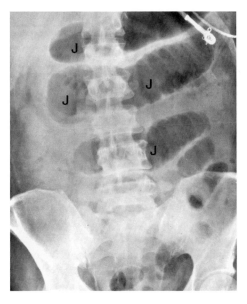

FIG. 8-E-13 (*Panel B*) Two days later, a follow-up abdominal plain film shows a gas pattern in several separated loops of the jejunum (J) at midabdomen, indicative of enteric ischemia.

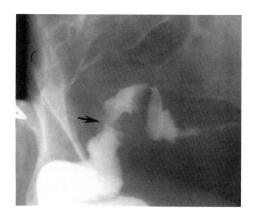

FIG. 8-E-16 (*Panel B*) Barium enema shows a narrowing (arrow) with an irregular contour at the rectosigmoid region, suggesting sigmoid carcinoma as the cause of colonic obstruction.

8-14. This patient has marked gaseous distension of the stomach, duodenum, and jejunum on the supine film, but no gas is seen in the colon, suggesting mechanical small bowel obstruction. Gastric outlet or duodenal obstruction is unlikely because many jejunal loops are dilated. At surgery, an obstructing jejunal adhesion was found (*D* is the correct answer to Question 8-14).

8-15. In this case, the patient has a huge distended and folded colonic loop in the midabdomen and pelvis (the "coffee bean" sign). The most likely consideration is a sigmoid volvulus (*C* is the correct answer to Question 8-15).

8-16. In this case, the transverse colon and descending colon are distended, with no gas in the sigmoid colon and rectum. The small bowel is not distended. Mechanical obstruction of the colon distal to the level of descending colon is likely (*B* is the correct answer to Question 8-16). Barium enema (Fig. 8-E-16*B*) shows an irregular narrowing (arrow) at the rectosigmoid region, indicative of sigmoid carcinoma.

Discussion:

Generalized or diffuse distribution of gas, both in the small bowel and in the colon, is more indicative of a functional ileus. The most common causes of functional ileus are postoperative status, neuromuscular diseases, ischemia, and intrinsic or extrinsic inflammations. Air-fluid levels may be seen in patients with functional ileus when plain films are obtained with the patient in upright position.

Limited distribution of abnormal gas in the intestine favors a mechanical obstruction. Air-fluid levels may be seen in patients with mechanical obstruction as well when an upright abdominal radiograph is obtained (Fig. 8-E-14*B*). The most common causes of mechanical obstruction in the small bowel are adhesions, internal or external hernias, neoplasms, or intussusceptions. Ileocolic intussusception is common in children.

When the small bowel is filled with a large amount of fluid, a row of small gas bubbles may be trapped between the valvulae conniventes; this is called the "string of beads" or "string of pearls" sign and is seen on the decubitus or upright view of the abdomen (Fig. 8-E-14*B*). A fluid-filled, closed-loop small bowel obstruction may appear as an oval mass in the abdomen and is known as the pseudotumor sign (Fig. 8-E-14*C*). These signs suggest a mechanical obstruction and possible strangulation.

Sigmoid volvulus may twist along the mesenteric axis and the long axis of the bowel. The twisted and overdistended sigmoid colon may appear as an inverted U shape or a coffee bean shape, without haustra or septa, at the upper pelvis and abdomen crossing the transverse colon (Fig. 8-E-15*B*). The colon above the sigmoid may be distended; however, the small bowel is rarely distended in a patient with sigmoid volvulus. Barium enema may show a beaking sign adjacent to the twisted point. Blood supply insufficiency may occur if volvulus cannot be corrected.

A small-bowel volvulus may be caused by internal hernia or adhesion similar to that of sigmoid volvulus. Small-bowel volvulus may be located outside the pelvis with no proximal colonic dilatation. Cecal volvulus is the cause of 1 to 2 percent of intestinal obstructions. Most often a cecal volvulus is twisted and relocated in the midabdomen or left upper quadrant (Fig. 8-E-15*C*).

FIG. 8-E-14 (*Panel B*) Two rows of air bubbles (*arrowheads*) with fluid levels in the left midabdomen are indicative of mechanical obstruction in the small intestine. (*Panel C*) Small bowel obstruction shows a huge mass (*arrowheads,* pseudotumor sign) in the midabdomen with several adjacent fluid levels. (*From Chen MYM et al: Radiology of the Small Bowel. New York, Igaku-Shoin, 1992; used with permission.*)

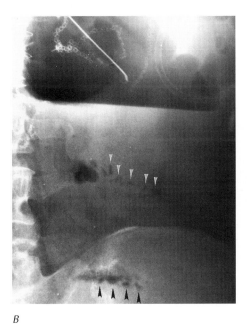

B

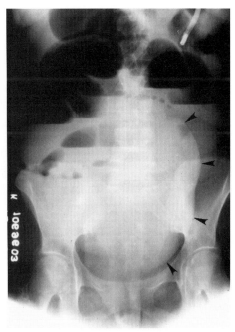

C

FIG. 8-E-15 (*Panel B*) Sigmoid volvulus shows a coffee bean sign (*arrowheads*) without haustra and septa. (*Panel C*) A distended cecum and right colon (*arrowheads*) are seen at midabdomen. The terminal ileum (*curved arrow*) is located laterally to the cecal volvulus. Barium enema may delineate the twisted point in the ascending colon.

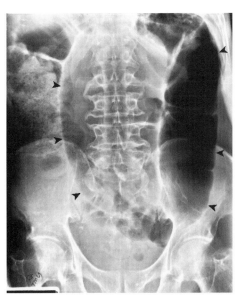
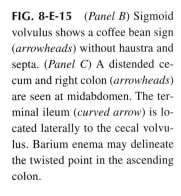

B

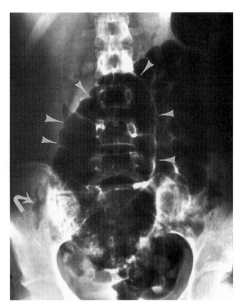

C

Mechanical obstruction of the colon is commonly caused by colonic neoplasm, volvulus, or inflammatory adhesion caused by diverticulitis of the left colon. All colonic segments proximal to the obstructive point are distended with gas or a combination of gas and feces in mechanical obstruction. When intestinal secretions and fecal matter fill the distended bowel loop, solid and liquid contents produce a mottled appearance. Whether the small bowel becomes distended as a result of a colonic obstruction depends on the duration and severity of the obstruction.

EXERCISE 8-5: INCREASED OR DECREASED DENSITY IN THE ABDOMEN

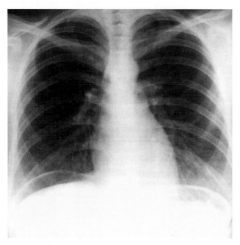

FIG. 8-E-17

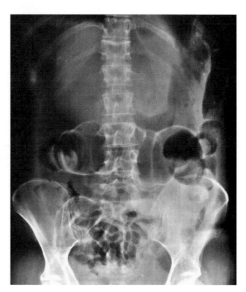

FIG. 8-E-18   *Panel A.*

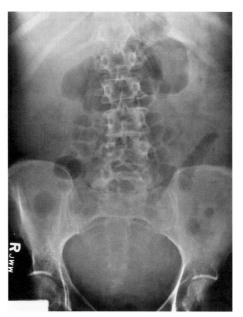

FIG. 8-E-19   *Panel A.*

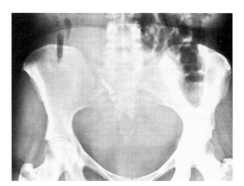

FIG. 8-E-20   *Panel A.*

Clinical Histories:

CASE 8-17
A 35-year-old man is seen who underwent laparotomy 2 days earlier (Fig. 8-E-17).

CASE 8-18
A 49-year-old woman presents with acute abdominal pain (Fig. 8-E-18*A*).

CASE 8-19
A 40-year-old woman presents with abdominal distension (Fig. 8-E-19*A*).

CASE 8-20
A 45-year-old woman is seen who had a motor vehicle accident (Fig. 8-E-20*A*).

Questions:

8-17. In Case 8-17, the most likely diagnosis is
A. tension pneumothorax.
B. pneumoperitoneum.
C. colon interposition.
D. bullous emphysema.
E. basilar pneumonia.

8-18. In Case 8-18, the most likely diagnosis would be
A. functional ileus of the bowel.
B. mechanical obstruction of the small bowel.
C. pneumoperitoneum.
D. ascites.
E. mechanical obstruction of the colon.

8-19. In Case 8-19, the most likely conclusion is
A. mechanical obstruction in the small bowel.
B. functional ileus.
C. gallstone ileus.
D. ascites.
E. pneumoperitoneum.

8-20. In Case 8-20, the most likely diagnosis would be
A. uterine fibroma.
B. ascites.
C. pelvic teratoma.
D. hemoperitoneum.
E. mechanical obstruction.

Radiologic Findings:

8-17. In this case, crescent-shaped lucencies beneath both hemidiaphragms outline the liver on the right and the spleen on the left in the PA chest film, suggesting pneumoperitoneum (*B* is the correct answer to Question 8-17).

8-18. In this case, both the inner and outer walls of the transverse colon are seen (arrows) (Fig. 8-E-18*B*). This double-wall sign is seen on the supine film of the abdomen because there is air within the intestinal lumen and in the peritoneal cavity, caused by rupture of the viscus (*C* is the correct answer to Question 8-18).

8-19. In this case, the hepatic angle (arrowheads) and the descending colon (*D*) are displaced medially, the small bowel (*S*) is located centrally in the abdomen, and there is increased density in the pelvis, suggesting ascites (Fig. 8-E-19*B*) (*D* is the correct answer to Question 8-19).

8-20. In this case, the soft-tissue density with no gas pattern in the pelvis is consistent with hemoperitoneum in this motor vehicle accident victim (*D* is the correct answer to Question 8-20).

Discussion:

In adults, the most common causes of pneumoperitoneum are postoperative status, ruptured abdominal viscus, and peritoneal dialysis. Residual air in the abdomen after surgery may persist for 1 to 2 weeks. Serial abdominal films, however, should show a gradual reduction in the amount of free peritoneal air. A persistent or increasing amount of air in postoperative serial films suggests a perforated viscus or ruptured surgical anastomosis. Spontaneous pneumoperitoneum is commonly caused by the perforation of a

FIG. 8-E-18 (*Panel B*) In a patient with pneumoperitoneum, the double-wall sign shows inner and outer walls of the transverse colon (*arrows*) delineated by air in the colon and in the peritoneal cavity. (*Panel C*) False double-wall sign. Both inner and outer walls of the ascending colon (*arrowheads*) are outlined by air inside the colon and fat shadow outside. (*Courtesy of Stanley Bohrer, M.D., Winston-Salem, N.C.*)

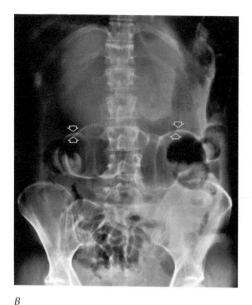

B

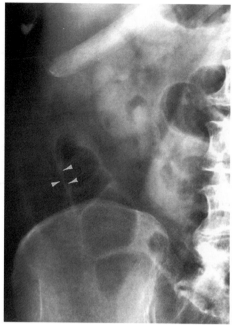

C

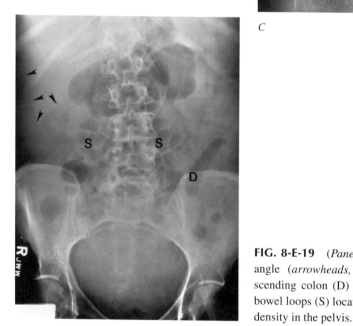

FIG. 8-E-19 (*Panel B*) Ascites shows hepatic angle (*arrowheads,* Helmer's sign) and descending colon (D) displacing medially, small bowel loops (S) located centrally, and increased density in the pelvis.

duodenal ulcer. Less common causes include pneumomediastinum, pulmonary emphysema, pneumatosis intestinalis, and entrance of air per vagina.

Pneumoperitoneum is most readily detected on the upright film of the chest, even if only a small amount of air is present. The left lateral decubitus view is preferred for accumulating a small amount of free air between the right lateral margin of the liver and the peritoneal surface. Normally, the interface between the air and inner intestinal wall is visible, but the serosal surface is not appreciated because its density is similar to that of the adjacent peritoneal contents. When gas is present in the peritoneal cavity, however, both inner and outer walls will be delineated; this is called the *double-wall sign* or *Rigler's sign* (Fig. 8-E-18*B*). A visible serosal margin of bowel also can be simulated by normal adjacent omental fat or adjacent contiguous loops of small or large bowel (Fig. 8-E-18*C*). If in doubt, the upright or left lateral decubitus film may confirm pneumoperitoneum. CT is more sensitive than plain film in assessing pneumoperitoneum. Colon interposition occurs on the right between the liver and hemidiaphragm, and haustrations are usually recognized, which aid differentiation from pneumoperitoneum.

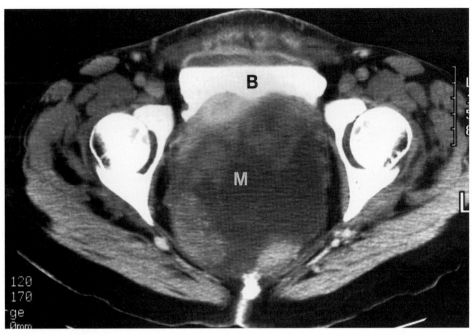

FIG. 8-E-20 (*Panel B*) CT shows a large soft-tissue mass (M) shadow with different attenuation in the pelvis, pushing the bladder (B) anteriorly. Hemoperitoneum was the diagnosis in this patient with a history of trauma.

Although plain film of the abdomen is not sensitive in assessing small amounts of intraperitoneal fluid, the plain film can demonstrate moderate and severe fluid collections. In ascites, the hepatic angle may be obscured or displaced medially (Helmer's sign) (Fig. 8-E-19*B*). The ascending or descending colon may be displaced medially by fluid in the paracolic gutter. A large amount of fluid may accumulate in the pelvis, causing increased density and symmetrical bulges (dog-ears sign). Other signs, such as separation of the small-bowel loops and overall higher density in the abdomen, are also seen, but not often. CT and ultrasonography more accurately assess intraperitoneal fluid and coexisting masses.

Blood and pus have a similar density to that of ascitic fluid in the peritoneal cavity; therefore, hemoperitoneum may produce signs similar to those found in ascites. High density in the pelvis is a sign of hemoperitoneum in patients with a history of trauma. CT better evaluates hemoperitoneum (Fig. 8-E-20*B*).

EXERCISE 8-6: EXTRALUMINAL GAS PATTERN

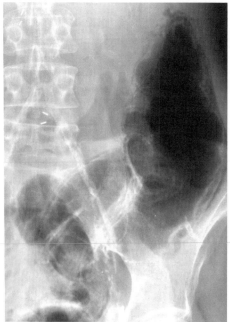

FIG. 8-E-21

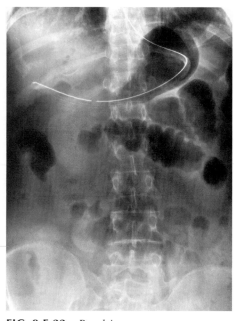

FIG. 8-E-22   *Panel A.*

Clinical Histories:

CASE 8-21
A 42-year-old man presents with mild abdominal pain (Fig. 8-E-21).

CASE 8-22
A 66-year-old woman is admitted with vague abdominal pain and vomiting (Fig. 8-E-22A).

CASE 8-23
A 77-year-old woman presents with fever and a 1-week history of abdominal pain (Fig. 8-E-23A).

CASE 8-24
A 64-year-old man presents with fever, abdominal pain, and distension (Fig. 8-E-24).

Questions:

8-21. In Case 8-21, the most likely diagnosis would be
    A.   mechanical obstruction of the colon.
    B.   pneumoperitoneum.
    C.   pneumatosis cystoides intestinalis.
    D.   colonic diverticulitis.
    E.   pelvic abscess.

8-22. In Case 8-22, the most likely diagnosis would be
    A.   functional ileus.
    B.   mechanical obstruction.
    C.   abscess.
    D.   gallstone ileus with pneumobilia.
    E.   hepatic portal vein gas.

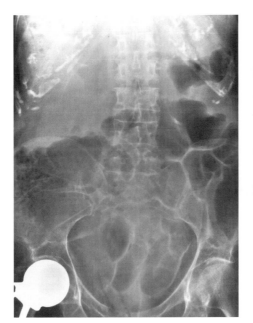

FIG. 8-E-23 *Panel A.*

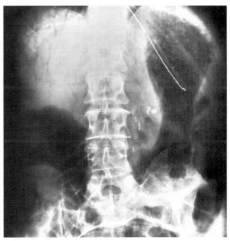

FIG. 8-E-24

8-23. In Case 8-23, the most likely conclusion is
  A. mechanical obstruction of the small bowel.
  B. gallstone ileus with gas in the biliary tree.
  C. hepatic portal venous gas.
  D. right subdiaphragmatic abscess.
  E. pneumoperitoneum.

8-24. In Case 8-24, the most likely diagnosis would be
  A. gallstone ileus with gas in the biliary tree.
  B. hepatic portal venous gas.
  C. subdiaphragmatic abscess.
  D. pneumoperitoneum.
  E. functional ileus.

Radiologic Findings: 8-21. In this case, linear air streaks are seen along the descending and sigmoid colon in a patient without serious symptoms. These streaks indicate pneumatosis cystoides intestinalis (*C* is the correct answer to Question 8-21).

8-22. In this case, a distended proximal jejunum and a few air bubbles are seen in the right upper quadrant, indicating gallstone ileus with mechanical obstruction and air in the biliary tree (Fig. 8-E-22*B*). An upper gastrointestinal study demonstrates a distended proximal small bowel, a fistula (Fig. 8-E-22*C*) between the biliary tree and the duodenum, and three gallstones in the small bowel (Fig. 8-E-22*D*) (*D* is the correct answer to Question 8-22).

8-23. In this case, multiple air bubbles in the right upper quadrant in a patient with fever are consistent with a subdiaphragmatic abscess (Fig. 8-E-23*B*). Bilateral linear rib calcifications and right hip replacement are also seen (*D* is the correct answer to Question 8-23).

8-24. In this case, a fine arborizing linear gas pattern in the right upper quadrant extends to the periphery of the liver, indicating portal venous gas (*B* is the correct answer to Question 8-24).

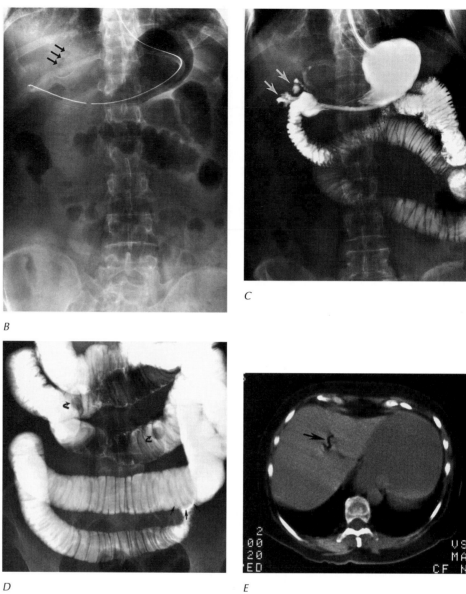

FIG. 8-E-22   (*Panel B*) Gallstone ileus in the same patient is seen as distended small-bowel loops and air bubbles at the right upper quadrant (*arrows*). (*Panel C*) Upper gastrointestinal series shows reflux of barium suspension into the biliary tree through a cholecystoduodenal fistula (*arrows*). (*Panel D*) Small-bowel examination shows three gallstones in the small bowel (*arrows*), with the distal stone (*straight arrows*) causing obstruction. (*Panel E*) CT study demonstrates air (*arrow*) in the biliary tree in the same patient. (*B–E from Chen MYM et al: CT of gallstone ileus. Appl. Radiol. 20:37–38, 1991; used with permission.*)

Discussion:

Pneumatosis cystoides intestinalis appears as linear streaks of gas or intramural cystic collections of gas in the small bowel or colon. The cysts range in size from 0.5 to 3 cm and may extend into the adjacent mesentery. Pneumatosis intestinalis is an incidental finding in most patients, usually with a self-limited benign course; simple bowel obstruction, volvulus, and air from the mediastinum or retroperitoneum are commonly associated. Pneumatosis intestinalis may be caused by ischemic and necrotizing enterocolitis in patients with leukemia or non-Hodgkin lymphoma and in those who have had bone marrow transplantation.

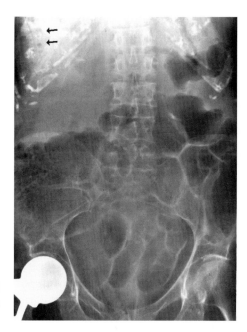

FIG. 8-E-23 (*Panel B*) Multiple air bubbles (*arrows*) in the right upper quadrant indicate a subdiaphragmatic abscess.

Gallstone ileus, the mechanical obstruction of the small bowel by an impacted gallstone, is seen commonly in elderly women. Clinical presentation in gallstone ileus is nonspecific, and the mortality rate is high (15 percent). A gallstone enters the intestinal lumen via a cholecystoenteric fistula (Fig. 8-E-22*C*). Major radiographic signs include small-bowel obstruction, air in the biliary tree, and an ectopic gallstone seen on plain abdominal film, upper gastrointestinal series, or CT study (Fig. 8-E-22*B–E*).

Abscess in the subphrenic and subhepatic spaces is a serious problem, with a mortality rate of 30 percent. Subphrenic abscess may arise spontaneously or as a complication of abdominal surgery, pancreatitis, diverticulitis, or appendicitis. A cluster of gas may be seen on plain film in 70 percent of abscesses. Left-sided abscess is difficult to discern because gas in the splenic flexure, stomach, or jejunum may obscure gas within the abscess. Other radiographic findings include elevation of the adjacent hemidiaphragm, pleural effusion, and basilar atelectasis.

In the right upper quadrant, when multiple tubular lucencies are seen reaching the lateral hepatic margins, portal venous gas is a likely consideration. Biliary tree gas is located in the central hepatic zone near the porta hepatis. Benign portal venous gas has been noted in sigmoid diverticulosis, nonobstructed splenic flexure carcinoma, ulcerative colitis, and bronchopneumonia. Mesenteric vascular insufficiency and necrotizing intestinal infection are common causes of hepatic portal venous gas. In children, necrotizing enterocolitis produces intramural gas within mesenteric veins to the liver; the mortality rate in patients with the sign of hepatic portal venous gas is higher than in those without portal venous gas.

BIBLIOGRAPHY

Baker SR: *The Abdominal Plain Film.* Norwalk, Conn, Appleton & Lange, 1990.

Gore RM et al (eds): *Textbook of Gastrointestinal Radiology.* Philadelphia, Saunders, 1994.

McCort JJ (ed): *Abdominal Radiology.* Baltimore, Williams & Wilkins, 1981.

Meyers MA: *Dynamic Radiology of the Abdomen: Normal and Pathologic Anatomy,* 4th ed. New York, Springer-Verlag, 1994.

Skucas J, Spataro RF: *Radiology of the Acute Abdomen.* New York, Churchill-Livingstone, 1986.

9

RADIOLOGY OF THE URINARY TRACT

Ronald J. Zagoria

Urinary tract radiology encompasses a broad array of imaging techniques that can yield both anatomic and functional information. Techniques such as standard radiography and intravenous urography (IVU) have been complemented by the development and refinement of newer techniques such as ultrasonography (US), computed tomography (CT), and magnetic resonance (MR) imaging. Other imaging techniques, including angiography, cystography, and urethrography, are useful to evaluate specific areas in the urinary tract and generally are used as an adjunct to the previously described radiologic techniques. Nuclear medicine techniques are particularly useful for evaluating renal function, but a description of these techniques is beyond the scope of this chapter.

This chapter describes the radiologic techniques commonly used for urinary tract imaging. The selection of appropriate techniques for various different clinical situations is discussed. Case presentations illustrative of some of these imaging principles are presented later in this chapter.

TECHNIQUES AND NORMAL ANATOMY

Plain-Film Radiography

The standard abdominal radiograph can be extremely useful in initial evaluation of the urinary tract in patients with suspected abnormalities. Although the soft tissues of the urinary tract are usually only faintly discernible, urinary tract stones, a common urinary tract abnormality, are usually visible on abdominal radiographs as focal radiopacities (Fig. 9-1). Approximately 90 percent of urinary tract calculi are radiopaque on an abdominal radiograph. Urinary tract calculi can be visualized within the kidney, ureters, or bladder. Even though most urinary tract stones are radiopaque and are a common cause of signs and symptoms, some care must be taken in the diagnosis of urolithiasis on the basis of a single abdominal radiograph. There are many other causes of abdominal radiopacities, including gallstones, calcified lymph nodes, vascular calcifications, ingested tablets, and bowel contents. When radiopacities project over the kidneys on an abdominal radiograph, oblique views can be used to confirm the position of these opacities within the kidney. Once a renal position has been confirmed, further imaging may be useful to better locate these radiopacities. A calcification within a calyx is presumed to represent a stone, whereas calcification in the renal parenchyma indicates other possible causes such as neoplasm, arterial aneurysm, or urinary tract infection.

In addition to detection of urinary tract calculi, abdominal plain films should be scrutinized for other abnormalities. Signs and symptoms of cholelithiasis, appendicitis, bowel obstruction, and other abdominal diseases may mimic some symptoms of urinary tract disease. Evidence of extraurinary tract abnormalities may be gleaned from

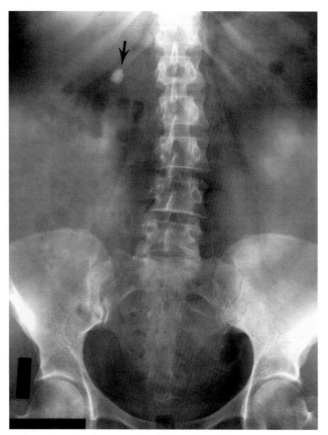

FIG. 9-1 Abdominal radiograph demonstrates a large round kidney stone (*arrow*) in the right upper quadrant.

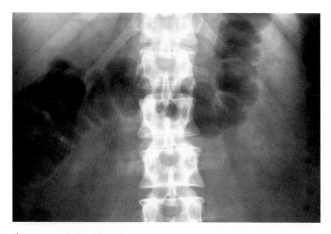

A

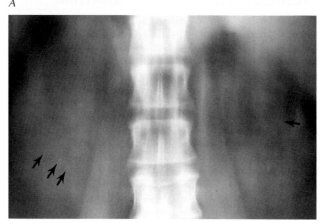

B

FIG. 9-2 (*A*) Standard radiograph of the upper abdomen demonstrates several small calcifications in the left kidney. The right kidney is largely obscured by overlying gas in the colon. (*B*) Single nephrotomogram shows the renal outlines more clearly, since the obscuration from the overlying bowel gas is minimized. Additional renal calculi are now clearly visible in both kidneys (*arrows*).

the plain abdominal radiograph and may provide clues to urinary tract disease. For instance, vertebral anomalies are commonly associated with congenital urinary tract disorders. In addition, abnormalities causing neurologic disease often affect urinary tract function. Diseases in this category include myelomeningocele, caudal regression syndrome, spinal cord trauma, sacrococcygeal teratoma, and others. Evidence of these conditions is often present on the plain abdominal radiograph, and these findings may explain urinary tract disease.

Nephrotomography

Plain-film tomography of the kidney is referred to as *nephrotomography*. This radiographic technique employs linear motion of the x-ray source and the radiographic film during a prolonged x-ray exposure. This results in clear depiction of the kidneys and blurring of the superimposed structures, such as overlying bowel gas (Fig. 9-2). Although slightly greater radiation exposure is required for this technique than for standard radiography, it is particularly useful for the detection of small radiopaque urinary tract calculi. Nephrotomography is often employed as a baseline examination in patients with urolithiasis when they are treated medically, and follow-up radiographs will be used to enumerate and measure renal stones. Nephroto-

mography also can be used as an adjunct to contrast studies, such as intravenous urography, when better definition of the renal outlines is desired.

Intravenous Urography

The intravenous urogram (IVU) remains a standard for urinary tract imaging. Radiographic contrast material is injected into a peripheral vein. This contrast material contains iodine molecules, which are radiopaque. Virtually all this contrast material is rapidly excreted with urine as a result of glomerular filtration of the iodine-containing molecules. Opacification of the kidneys, ureters, and bladder usually occurs over a span of 15 to 20 min (Fig. 9-3*A–E*). This opacification makes the urinary tract conspicuous on standard radiographs exposed after injection of the contrast material. Detailed images of the urinary tract can be obtained during this period while high concentrations of the

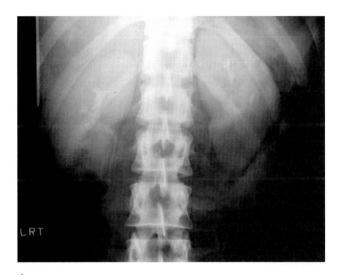

A

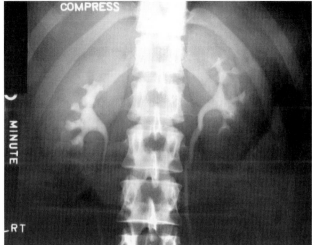

C

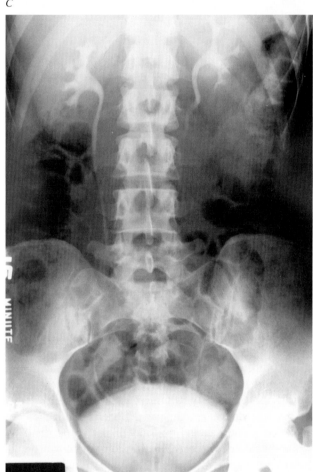

B

D

FIG. 9-3 (*A*) This abdominal radiograph taken 1 min after the injection of intravenous contrast material demonstrates opacification of both kidneys. The renal outlines are well defined as a result of opacification by the excreted contrast material. There is early opacification of the calyces and upper ureters. (*B*) A 5-min abdominal radiograph demonstrates good opacification of the calyces. Dilute contrast material is noted in the bladder, and there is good opacification of a large portion of both ureters. (*C*) This coned-down view of the kidneys was taken after applying compression to the lower abdomen to better distend the calyces. The

calyces and upper ureters are well opacified and appear normal. (*D*) This 15-min abdominal radiograph demonstrates further opacification of the bladder lumen. The nephrograms have faded significantly since earlier radiographs, but there is good opacification of the ureters. (*E*) This coned-down view of the pelvis was taken after voiding. The bladder mucosa is collapsed, and a small amount of residual contrast media is in the bladder. Curvilinear lucencies in the bladder are caused by mucosal folds and are normal. A portion of the lower right ureter is also opacified.

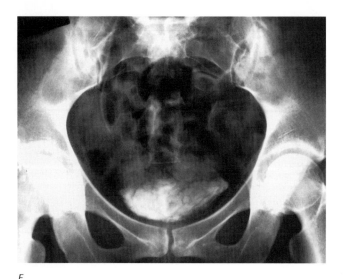

E

FIG. 9-3 (*Continued*)

contrast material are being excreted in the urine. Under normal circumstances, the IVU will allow detailed evaluation of the renal parenchyma, the calyces and renal pelvis, the ureters, and the bladder. The size, shape, contours, and temporal symmetry of the opacified kidney should be evaluated on each IVU. Normally, both kidneys are of similar length, although the left kidney is often slightly larger than the right kidney. The size of the kidneys as seen on IVU depends to some degree on the actual renal size, hydration status, renal rotation, body habitus, and filming techniques. While many variations in renal size exist, virtually all normal kidneys should be equal or greater in length than three adjacent lumbar vertebral bodies, including their intervening inner spaces. Additionally, normal kidneys are rarely longer than four adjacent lumbar vertebral bodies with their intervening disk spaces included. Symmetry is also important when evaluating renal size. While minimal variations in the length of the two kidneys are normal, a discrepancy in length between the two kidneys that exceeds 2 cm suggests an underlying urinary tract abnormality.

A line drawn around the peripheral margin of the opacified kidney should be smooth in contour, and its shape should be reniform. Mild lobation is common and is considered a congenital anomaly related to fusion of renal lobules during kidney development. Calyces are generally centered within these lobules, and the thickness of the renal parenchyma should be normal, with a width of approximately 15 to 20 mm. Indentations in other locations or those associated with parenchymal thinning suggest scarring related to remote infections or ischemia. Some other variations in normal contour can be seen, particularly on the left. The upper portion of the left kidney is often flattened during its development because of the adjacent spleen. Flattening also can result in formation of a "dromedary hump" on the lower lateral aspect of the left kidney. This hump of normal renal parenchyma will enhance ho-

mogeneously and, other than its shape, will appear as normal renal parenchyma. In addition, the overall thickness of this area of the kidney should be similar to that of other areas of the same kidney. This can be confirmed by measuring the distance from the edge of this hump to the calyx centered within this area and comparing it with other areas of that kidney. If the width in this area is excessive or the contrast-enhancement characteristics are atypical, then a mass lesion in this area is indicated. These rules also hold for evaluation of other areas of the renal parenchyma. Simultaneous homogeneous enhancement of the renal parenchyma of both kidneys should occur during IVU (see Fig. 9-3*A,B*). Delay in global enhancement of a single kidney suggests an abnormality of blood supply to that entire kidney. Focal abnormalities suggest space-occupying lesions or local inflammation.

Renal calyces and the renal pelvis usually opacify within the first 5 min after contrast material injection. Normally, the calyces are cup-shaped structures draining the renal medulla. Calyces should be spread out evenly so that all areas of renal parenchyma appear to have a subtending calyx. Minor calyces can have various normal appearances. When seen in profile, minor calyceal tips are usually cup-shaped with sharply defined fornices at each edge. Calyces may be seen on end or in different obliquities. When seen on end, an opacified calyx generally appears as a white circle more medially located than the calyces seen in profile. Additionally, fused or compound calyces are often present in normal kidneys. Compound calyces represent a conglomeration of two or more calyces draining into a single infundibulum. These are larger than simple calyces, and their shape varies according to the number of calyces compounded. Compound calyces occur more frequently in the upper and lower poles of the kidney than in the midportion of the kidney. Opacification of the calyces should be homogeneous, without filling defects or focal areas of caliber change (see Fig. 9-3). Minor calyces then drain urine and contrast material into their associated infundibulum, also known as a *major calyx,* and these empty into the renal pelvis. The normal size and shape of the renal pelvis can vary greatly. In general, the renal pelvis is prominent and triangular, with the apex of the triangle occurring at the ureteropelvic junction.

The ureter, a dynamic contracting organ, connects the renal pelvis and the bladder. From the kidney it courses obliquely over the ventral surface of the psoas muscle and extends caudally to the pelvis. On the IVU, the ureter generally is superimposed on the transverse processes of the lumbar vertebral bodies. As it enters the pelvis, the ureter should course slightly more medially before it extends posterolaterally to enter the bladder. Deviations in the normal course of the ureter suggest retroperitoneal or pelvic abnormalities. Aortic aneurysms, lymphadenopathy, retroperitoneal or pelvic tumors, and other disease processes of the retroperitoneum can deviate the ureters with or without causing obstruction of the urinary tract. Complete evaluation of the ureters and calyces also includes exclusion of filling defects, displacing the normal radiopaque contrast column, abnormalities of ureteral caliber, and temporal symmetry of ureteral opacification. Delayed opacification of one ureter suggests ureteral obstruction, and delayed films often will confirm this diagnosis as well as elucidate the level of obstruction. The presence of a filling defect within the contrast column suggests an abnormality. The etiology varies, but the most common cause is urolithiasis. However, urinary tract tumors, such as transitional cell carcinoma, often present as filling defects, and these can mimic the appearance of urinary tract stones.

The caliber of each ureter and of the collecting system should be evaluated during IVU. Although some narrowing is normal where the ureter joins both the renal pelvis and the bladder and where the ureter crosses the iliac artery, other signs of obstruction are not associated with these normal anatomic narrowings. Narrowing with evidence of obstruction or narrowing in areas other than those explained by normal anatomic structures indicates underlying urinary tract disease. Narrowing can be due to tumor infiltration, cicatrization, or encasement of the ureter from adjacent retroperitoneal or pelvic processes. Focal ureteral dilatation also suggests abnormalities in most cases. A ureteral spindle is a normal variant and should not be confused with disease. This term describes a focal dilatation of the ureter just before it crosses the iliac artery entering the pelvis. This transient phenomenon is often seen and is due to peristalsis of a bolus of urine and contrast material that is transiently delayed as it crosses the iliac vessels. Although this phenomenon may recur, it should not be present on every film of this area during IVU. Other focal areas of dilatation suggest focal pathology. Dilatation can be due to intraluminal mass, such as a stone or neoplasm, to increased intraluminal pressure, as seen with obstruction, or to increased urine volumes. Supranormal urine volumes can be seen in patients with chronic vesicoureteral reflux, functional ureteral abnormalities resulting in impaired peristalsis, and high-urinary-output states such as diabetes insipidus.

Later in the IVU series the bladder will be well opacified and can be evaluated. Normally, the bladder has a smooth contour with homogeneous enhancement (see Fig. 9-3D). Filling defects suggest abnormalities similar to those seen in the ureter and upper tract. Diffuse bladder irregularity, often with formation of numerous bladder diverticula or cellules, can be seen in patients with chronic bladder outlet obstruction. This may be due to mechanical or functional bladder obstruction. The size of the bladder can be grossly evaluated from the urogram. An extremely large bladder capacity usually suggests a flaccid bladder seen in conjunction with peripheral neuropathy.

In summary, the IVU gives detailed demonstration of the kidneys, calyces, renal pelvis, ureter, and bladder. It is therefore an excellent screening evaluation for patients with suspected urinary tract disease. This test is readily available, and the incidence of serious side effects associated with the administration of the intravenous contrast material is low.

Ultrasonography

Sonography is a useful technique for evaluating the kidneys and the bladder. Normal ureters are not visible by sonography because of their small size and intervening structures. Normally, renal parenchyma has an echo pattern similar to that of other solid abdominal organs. Its echogenicity should be equal to or slightly less than that of the adjacent liver or spleen. The echogenicity of the renal parenchyma should be homogeneous, and the contours and shape of the kidney should be evaluated in a fashion similar to that used with IVU (Fig. 9-4). The renal sinus, which contains the renal pelvis and calyces, fibrofatty tissue, and vascular and lymphatic structures, has a higher echogenicity than does the normal renal parenchyma. The renal sinus is located centrally within the kidney. Normally, the collecting system is invisible or barely visible in the renal sinus. When visible, it is a fluid-containing anechoic structure with a branching pattern similar to that seen for the collecting system on the IVU examination. When the collecting system is dilated, it is readily visible by ultrasound (US).

Sonography does not require the injection of contrast material, and no ionizing radiation is employed. It allows excellent visualization of the renal parenchyma and of the bladder lumen filled with urine. It also is useful in evaluating the calyces when they are dilated. In addition, most

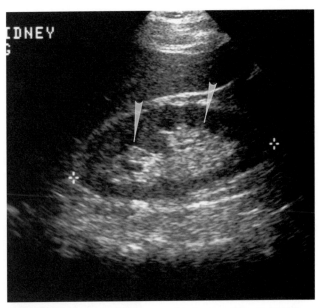

FIG. 9-4 A sagittal ultrasonographic image of the right kidney demonstrates homogeneous renal parenchyma surrounding the more echogenic renal sinus (*arrowheads*). The intrarenal collecting system is not visible, which is normal for a nondilated system.

renal calcifications, including calculi, are visible with US. They appear as hyperechoic foci with posterior shadowing. For these reasons, sonography is very useful in urinary tract evaluation, particularly in the detection and characterization of renal masses. The most common renal mass, the simple cyst, can be diagnosed with US with nearly 100 percent accuracy. Also, sonography is a useful technique in the triage of patients with renal failure to determine appropriate treatment. Patients with prerenal or renal causes for renal insufficiency generally require medical management. Alternatively, postrenal causes for renal insufficiency are generally managed with some form of interventional drainage. Postrenal causes include obstructive processes involving the urethra, bladder, or both ureters. These are diagnosed by US when bilateral hydronephrosis is present in a patient with renal insufficiency. The absence of this finding suggests that renal insufficiency is due to a renal or prerenal cause.

Ultrasonography is also useful as an adjunct to other urinary tract imaging procedures such as IVU. Filling defects or renal mass lesions seen with IVU often can be better characterized by US. For instance, although a radiolucent stone is indistinguishable from some neoplasms with IVU, urolithiasis is a characteristic US pattern different from that of other radiolucent filling defects. US is often applied in renal imaging for pediatric patients, since long-term follow-up is often necessary in these patients and the risk of repeated exposure to ionizing radiation may be considerable.

Computed Tomography

Computed tomography (CT) is a powerful tool for evaluation of the urinary tract and surrounding structures. It can be performed with and without the injection of intravenous contrast material, and it does use ionizing radiation. For optimal diagnosis of urinary tract abnormalities other than stones, intravenous contrast material is generally used during CT scan. Major advantages of CT include high resolution, high sensitivity for density differences among various tissues, ability to evaluate all the surrounding structures, and rapidity of the examination. Recent refinements in CT include the development of helical or spiral CT techniques. These techniques have improved acquisition of three-dimensional reconstructions of the urinary tract and other organ systems, as well as CT angiography studies.

Although the expense and cross-sectional imaging style of CT limit it to some extent as a screening technique, its strengths have greatly improved the diagnosis of some urinary tract abnormalities. With intravenous injection of contrast material, even millimetric lesions in the renal parenchyma are detectable with thin-section CT scanning. CT scanning also allows characterization of renal masses with a high accuracy for the diagnosis of simple cysts and renal neoplasms. Lesions less than 3 cm in diameter are often undetectable with IVU, yet these are readily detected with CT (Fig. 9-5). In addition, CT is an excellent tool for planning surgical management of renal neoplasms. Staging accuracy approaching 100 percent is possible with the use of meticulous CT technique in patients with renal adenocarcinomas. Other renal parenchymal lesions that are readily evaluated with CT include complicated renal infections such as renal abscess and xanthogranulomatous pyelonephritis. Ureteral dilatation and adjacent retroperitoneal pathology are readily detectable with CT. Bladder wall thickening and focal bladder wall lesions also can be detected with CT in many cases.

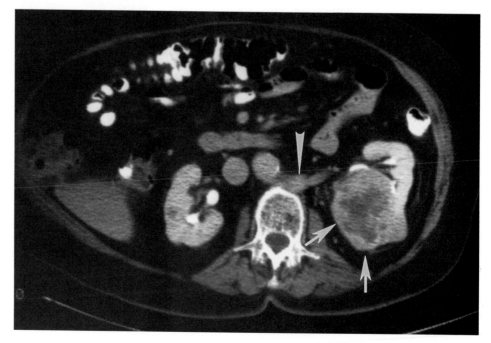

FIG. 9-5 CT scan through the midportion of the kidneys demonstrates a heterogeneous mass (*arrows*) arising from the posterior portion of the left kidney. The right kidney appears normal. Incidentally noted is a retroaortic left renal vein (*arrowhead*), a vascular anomaly.

Magnetic Resonance Imaging

The spatial resolution for magnetic resonance (MR) imaging of the urinary tract is slightly less than that of CT scanning. However, tissue contrast with MR imaging is superior to that of CT (Fig. 9-6). As a result, overall lesion detection is similar to that of CT for renal parenchymal lesions. The overall lesion detection rate and staging accuracy for MR imaging are similar to those with CT for renal neoplasms and benign renal parenchymal lesions. MR imaging has the advantage of not requiring intravenous contrast material for patients who have risk factors precluding its use in CT, and MR imaging uses no ionizing radiation. Disadvantages of the MR imaging examination as compared with CT include longer examination time, increased artifacts due to respiratory and bowel motion, and lack of bowel contrast agent, which sometimes precludes differentiation of bowel from retroperitoneal structures. However, MR imaging is widely accepted as a safe and effective tool for characterizing and staging renal masses when findings with other imaging techniques are inconclusive. CT and MR imaging have similar applications for urinary tract evaluation, but MR imaging is somewhat superior for imaging vascular structures such as the renal vein and inferior vena cava. This vascular imaging ability and the multiplanar imaging utilized with MR imaging make it an excellent technique for evaluating vascular structures in patients with renal malignancies that tend to extend into the renal vein, such as renal adenocarcinoma.

Arteriography

Renal arteriography has limited indications for urinary tract imaging. It is used primarily to evaluate vascular abnormalities of the urinary tract or to evaluate vascular anatomy for surgical planning. Arteriography requires puncture and catheterization of the arterial system. Selective catheterization of the renal artery may be necessary. Renal arteriography yields exquisite pictures of the renal arterial system, and it can be used for therapeutic management of some vascular lesions (Fig. 9-7). Currently, arteriography is indicated for the evaluation of suspected renovascular hypertension. Stenosis of the main renal artery or one of its branches can be demonstrated with renal arteriography. In many cases, balloon angioplasty can be performed to treat the stenosis. Other vascular lesions, such as arteriovenous fistulas or malformations, can be demonstrated by means of renal arteriography. Transcatheter embolotherapy is an accepted technique for treating some arteriovenous connections. Embolotherapy also can be used as a palliative measure in patients with advanced renal malignancy when control of local symptoms is desired. Finally, renal arteriography is often used for vascular mapping prior to surgery. The number and position of renal arteries supplying each kidney are readily determined with arteriographic images. In addition, selective and superselective catheterization can demonstrate vascular supply to tumors when renal-sparing surgery is being planned. Because of the invasive nature of arteriography and the imaging strengths of cross-sectional imaging, the use of arteriography is of limited usefulness in the urinary tract.

Cystography

A cystogram is performed for radiographic evaluation of the bladder. The bladder is filled with dilute contrast material through a bladder catheter. Images of the bladder are then obtained and evaluated. In addition, bladder capacity can be assessed by measuring the volume of contrast material needed to fill the bladder. Normally, the bladder will be smooth-walled and rounded when filled (Fig. 9-8). There should be no reflux of contrast material into the ureters. No filling defect should be present within the lumen of the bladder other than the bladder catheter itself. Normally, a patient can completely evacuate the bladder upon voiding.

The cystogram can be coupled with radiographic evaluation of the urethra during voiding. This study, called a *voiding cystourethrogram,* allows evaluation of the bladder with a cystogram, followed by images of the urethra obtained during voiding of the contrast material from the bladder. The urethra can be evaluated for filling defects, strictures, diverticula, evidence of inflammation, or obstruction.

Retrograde Urethrography

The retrograde urethrogram is another imaging study for evaluation of the urethra. A catheter is introduced cutaneously into the urethra, and dilute contrast material is injected through the catheter directly into the urethra while radiographic images are exposed. Normally, in male patients, the anterior urethra (penile and bulbous segments) is well distended during retrograde urethrography. There is some resistance to retrograde flow imposed by the external urethral sphincter. Ideally, the urethra should be distended enough so that some contrast material does reflux beyond the external sphincter into the bladder. This will confirm continuity of the urethra with the bladder and allow some evaluation of the posterior (membranous and prostatic segments) urethra. The opacified urethra is evaluated for extravasation, diverticula, strictures, filling defects, or obstruction. Normally, the male urethra is smooth-walled with mild dilatation in the bulbous segment (Fig. 9-9). There is tapering of the urethra at the external sphincter. With filling of the posterior urethra, a linear filling defect, representing the verumontanum, is seen posteriorly in the prostatic urethra. No other filling defects are normally seen within the urethra. Relative narrowing at the junction of the urethra and the bladder represents the bladder neck. No other areas of narrowing should be seen in the normal urethra. Outpouchings from the urethra may represent congenital or acquired urethral diverticula, dilated periurethral

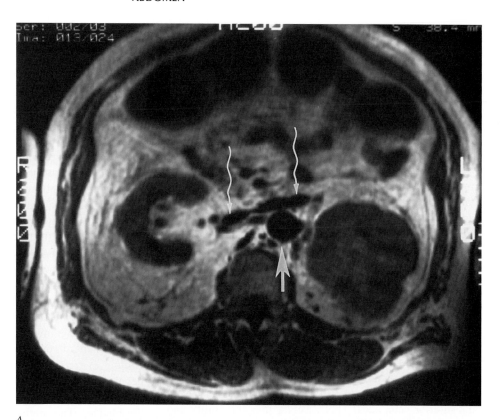

A

FIG. 9-6 (*A*) T2-weighted transverse MR image through the mid-portion of the kidneys demonstrates a normal right kidney. The renal parenchyma is horseshoe-shaped and homogeneous. The renal sinus has high signal intensity because of its high fat content. The left kidney contains a heterogeneous solid mass. Vascular structures such as the aorta (*arrow*) and the left renal vein as it enters the inferior vena cava (*curved arrows*) are clearly seen. (*B*) Gradient-recall-echo MR image of the kidneys at the same level as part *A* demonstrates the high signal emitted by flowing blood. The aorta and inferior vena cava appear as white structures just anterior to the spine. The superior mesenteric artery (*arrow*) and the left renal vein (*arrowhead*) are also well visualized. Seen again is the heterogeneous left renal mass, which was found to be a renal adenocarcinoma.

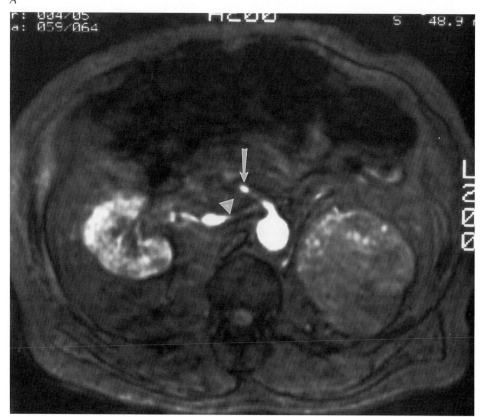

B

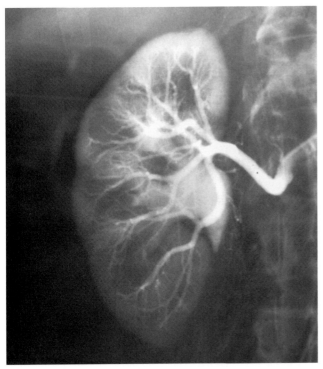

FIG. 9-7 Normal arteriogram of the right kidney demonstrates opacification of the main renal artery, with a normal branching pattern and good opacification of the interlobar and segmental renal arteries.

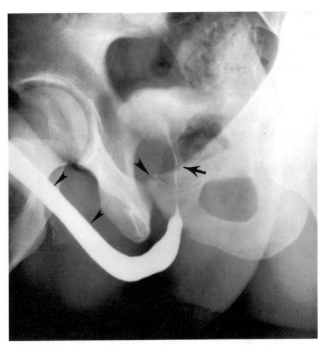

FIG. 9-9 This retrograde urethrogram appears normal in this trauma patient with a left pubic fracture (*large arrowhead*). The anterior urethra is well distended (*small arrowheads*). There is contrast material flowing through the posterior urethra into the bladder. The linear filling defect in the contrast column is due to the verumontanum (*arrow*).

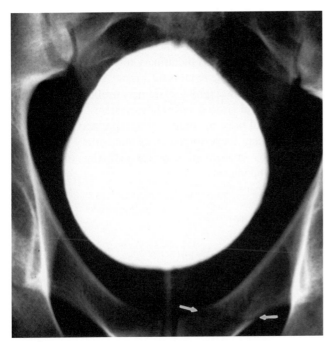

FIG. 9-8 This cystogram obtained in a trauma patient shows an oblique fracture of the left superior pubic ramus (*arrows*). The bladder appears normal, without extravasation. The bladder is round and has smooth margins. There is some uplifting of the bladder base above the pubic symphysis resulting from pelvic hematoma caused by the fracture.

glands, or residual spaces from previous urethral and periurethral infection. Leakage of contrast material outside the urethral lumen indicates urethral laceration or transection and may have either iatrogenic or traumatic causes. Retrograde urethrography is useful for radiographic evaluation of the urethra when an isolated urethral abnormality is suspected or when evaluation of the urethra is to be adjunct to other urinary tract imaging procedures.

TECHNIQUE SELECTION

Many techniques, as outlined in this chapter, have applications in urinary tract imaging; however, judicious use of these techniques is recommended. Common indications leading to urinary tract imaging include abdominal or flank pain and hematuria. Evaluation is properly initiated with an abdominal radiograph, with which approximately 90 percent of urinary tract calculi will be visible. Oblique views or nephrotomograms can be helpful to confirm the position of radiopacities within the urinary tract and to detect some radiopacities that may be obscured by overlying shadows. The IVU is an excellent screening examination for patients with suspected urinary tract abnormalities. The urogram allows excellent visualization and evaluation of the renal parenchyma, collecting system, ureters, and bladder and is the best noninvasive technique for evaluation of the ureters and intrarenal collecting system. For evaluation of the renal parenchyma, IVU will demonstrate most renal masses, although masses smaller than 3 cm may go undetected. Detection of an abnormality on the urogram may complete the imaging evaluation. For example, an obstructing ureteral stone can be treated appropriately after IVU diagnosis without the need for further imaging.

Detection of some lesions with IVU, such as a renal mass or a radiolucent filling defect in the ureter, will necessitate further evaluation. If a renal mass that appears to represent a cyst is detected with IVU, the US can be used to confirm that it represents a benign, simple cyst. Alternatively, a complex-appearing renal mass should be evaluated further with CT or MR imaging to characterize and stage the lesion, since it is likely to be a neoplasm. Filling defects in the ureter or collecting system also need further evaluation. If a nonimaging approach is desired, endoscopy can be performed, and often a tissue diagnosis can be obtained. Alternatively, US or CT can be used to detect mineralization in a filling defect that appears radiolucent with IVU. The most common etiology of a radiolucent filling defect seen with IVU is a uric acid stone. Such stones are readily diagnosed with US when they are in the renal pelvis or calyxes or with CT in any location in the urinary tract.

Other findings seen with IVU that may necessitate further examination include strictures or deviation of the ureter. Ureteric strictures that appear to have an extrinsic etiology and ureteral deviation should be followed with CT scanning of the abdomen to detect retroperitoneal disease. Intrinsic strictures are best evaluated with endoscopy and biopsy.

Other applications for IVU include screening the upper urinary tract to rule out serious traumatic injury and evaluating the urinary tract for pathologic conditions in patients with recurrent urinary tract infections. Patients involved in serious motor vehicle accidents often have significant hematuria. Radiologic evaluation of the urinary tract is indicated in these patients. The upper tracts can be readily evaluated with a CT scan when it is obtained in the trauma setting. If CT scanning is not otherwise indicated, serious abnormalities of the upper urinary tracts, the kidneys, and the ureters can be excluded with a standard IVU. A trauma-related abnormality seen with IVU requires further evaluation, usually with CT scanning. The bladder and urethra can now be reliably evaluated in the trauma setting with IVU. Evaluation of the urethra in the male trauma patient requires a retrograde urethrogram prior to bladder catheterization. Stretching of the urethra or urethral lacerations can be readily detected with this technique. The cystogram is the best technique for evaluating the bladder in trauma patients. Intraperitoneal or extraperitoneal bladder rupture can be readily detected and characterized with a simple cystogram. These three techniques also may be useful in patients with recurrent urinary tract infections to localize areas of urinary tract obstruction or stasis, which can lead to propagation of bacteria. Most simple, isolated urinary tract infections are idiopathic, and no underlying anatomic abnormality will be detected.

The evaluation of patients with recurrent urinary tract infections also can include US. This a noninvasive technique for evaluating the renal parenchyma to detect evidence of renal scarring and parenchymal loss. Nuclear medicine scans can give functional information for follow-up of patients with suspected postinfectious atrophy.

Patients presenting with newly diagnosed renal failure should first be evaluated radiologically with US. This test can exclude postrenal, obstructive causes of renal failure. The group of patients with an obstructive cause can be triaged to appropriate management with urinary tract drainage. Renal US also can be used to detect patients with diffuse renal parenchymal diseases that can cause renal insufficiency. These include medical renal diseases such as chronic glomerulonephritis and autosomal dominant polycystic kidney disease. If the urinary tract appears normal, a prerenal cause for the renal insufficiency should be sought.

Finally, angiography is extremely useful in the evaluation of the renal arterial and venous systems. Angiography is often useful prior to surgery or as a prelude to interventional treatment for lesions such as renal artery stenosis or arteriovenous malformation or for palliation of symptomatic renal neoplasms.

EXERCISE 9-1: RENAL MASSES

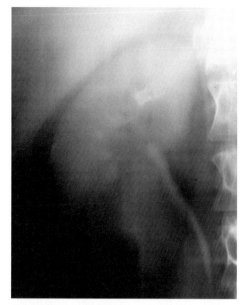

FIG. 9-E-1 *Panel A.*

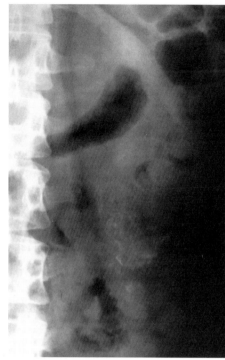

FIG. 9-E-2 *Panel A.*

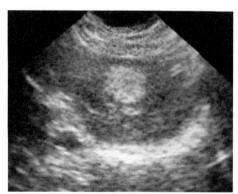

FIG. 9-E-3 *Panel A.*

Clinical Histories:

CASE 9-1
A 65-year-old woman presents with a pelvic mass and is having an intravenous urogram to evaluate her ureters for possible obstruction related to this mass. A coned-down view of the right kidney is shown (Fig. 9-E-1*A*).

CASE 9-2
A 45-year-old woman presents with left flank pain and microscopic hematuria. A coned-down view of the left upper abdomen is shown (Fig. 9-E-2*A*).

CASE 9-3
A 40-year-old woman presents with intermittent postprandial right upper quadrant pain. A transverse sonogram of the right kidney is shown (Fig. 9-E-3*A*).

Questions:

9-1. In Case 9-1, the mass in the lower pole of the right kidney is most likely
A. a renal abscess.
B. a simple renal cyst.
C. a renal adenocarcinoma.
D. a renal abscess.
E. metastatic disease from an ovarian neoplasm.

9-2. Regarding Case 9-2, which of the following statements is *not* true?
A. There is evidence of a mass arising from the left kidney.
B. The left kidney most likely contains a simple cyst.
C. Cysts are the most common renal mass.
D. Renal masses that calcify are usually malignant.
E. A renal mass containing calcifications should be further evaluated with CT or MR imaging.

9-3. Regarding the lesion demonstrated on the sonogram in Case 9-3, all the following are true except which one?
A. This lesion could be better characterized with CT.
B. This lesion most likely contains fat.
C. This renal mass may be malignant.
D. After diagnosis, this lesion is best followed up with sonography.
E. Masses like the one shown here usually cause upper abdominal pain.

Radiologic Findings:

9-1. In this case, a round, nonenhancing, water-density mass extends from the lower pole of the right kidney. There is no thickening of the peripheral margin of this mass. This mass has all the urographic features of a simple renal cyst (*B* is the correct answer to Question 9-1). Although urography is quite accurate in the diagnosis of simple renal cysts when all the above-mentioned features are present, sonography would be useful to better evaluate the architecture of this renal mass and confirm the diagnosis. A sonogram of this kidney (Fig. 9-E-1*B*) demonstrates a round lower-pole mass that contains no significant internal echoes. There is enhancement of sound transmission behind the mass, demonstrated by relatively increased echogenicity posterior to the renal mass. This enhanced sound transmission indicates the cystic nature of this mass. There is a well-defined back wall of this cyst. These features are diagnostic of a simple renal cyst.

9-2. The radiograph in this case demonstrates numerous calcifications overlapping the lower pole of the left kidney and extending inferiorly. A mass that arises in the kidney and that calcifies is usually malignant (*B* is the correct answer to Question 9-2). A CT scan of this kidney obtained 1 day later demonstrates an inhomogeneous left renal mass that contains the calcifications (Fig. 9-E-2*B*). This mass is typical of a renal adenocarcinoma.

9-3. In this case, a small hyperechoic mass is seen in the right kidney. This mass was detected incidentally during examination of the gallbladder. While this mass is most likely a benign tumor, further evaluation to confirm this diagnosis would be necessary. However, masses this small, whether benign or malignant, are rarely symptomatic (*E* is the correct answer to Question 9-3). A CT scan through this area demonstrates that the mass contains fat, typical of an angiomyolipoma of the kidney (Fig. 9-E-3*B*).

Discussion:

Cases 9-1 to 9-3 demonstrate renal masses. Most renal masses grow by expansion, deviating and compressing normal renal parenchyma, as in Case 9-1. Extrinsic masses, such as adrenal tumors, generally deviate the entire kidney, altering its axis but without significantly affecting its contour. Simple renal cysts, the most common renal tumor, typically appear as water-density masses that do not enhance with contrast material injection.

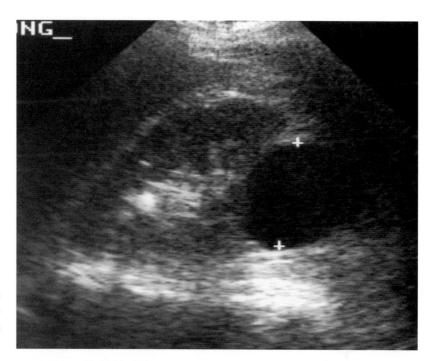

FIG. 9-E-1 *Panel B.* Sagittal sonogram of the right kidney demonstrates findings diagnostic of a simple renal cyst corresponding to the lower-pole mass on the IVU.

FIG. 9-E-2 *Panel B.* CT scan of the left kidney demonstrates a heterogeneous mass that has grown to fill the renal sinus of the lower portion of the left kidney. Punctate calcifications are seen around the periphery and within the center of this mass, which was found to be a renal adenocarcinoma. There is lymphadenopathy just lateral to the aorta and anterior to the vertebral body.

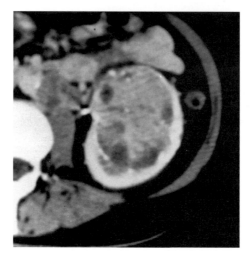

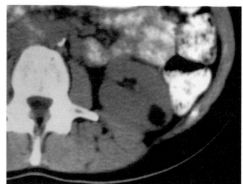

FIG. 9-E-3 *Panel B.* CT scan of the left kidney demonstrates that the mass seen on sonography is composed mainly of fat. The density of this mass is the same as that seen in surrounding perinephric and subcutaneous fat.

These masses, which may become quite sizable, are completely benign and generally are asymptomatic. They are also quite common, since approximately 50 percent of people over age 50 have at least one simple renal cyst. Most renal neoplasms, primary and metastatic, and renal infections demonstrate some enhancement at their margins. This finding suggests a cyst complicated by infection or a cystic neoplasm. In either case, with findings of a simple or complex cystic mass, sonography is useful to further evaluate the lesion. The sonographic findings of an echolucent round mass, with enhancement of sound transmission, and a well-defined back wall are diagnostic of a simple cyst. A renal abscess is usually associated with clinical findings of infection. By urography or sonography, a renal abscess is generally a thick-walled, irregular cystic mass, different from a simple renal cyst. Renal adenocarcinomas are predominately cystic in approximately 20 percent of cases, but again, they usually have thick walls with some degree of wall enhancement by urography and internal echoes with sonography.

While cysts are the most common renal mass, they calcify infrequently. When they do calcify, the calcium generally has a thin eggshell pattern at the mass margin. Renal adenocarcinomas calcify in up to 30 percent of patients. Of all renal masses with calcium, over half are malignant. Therefore, the detection of a calcified renal mass should lead one to suspect a renal adenocarcinoma. The next step would be further evaluation with CT or MR imaging to confirm this diagnosis and to stage the lesion for treatment planning. Renal adenocarcinomas can be staged accurately with either contrast-infused CT or with MR imaging of the abdomen and pelvis.

Case 9-3 illustrates a well-circumscribed fat-containing renal mass detected with sonography and confirmed by CT. A fat-containing renal mass is virtually diagnostic of an angiomyolipoma, a type of renal hamartoma. These benign masses are usually encountered incidentally, and small lesions are usually asymptomatic. Angiomyolipomas greater than 4 cm in diameter have been associated with a higher incidence of complications, including acute hemorrhage, or symptoms secondary to mass effect from the lesion. Therefore, once diagnosed, these lesions should be evaluated occasionally with sonography, since they may grow and put the patient at risk for serious complications. This case does illustrate one potential pitfall of renal sonography. Even though the sonographic features of this lesion, particularly its marked echogenicity, suggest that it contains fat, this must be confirmed with CT or MR imaging at the time of initial diagnosis. It has been shown that many small renal adenocarcinomas can be hyperechoic, mimicking angiomyolipomas. However, these small adenocarcinomas do not contain fat, and therefore, their appearance on CT or MR images will distinguish them from most angiomyolipomas.

Approximately 80 percent of angiomyolipomas are isolated lesions that are often discovered incidentally; the remaining lesions are associated with tuberous sclerosis. Tuberous sclerosis is a multisystem disease with central nervous system and abdominal manifestations. Patients with tuberous sclerosis are usually mentally retarded. They also have seizures and a characteristic facial skin lesion, adenoma sebaceum. Intracerebral calcifications usually occur as a result of multiple small hamartomas in the brain. Approximately 80 percent of these patients have renal angiomyolipomas, which are usually multiple and often quite large.

EXERCISE 9-2: RENAL DISEASES

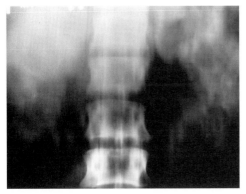

FIG. 9-E-4 *Panel A.*

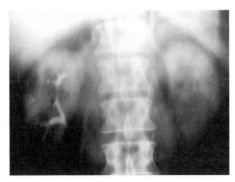

FIG. 9-E-5 *Panel A.*

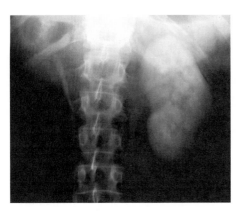

FIG. 9-E-6

Clinical Histories:

CASE 9-4
A 35-year-old man presents with hematuria and upper abdominal pain. A 1-min nephrotomogram film from an IVU is shown (Fig. 9-E-4*A*).

CASE 9-5
A 38-year-old woman presents with intermittent abdominal pain. She has previously had surgery for a pelvic malignancy. A 1-min film from an IVU is shown (Fig. 9-E-5*A*).

CASE 9-6
A 50-year-old man is being evaluated for microscopic hematuria. A 45-min film from an IVU is shown (Fig. 9-E-6).

Questions:

9-4. The IVU abnormalities shown in this case are most likely caused by which one of the following?
  A. Acute glomerulonephritis
  B. Metastatic disease involving the kidneys
  C. Autosomal dominant polycystic kidney disease (ADPKD)
  D. Renal adenocarcinoma
  E. Acute pyelonephritis

9-5. The abnormality depicted in this case is best described as which one of the following?
   A.   Unilateral large, smooth kidney
   B.   Unilateral large, irregular kidney
   C.   Unilateral small, smooth kidney
   D.   Unilateral small, irregular kidney
   E.   Unilateral renal hypoplasia

9-6. Based on the film shown, the most likely diagnosis in this case is which one of the following?
   A.   Chronic atrophic pyelonephritis
   B.   Renal artery stenosis
   C.   Renal hypoplasia
   D.   Acute pyelonephritis
   E.   Acute ureteral obstruction

Radiologic Findings:

9-4. The nephrotomogram shown in this case demonstrates inhomogeneous renal parenchyma bilaterally. There are numerous nonenhancing round lesions in each kidney, leading to an appearance that has been described as the "Swiss cheese nephrogram." This indicates the presence of multiple cysts in each kidney (*C* is the correct answer to Question 9-4).

9-5. This single film from an IVU demonstrates a size discrepancy between the two kidneys. Both kidneys have a smooth, reniform shape. The normal kidney ranges from three to four lumbar vertebral bodies in length. Using this rule, one finds that the right kidney is normal in size and the left kidney is small (*C* is the correct answer to Question 9-5).

9-6. The delayed film shown in this case demonstrates findings typical of acute ureteral obstruction (*E* is the correct answer to Question 9-6). Here the left kidney is mildly enlarged with a persistent nephrogram. There is delayed filling of the ureter.

Discussion:

ADPKD, sometimes referred to as *adult polycystic kidney disease,* is one of the more common inherited renal disorders. In most cases, this follows a straight dominant inheritance pattern. Therefore, at least one parent of each patient with ADPKD will have had this disorder. These patients are usually asymptomatic until their third or fourth decade of life. At that time, they often present with abdominal pain, infected cysts, hematuria, hypertension, or renal insufficiency. The diagnosis can be made with renal sonography or CT. Figure 9-E-4*B* shows a CT scan from another patient with ADPKD, and it demonstrates multiple simple renal cysts. Often some of these cysts become complicated with infection or acute hemorrhage. This can lead to calcification in the wall of some of the cysts and the collection of high attenuation material in some of the cysts. In addition, patients with ADPKD often develop cysts in other solid organs, including the liver, spleen, and pancreas. There does not appear to be any increased risk of renal malignancy associated with ADPKD. There is a well-known association with intracranial berry aneurysm formation. Approximately 15 percent of ADPKD patients develop these aneurysms, which can lead to life-threatening intracranial hemorrhage. Renal adenocarcinomas, which were mentioned earlier in this chapter, are usually unifocal and solid. Acute pyelonephritis, a unilateral process, and acute glomerulonephritis, which is bilateral, do not lead to the development of multiple renal cysts. Metastatic disease could manifest as multiple solid renal masses, but this would be rare in a 35-year-old man.

Case 9-5 illustrates the importance of appreciating size discrepancies when evaluating IVUs. It is also important to evaluate the renal contour and to categorize the pattern into the proper diagnostic set. This case illustrates a unilateral small, smooth kidney. By far the most common etiology of this appearance is renal artery stenosis. Figure 9-E-5*B*

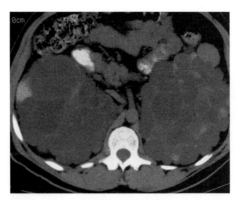

FIG. 9-E-4 *Panel B.* This CT scan from another patient with ADPKD demonstrates innumerable renal cysts. Although most of these are water-density cysts, some contain high-attenuation material related to recent hemorrhage or infection. No normal renal parenchyma is visible.

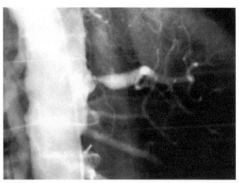

FIG. 9-E-5 *Panel B.* Aortogram in the same patient demonstrates a high-grade stenosis at the origin of the left renal artery and poststenotic dilatation of the main renal artery caused by turbulent flow through the stenotic segment.

is a single film from a renal arteriogram in this patient. It demonstrates a tight osteal stenosis of the left renal artery, with poststenotic dilatation of the renal artery segment just beyond the stenosis. This patient had hypertension, which was difficult to control with routine antihypertensive agents. Less common etiologies of this IVU pattern include congenital renal hypoplasia and previous radiation treatment of the kidney. Renal hypoplasia is a rare condition in which the kidney is not only small and smooth but contains a small number of calyces (five or fewer). Although previous radiation treatment to this kidney is also a possibility, it is rarely seen clinically. Patients who have had long-standing ureteral obstruction that is later relieved also can develop a similar appearance following renal parenchymal atrophy. This global atrophy is not common today, since most ureteral obstructions are treated within the first few weeks, prior to the development of irreversible renal damage.

Another common cause of unilateral renal atrophy is chronic atrophic pyelonephritis. This entity results from renal parenchymal scarring related to chronic bacterial pyelonephritis. In patients with this condition, the small kidney is also irregular in contour as a result of multifocal involvement of the renal parenchyma, which later leads to scarring. The renal atrophy remains long after the cessation of the acute renal infection. Generally, chronic atrophic pyelonephritis results from repeated episodes of pyelonephritis that occur during childhood as a result of chronic vesicoureteral reflux, which is not a rare finding in children.

Case 9-6 illustrates a typical acute ureteral obstruction. Because of the high pressure in the renal collecting system resulting from ureteral obstruction, there is persistence of contrast material in the intrarenal tubules. There is also renal edema secondary to this obstruction. Hydronephrosis is mild, since this is an acute obstruction. If the obstruction persists for months or longer, severe hydronephrosis and parenchymal atrophy will develop. Other clinical entities, including renal vein thrombosis and acute pyelonephritis, can lead to renal enlargement with a persistent nephrogram. Hydronephrosis is generally absent in these situations; therefore, it is essential that delayed films demonstrating hydronephrosis be obtained to exclude these alternative diagnoses. Acute pyelonephritis is diagnosed clinically, and IVU should not be performed in most patients with this condition. Imaging with either US or CT can be useful in patients with atypical pyelonephritis or pyelonephritis refractory to standard therapy. In these cases, complicating features such as renal abscess must be considered.

EXERCISE 9-3: RENAL DISEASES

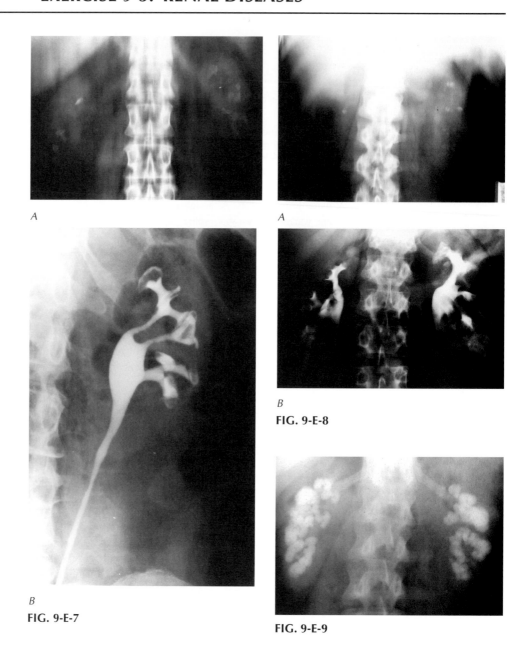

A

B
FIG. 9-E-7

A

B
FIG. 9-E-8

FIG. 9-E-9

Clinical Histories:

CASE 9-7

A 45-year-old patient presents with renal insufficiency and hematuria. A scout tomogram and film from a retrograde pyelogram are shown (Fig. 9-E-7).

CASE 9-8

A 35-year-old man presents with recurrent urolithiasis. A scout radiograph and a coned-down view of the kidneys from an IVU are shown (Fig. 9-E-8).

CASE 9-9

A 40-year-old man presents with recurrent urolithiasis. A scout radiograph is shown (Fig. 9-E-9).

Questions:

9-7. On the basis of the two films shown, the most likely diagnosis is
A. nephrolithiasis.
B. atherosclerosis.
C. papillary necrosis.
D. transitional cell carcinoma.
E. renal tuberculosis.

9-8. The abnormalities shown involve which part of the kidney?
A. Renal cortex
B. Renal medulla
C. Minor calyces
D. Major calyces
E. Small renal blood vessels

9-9. The pattern of calcification shown in this case suggests which type of disease?
A. Recurrent bacterial infections
B. Severe systemic hypotension
C. Bilateral ureteral obstruction
D. Systemic metabolic disease
E. Bilateral renal malignancies

Radiologic Findings:

9-7. The preliminary radiograph shown in this case demonstrates bilateral renal calcifications. These calcifications have a curvilinear appearance in the shape of rings and triangles. These calcifications project over the area of the renal medulla. The retrograde pyelogram demonstrates that some of these calcifications are within the calyces, whereas others are outlined by contrast material and are in cavities in the tips of the medulla. This indicates that the calcifications are in fact sloughed papillary tips that result from papillary necrosis (*C* is the correct answer to Question 9-7). Although nephrolithiasis can have a branched appearance, the stones would be restricted to the intrarenal collecting system and would not extend into the renal medulla. In addition, the ring-shaped and triangular curvilinear calcifications are typical of dystrophic calcifications in necrotic papillae. Transitional cell carcinoma is not commonly bilateral and rarely calcifies. When transitional cell carcinomas do calcify, the calcifications are usually punctate, not linear. Renal tuberculosis can be associated with papillary necrosis and intrarenal calcifications. However, it is rarely bilateral and is generally focal, involving only one or two renal pyramids before extending into the collecting system and down the ureter. Atherosclerotic calcifications can involve the intimal lining of the small renal blood vessels. These calcifications are linear, they have a branching pattern, and they follow the pathways of the normal renal arteries. This pattern is distinctly different from the pattern seen in this case.

9-8. The two films shown in this case demonstrate bilateral multifocal areas of calcification. The position in the renal medulla is confirmed by the intravenous urogram (*B* is the correct answer to Question 9-8). Some of the calcified areas seen on the preliminary radiograph appear to enlarge after the injection of contrast material. Not all renal pyramids are involved. Medullary calcifications can be referred to as *medullary nephrocalcinosis*. Renal cortical nephrocalcinosis has a distinctly different appearance. When the cortex calcifies, its appearance is analogous to that of an eggshell, a peripheral rim of calcium. The calcifications in abnormal renal pyramids are separate from the major and minor calyces, and they therefore do not represent nephrolithiasis.

9-9. This preliminary radiograph in this case again demonstrates medullary nephrocalcinosis. In this case, the calcifications are somewhat symmetrical and appear to involve all pyramids in the kidneys. This appearance suggests a systemic disease and is consistent with a metabolic disorder such as renal tubular acidosis (*D* is the correct answer to Question 9-9). Severe hypotension is associated with nephrocalcinosis, but it is a cortical pattern, since the cortex is more sensitive to acute ischemic insult. The diffuse bilateral appearance of this process suggests a systemic disorder rather than a process such as recurrent pyelonephritis or ureteral obstruction, which could lead to dystrophic calcifications in focal areas of the kidney. Renal cell carcinoma can be bilateral, and up to 30 percent of these tumors calcify. However, there is no evidence of a mass lesion in this case, and even bilateral multifocal adenocarcinomas would not contain the diffuse and symmetrical calcifications seen here.

Discussion:

Renal papillary necrosis can have numerous causes. Various renal insults, including pyelonephritis, ureteral obstruction, tuberculosis, and fat emboli, can lead to papillary necrosis. In addition, systemic disorders such as diabetes, sickle cell disease, and excessive use of analgesics can lead to papillary necrosis. The patient shown in Case 9-7 had long-standing rheumatoid arthritis and a history of high-dose analgesic use over a prolonged period of time. The common thread connecting all causes of papillary necrosis seems to be small-vessel disease leading to medullary ischemia and finally to necrosis. In many cases of papillary necrosis, only the central portion of the papillary tip is involved, and this causes a central cavity extending from a minor calyx into the medulla. On urography, this can appear as a "ball-on-tee." Severe papillary necrosis can lead to renal insufficiency and renal failure. Therefore, accurate diagnosis may prevent worsening of renal function.

Medullary nephrocalcinosis is caused most commonly by one of three general entities: systemic hypercalcemia, renal tubular acidosis, and medullary sponge kidney. The first two disorders, which are systemic and involve virtually all renal pyramids, lead to bilateral symmetrical medullary nephrocalcinosis. Medullary sponge kidney is a benign inherited disorder seen in up to 0.5 percent of patients undergoing urography. This disorder is commonly multifocal and bilateral, but it rarely involves all the renal pyramids. Its etiology is unexplained, but it causes focal areas of ectatic distal tubules in the renal medulla. Within these tubules, small calcifications can form as a result of stasis of urine. On urograms, the dilated tubules appear as discrete linear or rounded collections of contrast material that blend with the medullary calcifications and appear to enlarge them. This "growing calculus sign" is virtually diagnostic of medullary sponge kidney.

Other common causes of medullary nephrocalcinosis include renal tubular acidosis and hypercalcemia, usually with hypercalciuria. Renal tubular acidosis includes a spectrum of diseases, all characterized by abnormalities of hydrogen ion and bicarbonate excretion by the kidney. Medullary nephrocalcinosis is associated with type 1 renal tubular acidosis, which includes a distal tubular hydrogen ion transfer defect. In these patients, urine does not acidify below a pH of 5.8. Hypercalciuria and low urine citrate level result, leading to medullary nephrocalcinosis and nephrolithiasis.

Cortical nephrocalcinosis, a less common entity, is associated with distinct causes. Most commonly it is due to acute tubular necrosis, as is seen with severe systemic hypotension or ingestion of potent nephrotoxic agents. Cortical nephrocalcinosis is also seen commonly in patients with chronic glomerulonephritis. Less common causes include hyperoxaluria and a rare form of congenital nephritis, Alport's syndrome.

EXERCISE 9-4: URETER DISEASES

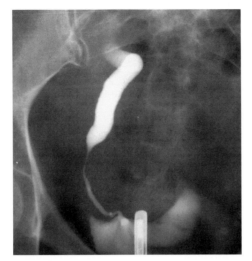

FIG. 9-E-10

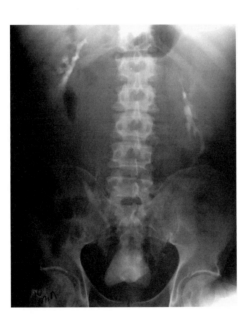

FIG. 9-E-11

FIG. 9-E-12 *Panel A.*

Clinical Histories:

CASE 9-10
A retrograde pyelogram is performed after an abnormal IVU in a woman with chronic pain in the right flank (Fig. 9-E-10).

CASE 9-11
A 50-year-old woman is seen who had one episode of gross hematuria. A coned-down view of the lower right ureter from an IVU is shown (Fig. 9-E-11).

CASE 9-12
A 55-year-old man presents with abdominal pain and weight loss. An abdominal film from an IVU is shown (Fig. 9-E-12*A*).

Questions:

9-10. The primary abnormality demonstrated here is which one of the following?
A. A dilated ureter
B. A narrowed ureter
C. A deviated ureter
D. Ureteral irregularity
E. A filling defect in the ureteral lumen

9-11. The radiographic appearance of this ureteral abnormality suggests all the following except which one?
A. This is most likely due to acute infection.
B. The abnormality involves the ureteral mucosa.
C. This abnormality is infiltrating the ureteral wall.
D. Other areas of urothelium are at risk for similar lesions.
E. Ureteroscopy will most likely be useful in further evaluation of this abnormality.

9-12. The IVU suggests that further imaging of this patient may be useful. Based on the findings shown, the imaging test most likely to yield a diagnosis is which one of the following?
A. Retrograde pyelogram
B. Renal sonography
C. Aortography
D. Functional radionuclide renal imaging
E. Computed tomography

Radiologic Findings:

9-10. This retrograde pyelogram demonstrates a markedly dilated ureter, indicative of chronic obstruction. This dilated ureter is a secondary finding; therefore, the cause of obstruction must be sought. This retrograde pyelogram also demonstrates an area of smooth tapered narrowing of the lower ureter just above the bladder. This is the abnormality that led to obstruction above it (*B* is the correct answer to Question 9-10). No filling defects are present within the opacified segment of the ureter, and the ureteral mucosa is smooth without irregularity. The ureter follows a normal course and is not deviated.

9-11. The film from an IVU in this case demonstrates an abrupt area of change in ureteral caliber. There is a short segment that is severely narrowed concentrically. Irregularity of the lumen of this segment suggests mucosal involvement. This abrupt, irregular narrowing suggests an intrinsic neoplasm arising from the ureter and infiltrating the ureteral wall. This concentric mass, which narrows the ureteral lumen and leads to obstruction, is typical of an invasive transitional cell carcinoma. Examination and biopsy with ureteroscopy would be a logical step to confirm the radiologic diagnosis and could be accomplished easily. Since transitional cell carcinomas are often multifocal, a search for other lesions along the ureteral lining should be performed. Acute infection can lead to ureteral edema, but it never leads to a focal, irregular, and concentric stricture of the ureter (*A* is the correct answer to Question 9-11).

9-12. The urogram in this case demonstrates an abnormal course of both ureters. The ureters are deviated laterally in the upper abdomen and medially in the pelvis. The ureters contain no filling defects and are of normal caliber. These findings suggest an extrinsic process and are typical of massive lymphadenopathy. The next logical step would be to evaluate the retroperitoneum thoroughly with CT (*E* is the correct answer to Question 9-12). A retrograde pyelogram is unnecessary, since the ureteral lumen is well opacified with the intravenous urogram, and would not yield any additional information. An aortic aneurysm can deviate the ureters laterally in the abdomen and should not lead to medial deviation in the pelvis; therefore, aortography is not likely to provide any useful diagnostic information in this case. There is no evidence of renal functional impairment, since contrast material is excreted normally and symmetrically. Global renal function is better assessed with laboratory analysis, and functional radionuclide renal imaging would not be useful in this case. Renal sonography could demonstrate lymphadenopathy, but obscuration by bowel gas would limit its usefulness, and sonography would be less useful to characterize the appearance and extent of these enlarged lymph nodes than would CT.

Discussion:

Although there are numerous causes for ureteral stricturing, the urographic appearance of the stricture often helps one arrive at the correct diagnosis expeditiously. Extrinsic processes, such as pelvic or retroperitoneal malignancies that engulf the ureter, typically cause a smooth, tapered narrowing of the ureter. These can be multifocal and bilateral. The patient shown in Case 9-10 was found to have carcinoma of the cervix, which had extended into the parametrium and encased the right ureter. The mucosa of the ureter may be compressed but is usually not infiltrated by these extrinsic processes. This leads to a smooth narrowing of the lumen without mucosal irregularity. Alternatively, intrinsic neoplasms, such as infiltrating transitional cell carcinomas, lead to abrupt, nontapered strictures, often with mucosal irregularity. These lesions arise in the mucosa and infiltrate the deeper layers of the ureteral wall. Infiltration of the ureteral wall often leads to the appearance of radiolucent "shoulders" indenting the normal contrast-filled lumen at the upper and lower aspects of the tumor. Transitional cell carcinomas are commonly multifocal. Up to 40 percent of patients with a ureteral lesion will be found to have another transitional cell carcinoma elsewhere in the urinary tract, most commonly in the bladder. Therefore, a meticulous search for synchronous lesions should be completed prior to treatment planning.

Based on the appearance of lesions involving the ureter, further diagnostic evaluation can be planned efficiently. Intrinsic lesions such as the transitional cell carcinoma demonstrated in Case 9-11 are best evaluated directly with ureteroscopy and biopsy. Since this lesion is intrinsic and involves the mucosa, it will be visible with an endoscope. However, extrinsic lesions such as those demonstrated in Cases 9-10 and 9-12 will not be amenable to diagnosis by ureteroscopy, since the lesions are extrinsic and only secondarily involve the ureter. In these cases, imaging with CT or MR imaging is most effective. These imaging techniques can be augmented with percutaneous needle

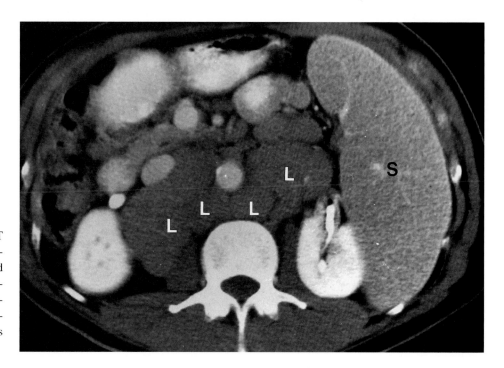

FIG. 9-E-12 *Panel B.* This CT scan of the upper abdomen demonstrates splenomegaly (S) and massive retroperitoneal lymphadenopathy (L). This lymphadenopathy accounts for the ureteral deviation seen on the intravenous urogram.

biopsy for a tissue diagnosis if the lesions are amenable to this approach. Case 9-12 demonstrates marked deviation of both ureters, typical of massive lymphadenopathy. This degree and symmetry of lymphadenopathy generally indicate chronic leukemia or lymphoma. The patient in Case 9-12 had chronic lymphocytic leukemia and was found to have extensive intraabdominal and pelvic lymphadenopathy (Fig. 9-E-12*B*). Any retroperitoneal mass can cause lateral deviation of the ureters. Other common retroperitoneal masses include abdominal aortic aneurysms, primary and metastatic retroperitoneal neoplasms, pancreatic pseudocysts or abscesses, hematomas and urinomas. CT or MR imaging of the abdomen will be useful in distinguishing among these various causes of ureteral deviation.

EXERCISE 9-5: BLADDER DISEASES

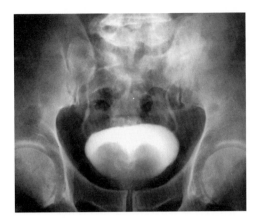

FIG. 9-E-13

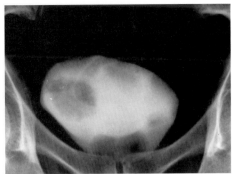

FIG. 9-E-14

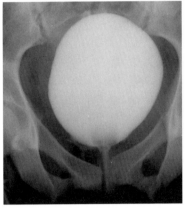

FIG. 9-E-15

A

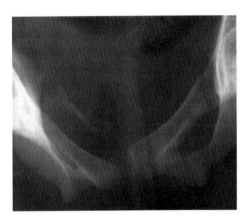

B

Clinical Histories:

CASE 9-13

A 65-year-old patient presents with microscopic hematuria. A coned-down view of the bladder from an IVU is shown (Fig. 9-E-13).

CASE 9-14

A 48-year-old man presents with intermittent gross hematuria. A coned-down view of the bladder from an IVU is shown (Fig. 9-E-14).

CASE 9-15

A 19-year-old woman is seen who was involved in a motor vehicle accident and has gross hematuria. Two films from a cystogram are shown (Fig. 9-E-15).

Questions:

9-13. Regarding the image shown in Case 9-13, all the following are true except which one?

    A. There is uplifting of the bladder base.

    B. The findings suggest a benign pathology.

    C. The demonstrated appearance is most often due to enlarged lymph nodes.

    D. The prostate gland is often involved.

    E. This appearance is commonly encountered with urography in elderly men.

9-14. The appearance depicted in Case 9-14 suggests that the most likely diagnosis is which of the following?
   A. Bladder hematoma
   B. Transitional cell carcinoma
   C. Acute cystitis
   D. Colon carcinoma invading the bladder
   E. Radiation cystitis

9-15. The radiographs shown in Case 9-15 are best described as showing which of the following?
   A. Normal bladder
   B. Bladder hematoma
   C. Bladder contusion
   D. Extraperitoneal bladder rupture
   E. Intraperitoneal bladder rupture

Radiologic Findings:

9-13. The radiograph shown in this case reveals symmetrical, smooth uplifting of the bladder base. This is commonly seen in elderly men and is most often due to benign prostatic hypertrophy (*C* is the correct answer to Question 9-13). Lymphadenopathy in this area is rare, and the typical appearance of lymphadenopathy is compression of the lateral aspects of the bladder.

9-14. The single radiograph in this case demonstrates a solitary filling defect in the contrast-filled bladder. This lesion arises near the right ureterovesical junction, and its surface is irregular. The most likely diagnosis in this case is transitional cell carcinoma (*B* is the correct answer to Question 9-14). Bladder hematomas can mimic neoplasms, but they are generally very smooth and are usually located near the midline on a supine radiograph. Cystitis causes mucosal edema and results in multiple nodular indentations on the bladder lumen. This is distinctly different from the radiographic appearance shown here. Carcinoma of the colon could invade the bladder, but this is uncommon. When colon carcinoma does invade the bladder, fistula formation and cystitis secondary to fecal contamination are common manifestations. It would be distinctly unusual for an invasive colon carcinoma to present as a solitary bladder mass in an otherwise normal bladder.

9-15. Two radiographs (Fig. 9-E-15) from an emergency cystogram in this young woman demonstrate fracture of the left superior and inferior pubic rami. There is a small amount of extravasation of contrast material near the bladder base, in the region of the fracture. This extravasation is seen on both radiographs and has a curvilinear shape. The location and appearance of this extravasation are typical of extraperitoneal bladder rupture (*D* is the correct answer to Question 9-15). Bladder contusion and hematoma commonly occur with pelvic trauma, but no extravasation of contrast material is seen with these injuries. Contrast extravasation associated with intraperitoneal bladder rupture has an appearance different from that of extraperitoneal extravasation. With intraperitoneal leakage of contrast material, the contrast material extends cephalad and outlines other intraperitoneal structures such as bowel loops and upper abdominal organs. The contrast material extravasated is homogeneous and disperses smoothly in the intraperitoneal cavity.

Discussion:

Cases 9-13 through 9-15 illustrate some of the bladder abnormalities seen with both urography and cystography. Hematuria is often evaluated with an IVU initially. Careful evaluation of the bladder often will lead to detection of an abnormality. A bladder base indentation is a common finding with urography. Benign prostatic hypertrophy is seen throughout the elderly male population. When the hypertrophied lobes extend cephalad, they tend to uplift the bladder base. Extension of the prostate above the pubic symphysis indicates prostatic enlargement. Prostatic hypertrophy can be present without bladder base uplifting; therefore, it is not a sensitive sign for prostatic enlargement. The most reliable urographic sign of prostatic enlargement is uplifting of the ureterovesicle junction, resulting in a J shape of the lower ureter. This may be seen even in the absence of an impression of the bladder base by the enlarged prostate gland. In addition, enlargement of the prostate is nonspecific, in that it can be due to benign or malignant processes in the prostate gland. Unless signs of metastatic disease are seen on the urogram, the distinction between benign and malignant enlargement cannot be made reliably with this study.

Transitional cell carcinoma is the most common neoplasm of the transitional epithelium. Approximately 90 percent of these tumors occur in the bladder, and the remainder occur in the upper tracts. Approximately two-thirds of transitional cell carcinomas are papillary, appearing as polyps in the urinary tract. On urography these are radiolucent filling defects. These masses often have a frondy mucosa with numerous interstices. Contrast material may outline these irregularities, and small stipples of contrast material may become trapped between the tumor fronds. This is a nearly diagnostic appearance for transitional cell carcinoma. The remaining one-third of transitional cell carcinomas are nonpapillary, or infiltrative. They tend to grow into deeper layers below the epithelium. These tumors lead to bladder wall thickening or malignant strictures. Obstruction of the ureter is also a common appearance for these invasive tumors when they arise near the ureterovesical junction. Transitional cell carcinomas are notorious for being multifocal. Meticulous review of the contrast images of the entire ureteral lining is mandatory to exclude synchronous lesions. In addition, radiographic follow-up is necessary to monitor patients for subsequent development of metachronous transitional cell carcinomas.

In patients with significant pelvic trauma, the bladder is at risk for significant injury. The spectrum of bladder injury extends from bladder contusion to bladder rupture. Bladder contusion is a diagnosis of exclusion, to be considered after more serious injuries have been ruled out. Bladder rupture can be extraperitoneal, intraperitoneal, or a combination of both. Extraperitoneal bladder rupture is the most common variety and is almost always associated with pelvic fractures. It is believed that bone shards puncture the bladder base and lead to extraperitoneal extravasation of urine. These ruptures are generally treated with simple catheter drainage of the bladder and follow-up cystography to confirm resolution. Intraperitoneal bladder rupture, whether alone or in combination with extraperitoneal bladder rupture, is a more serious process. Because the peritoneal cavity is a vast potential space, urine will readily flow through the rent in the bladder wall and into the peritoneal cavity. There, the peritoneal membrane will not only become inflamed but also will resorb many of the constituents present in the urine. Significant uremia can develop rapidly. Serious intraperitoneal bladder ruptures are treated surgically, in an emergent fashion. The distinction between intraperitoneal and extraperitoneal bladder rupture is clinically important. When contrast material extravasates into the extraperitoneal space, it infiltrates among the fascial layers around the base of the bladder. The result is a feathery or inhomogeneous "sunburst" pattern of extravasation as the fascia separates the contrast media into layers. Intraperitoneal rupture is quite different in appearance. In this case, the contrast material collections are often cloudlike and have a homogeneous, fluffy appearance. Contrast material may outline the bladder wall near the dome of the bladder, and other intraperitoneal structures are commonly outlined as well. This appearance is diagnostic of intraperitoneal bladder rupture.

BIBLIOGRAPHY

Bosniak MA: The current radiological approach to renal cysts. *Radiology* 158:1, 1986.
Bosniak MA, Ambos MA: Polycystic kidney disease. *Semin Roentgenol* 10:133, 1975.
Dyer RB, Zagoria RJ: Radiological patterns of mineralization as predictor of urinary stone etiology, associated pathology, and therapeutic outcome. *J Stone Dis* 4:272, 1992.

Hattery RR et al: Intravenous urographic technique. *Radiology* 167:593, 1988.

Mariani AJ et al: The significance of adult hematuria: 1000 hematuria evaluations including a risk-benefit and cost-effectiveness analysis. *J Urol* 141:350, 1988.

McCallum RW: The adult male urethra. *Radiol Clin North Am* 17:227, 1979.

McCallum RW: Lower urinary tract trauma. *Appl Radiol* 22:15, 1993.

McClennan BL: Diagnostic imaging evaluation of benign prostatic hyperplasia. *Urol Clin North Am* 17:517, 1990.

Mellins HZ: Cystic dilatations of the upper urinary tract: A radiologist's developmental model. *Radiology* 153:291, 1984.

Sandler CM et al: Bladder injury in blunt pelvic trauma. *Radiology* 158:633, 1986.

Schwartz G et al: Detection of renal calculi: The value of tomography. *AJR* 143:143, 1984.

Sutton JM: Evaluation of hematuria in adults. *JAMA* 263:2475, 1990.

Winalski CS et al: Ureteral neoplasms. *RadioGraphics* 10:271, 1990.

Yousem DM et al: Synchronous and metachronous transitional cell carcinoma of the urinary tract: Prevalence, incidence, and radiographic detection. *Radiology* 167:613, 1988.

Zagoria RJ et al: Staging of renal adenocarcinoma: Role of various imaging procedures. *AJR* 164:363, 1995.

10

GASTROINTESTINAL TRACT

David J. Ott

TECHNIQUES AND NORMAL IMAGING
  Luminal Contrast Examinations
  Other Imaging Modalities

TECHNIQUE SELECTION
  Patient Preparation
  Specific Contrast Examinations

EXERCISES
  10-1: Dysphagia
  10-2: Upper Gastrointestinal Bleeding
  10-3: Small Bowel Bleeding
  10-4: Small Bowel Obstruction
  10-5: Colonic Bleeding
  10-6: Colonic Obstruction

Imaging of the hollow organs of the gastrointestinal tract began a century ago with the use of heavy metal salts of bismuth and barium. By the first decades of this century, barium sulfate suspensions emerged as the contrast agent of choice for opacification and radiographic examination of the gastrointestinal tract. By the 1970s, other imaging modalities, including fiberoptic endoscopy and computed tomography (CT), were invented and developed into alternate ways of imaging the hollow gastrointestinal organs.

The emergence of the newer techniques has had a dramatic impact on the use of luminal contrast examinations of the gastrointestinal tract. In this chapter I will describe the current radiographic techniques available to examine the gastrointestinal tract with contrast materials, emphasizing the use of barium suspensions and illustrating normal anatomy. Patient preparation, selection of these techniques, and imaging options also will be discussed. Finally, a series of exercises will show the most common pathologic lesions of the gastrointestinal tract relative to specific clinical presentations.

TECHNIQUES AND NORMAL IMAGING

Luminal Contrast Examinations

Luminal contrast examinations of the gastrointestinal tract can be performed with a variety of contrast materials. Barium sulfate suspensions are the preferred material for most examinations. A number of barium sulfate suspensions are

available commercially, and many are formulated for specific examinations depending on their density and viscosity. Water-soluble contrast agents, which contain organically bound iodine, are used less often and primarily to demonstrate perforation of a hollow viscus or to evaluate the status of a surgical anastomosis in the gastrointestinal tract.

UPPER GASTROINTESTINAL TRACT

The organs that can be examined in the upper gastrointestinal tract include the pharynx, esophagus, stomach, and duodenum. The pharynx and esophagus may be evaluated separately or as part of more complete examinations of the upper gastrointestinal tract. Various techniques are available to assess the function and structure of the pharynx depending on the indications for the examination. Videotape recording of pharyngeal function and filming of pharyngeal structures are often combined for a more thorough examination. Also, materials of variable viscosity can be used in patients to determine dietary needs.

Pharyngeal function is complex and is best evaluated with motion-recording techniques that allow slow motion review of the recording. Filming of the pharynx is usually done with the patient in the frontal and lateral positions (Fig. 10-1). In the frontal view, the paired valleculae and piriform sinuses are separated. The lateral view of the pharynx superimposes these structures but permits better visualization of the base of the tongue, hyoid bone, and epiglottis anteriorly and the posterior pharyngeal wall and cervical spine posteriorly.

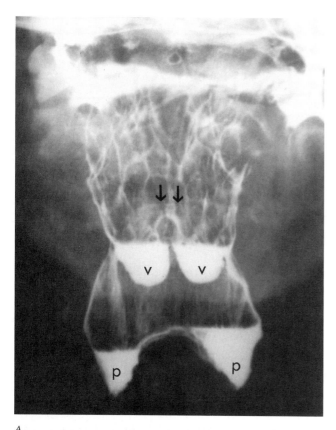

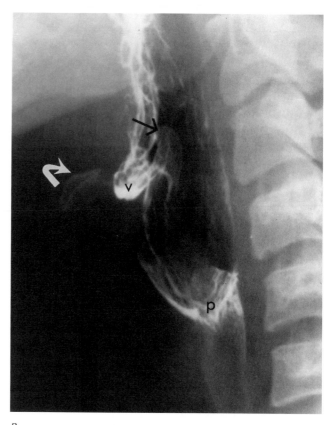

A

B

FIG. 10-1 Frontal (*A*) and lateral (*B*) views of the pharynx. In the frontal position, the paired valleculae (v) and piriform sinuses (p) have a symmetric appearance and are seen separately. On the lateral projection, the valleculae (v) and piriform sinuses (p) are superimposed. The upright epiglottis (*arrows,* both views) lies posterior to the valleculae, which are posterior to the hyoid bone (*curved arrow*).

The esophagus, stomach, and duodenum are usually examined together as part of the upper gastrointestinal series. A number of radiographic techniques are used and usually are combined to optimize the upper gastrointestinal examination. Techniques include observation of esophageal motility, which also may be recorded on videotape; filming of the organs with varying amounts of barium suspension, gas, or air; and obtaining views of the mucosal surfaces. An upper gastrointestinal examination may be done with a moderately dense barium suspension using the natural amount of air present in the upper gastrointestinal tract; this is usually called a *single-contrast upper gastrointestinal series* (Fig. 10-2). Another method involves the use of a high-density barium suspension plus gas-producing crystals and is called a *double-contrast upper gastrointestinal series* (Fig. 10-3).

The esophagus consists mainly of a tubular portion with a bell-shaped termination called the esophageal vestibule (Fig. 10-4). The esophagogastric junction normally lies within or below the esophageal hiatus. When the esophagogastric junction lies above the hiatus, hiatal hernia is present, which is the most common structural abnormality found on upper gastrointestinal examination. The esophageal mucosal surface has a smooth appearance when distended and shows smooth, thin longitudinal folds when the organ is collapsed. Esophageal peristalsis can be observed by having the patient swallow single volumes of barium suspension.

The stomach has a complex shape that varies considerably depending on the degree of distension. When the stomach is collapsed, the rugal folds are seen prominently and may mimic focal or diffuse gastric disorders. With gastric distension, the rugal folds are flattened, and the mucosal surface of the stomach is seen more effectively (Fig. 10-5). A fine reticulated mucosal pattern of the stomach called the areae gastricae may be appreciated, especially when high-density barium suspensions are used. Barium studies of the upper gastrointestinal tract evaluate gastric function poorly; radionuclide gastric emptying studies are more effective for this purpose.

The duodenum is attached to the stomach at the narrow pylorus and consists of the duodenal bulb and the descending and ascending portions, although a horizontal segment is often added (Fig. 10-6). The duodenum terminates at the duodenojejunal flexure, which is attached to the ligament of Treitz. The duodenal bulb has a triangular

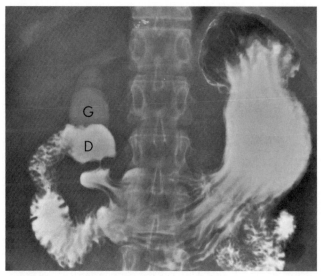

FIG. 10-2 Prone frontal radiograph of stomach and duodenum from a single-contrast upper gastrointestinal examination. The duodenal bulb (D) is attached to the gastric antrum by the pyloric channel. The gallbladder (G) is also opacified from an oral cholecystogram.

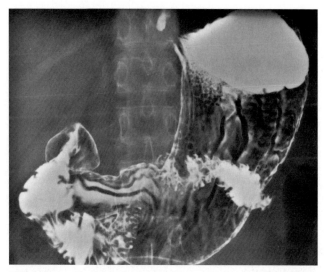

FIG. 10-3 Supine frontal film of the stomach and duodenum from a double-contrast upper gastrointestinal examination in which a high-density barium suspension and gas crystals (CO_2) are used. Compared with the preceding figure, the stomach is better distended primarily by the generated gas.

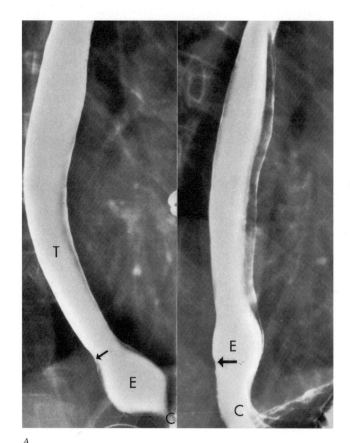

A

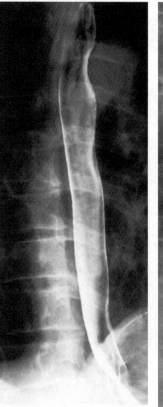

B

FIG. 10-4 (*A*) Full-column radiograph of the normal esophagus (*left*) with the patient drinking barium rapidly in the prone oblique position. The tubular esophagus (T) joins the esophageal vestibule (E) at the tubulovestibular junction (*arrow*). The lower end of the esophageal vestibule is constricted (C) at the level of the diaphragmatic hiatus. In another patient (*right*), the esophagogastric junction (*arrow*) lies above the level of the diaphrag-

matic hiatus (C), indicating the presence of hiatal hernia (E = esophageal vestibule). (*B*) Double-contrast (*left*) and mucosal relief (*right*) films of the esophagus. Multiple radiographic techniques are combined to evaluate the esophagus to optimize the efficacy of the examination. (*C*) Hiatal hernia (hh) protruding above the diaphragmatic hiatus and demarcated from the esophageal vestibule (v) at the esophagogastric junction (*arrows*).

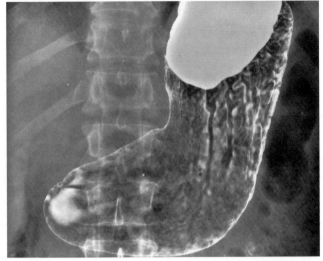

A

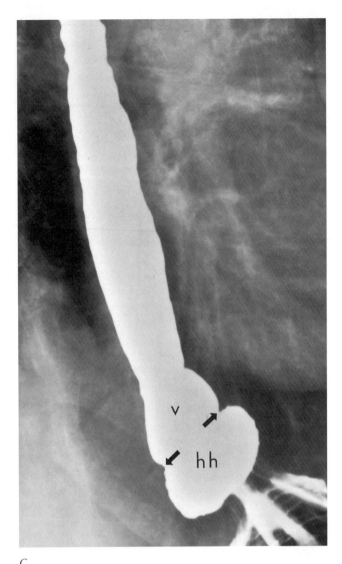

C

FIG. 10-4 (*Continued*)

or heart-shaped appearance, normally tapering to the apex of the bulb with its junction with the descending portion. The bulbar mucosal surface is normally smooth. The duodenum assumes a C-shaped configuration within the upper abdomen, and the mucosal folds have a circumferential and symmetric appearance throughout its length.

SMALL INTESTINE
The radiographic examination of the small bowel evaluates the mesenteric portion of the organ, which consists of the jejunum and ileum. The following three methods can be used to examine the small intestine: (1) peroral small bowel series, (2) enteroclysis, and (3) various retrograde techniques. The peroral small bowel series is used most commonly and is often done immediately following an upper gastrointestinal series. The patient ingests 16 to 24 oz of an appropriate barium suspension, and serial films of the abdomen are obtained in a timely order (Fig. 10-7). In ad-

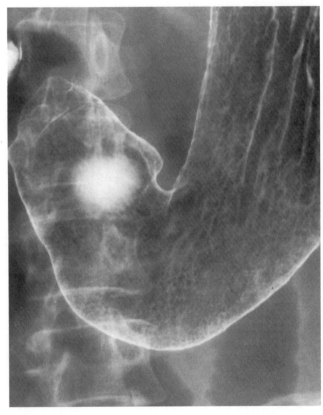

B

FIG. 10-5 (*A*) Double-contrast radiograph of the stomach with the patient in the supine position. In the body of the stomach, posterior wall rugal folds are seen as long lucent defects surrounded by the barium suspension, and anterior rugal folds are etched by a coating of the contrast material. (*B*) Double-contrast film of the lower gastric body and antrum. The areae gastricae are seen as a fine reticulated pattern, especially in the lowest portion of the stomach, while larger and linear rugal folds are present in the upper gastric body.

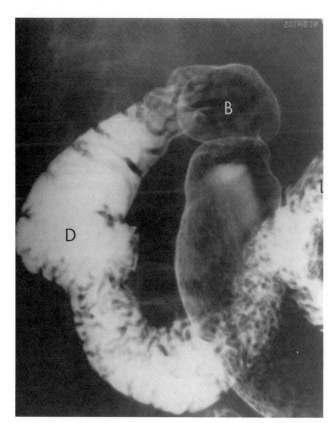

FIG. 10-6 Radiograph of the duodenum showing the duodenal bulb (B) attached to the gastric antrum. The descending duodenum (D) extends from the apex of the bulb to the inferior duodenal flexure. The horizontal and ascending portions of the duodenum terminate at the duodenojejunal junction (L), which is attached to the ligament of Treitz.

dition, smaller films with pressure on the abdomen (i.e., compression) are used to separate and visualize all the loops of the small bowel; the entire small bowel, including the terminal ileum, is filmed in this fashion.

Enteroclysis is an intubated examination of the small intestine and can be done by several techniques. The small intestine is intubated by a nasal or oral route with a small-bore enteric tube that is directed with fluoroscopic guidance into the distal duodenum or proximal jejunum (Fig. 10-8). In the single-contrast method, a dilute barium suspension is allowed to flow into the small bowel by gravity. Other techniques include the use of a dense and more viscous barium suspension along with water, air, or a methylcellulose solution to produce a "double-contrast" effect. Compared with the peroral small bowel examination, the enteroclysis techniques permit better control of small bowel distension and more exact visualization of small bowel loops.

Retrograde examination of the small bowel involves filling of the organ from the opposite direction. A number of techniques are used depending on the patient's anatomy (Fig. 10-9). Reflux of the small intestine through the ileocecal valve can be done as part of a barium enema. If the patient has an ileostomy, various devices can be introduced

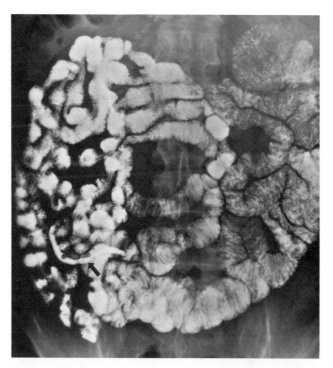

A

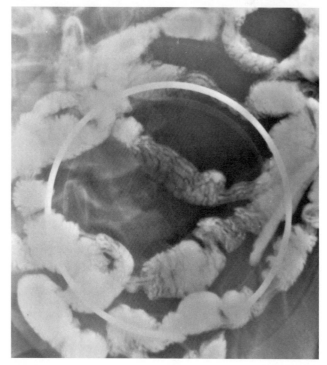

B

FIG. 10-7 (*A*) Large film of the abdomen from a peroral small bowel examination with the entire small intestine opacified with barium suspension. On the left side of the abdomen, the jejunum shows a more typical "feathery" pattern of the mucosal folds compared with the ileum, which is smaller in caliber and has fewer folds in the right lower abdomen. The appendix (arrow) is also visualized. (*B*) Compression film (balloon paddle is identified by the circular metallic ring) of the small bowel from a peroral examination with separation and clear visualization of the small bowel loops.

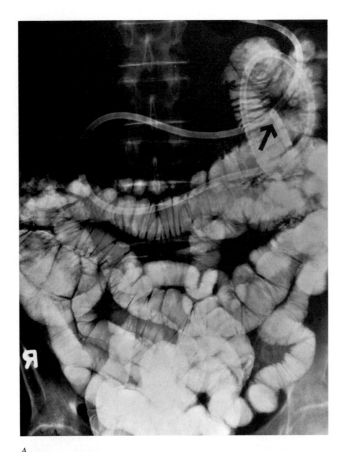

A

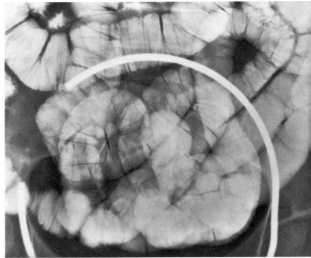

B

FIG. 10-8 (*A*) Large film of the abdomen from an enteroclysis examination of the small intestine. The small bowel is intubated with the tip of the tube (*arrow*) in the jejunum. Compared with the peroral examination, the small bowel loops are distended more fully, causing the mucosal folds to assume a transverse orientation. (*B*) Compression film (ring of balloon paddle) of the small bowel loops in the pelvis with the patient in a prone position. Although the loops are overlapped, the "see-through" effect using a dilute barium suspension permits their clear visualization.

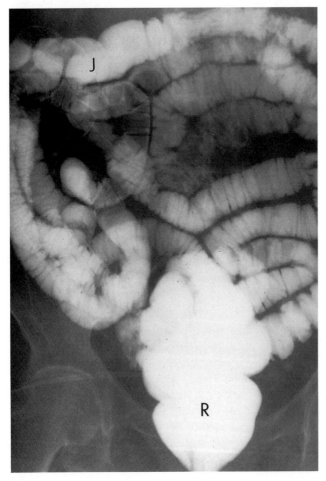

A

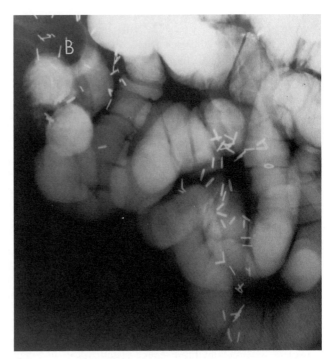

B

FIG. 10-9 (*A*) Reflux examination of most of the small intestine from a barium enema (R = rectum) in a patient following a right hemicolectomy for colon carcinoma who presents with rectal bleeding. The ileocolic junction (J) is located in the right upper abdomen. (*B*) Reflux study of the small bowel via an ileostomy in a patient following total colectomy for ulcerative colitis. A Foley catheter was inserted into the ileostomy and the balloon (B) distended with air to prevent leakage at the cutaneous site.

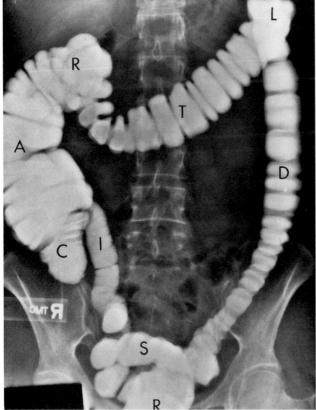

A

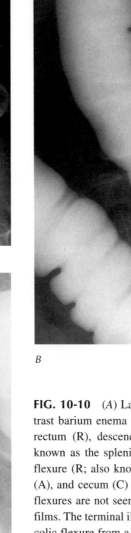

B

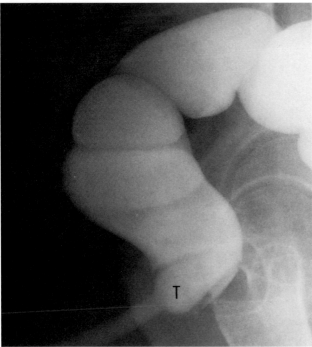

C

FIG. 10-10 (*A*) Large film of the abdomen from a single-contrast barium enema with the patient in the supine position. The rectum (R), descending colon (D), left colic flexure (L; also known as the splenic flexure), transverse colon (T), right colic flexure (R; also known as the hepatic flexure); ascending colon (A), and cecum (C) are visualized. The sigmoid colon and colic flexures are not seen well in this position and require additional films. The terminal ileum (I) has refluxed from the colon. (*B*) Left colic flexure from a single-contrast examination with the patient turned to the right shows clear separation of the upper descending colon and distal transverse colon. (*C*) Lateral radiograph of the rectum from a single-contrast barium enema. The rectal tip (T) is located in the lower rectum. The valves of Houston are seen as transverse folds crossing the lumen of the rectum.

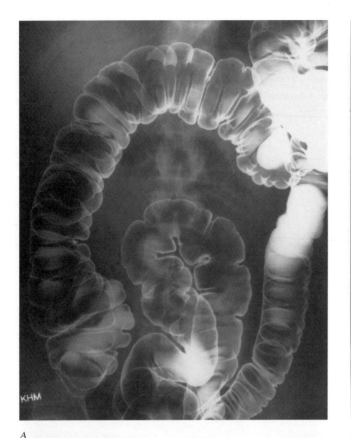

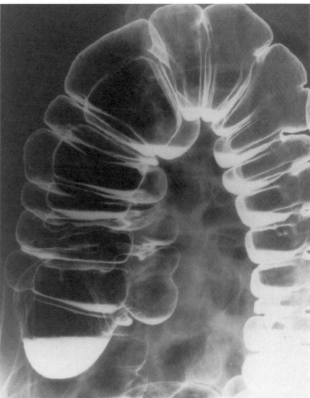

A

B

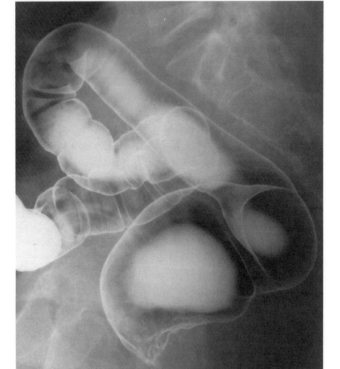

C

FIG. 10-11   (*A*) Large film of abdomen from a double-contrast barium enema with the patient in the supine position. The double-contrast effect is produced by coating the mucosal surface of the colon with a moderately dense, viscous barium suspension and distending the organ with air; a specially designed enema tip is needed for the examination. (*B*) Double-contrast radiograph of the right colic or hepatic flexure with the patient turned toward the left with separation of the ascending colon and proximal transverse colon to improve visualization. (*C*) Double-contrast film of the rectum and a portion of the sigmoid colon with the patient in a lateral position.

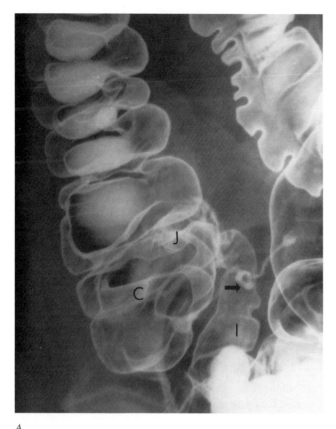

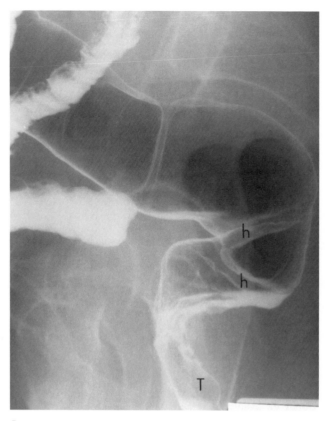

A

B

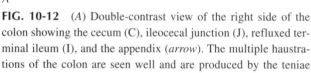

FIG. 10-12 (*A*) Double-contrast view of the right side of the colon showing the cecum (C), ileocecal junction (J), refluxed terminal ileum (I), and the appendix (*arrow*). The multiple haustrations of the colon are seen well and are produced by the teniae coli. (B) Double-contrast appearance of the rectum with the patient in the lateral position. The valves of Houston (h) are shown clearly. The rectal tip (T) has migrated into the anal canal.

into the ostomy site and a barium suspension instilled directly.

The length of the mesenteric small bowel in adults averages about 20 ft but varies considerably among individuals. The jejunum comprises just over a third of the length, and the ileum, the remainder, although no discrete transition is seen between the two segments. The normally distended small bowel has a caliber of 2 to 3 cm, being slightly larger, more orad in the jejunum. Depending on the degree of distension, the mucosal folds (valvulae conniventes) may have a feathery appearance or may be transversely oriented across the intestinal lumen with more complete distension. The mucosal folds are more numerous in the jejunum and gradually decrease in number and size in the ileum.

LARGE INTESTINE

The radiographic examination of the large bowel evaluates the entire organ from the rectum to the cecum. Reflux of barium suspension into the ileum and the appendix, if present, occurs commonly. As with upper gastrointestinal ex-

aminations, the colon can be evaluated by the following techniques: (1) single-contrast barium enema and (2) double-contrast barium enema. Both examinations require insertion of a rectal tip for instillation of the examining materials. The single-contrast barium enema is performed using a low-density barium suspension that flows into the colon through the rectal tip (Fig. 10-10). Small films with abdominal pressure applied to the area of interest are exposed as each segment of the colon is opacified. A series of larger films is also obtained with the patient in various frontal and oblique positions.

The double-contrast barium enema is performed with a special rectal tip that allows instillation and removal of a dense and more viscous barium suspension as well as instillation of air. The double-contrast effect is produced by the combined use of the barium suspension and the air (Fig. 10-11). As with the single-contrast method, all segments of the colon are examined with the patient in various positions, and both large and small films are obtained.

The large intestine consists of the rectum, sigmoid colon, descending colon, splenic flexure, transverse colon, hepatic flexure, ascending colon, and cecum. The length of the colon varies considerably among adults, depending mainly on the length and redundancy of the sigmoid colon and the colic flexures. The colon varies in caliber depending on location and the degree of luminal distension. The mucosal surface has a smooth appearance, and the colonic contour is indented by the haustra, which are less numerous in the descending portion of the colon (Fig. 10-12). The rectal valves of Houston are often seen, especially on the double-contrast barium enema. The ileocecal valve has a variety of appearances and may appear large if infiltrated with fat, mimicking a neoplasm.

Other Imaging Modalities

Fiberoptic gastrointestinal endoscopy and newer cross-sectional imaging techniques have had an impact on the number and types of traditional luminal contrast examinations performed on the gastrointestinal tract. In addition to endoscopy, these newer techniques include CT imaging, abdominal ultrasound, and magnetic resonance (MR) imaging. Each of these imaging modalities will be discussed briefly to illustrate their impact on luminal contrast radiology.

ENDOSCOPY

Upper gastrointestinal endoscopy visualizes the mucosal surfaces of the esophagus, stomach, and duodenum. The pharynx and often the distal portion of the duodenum are not evaluated. Also, endoscopy does not assess functional abnormalities of the pharynx, esophagus, and stomach. The major advantage of endoscopy compared with barium examination of the upper gastrointestinal tract is better demonstration of milder inflammatory processes, such as small peptic ulcers and erosions.

Endoscopy of the mesenteric portions of the small intestine has become possible in recent years, although the technology is evolving. A number of enteroscopes have been developed, and several techniques are available to examine the jejunum and ileum; however, complete endoscopic visualization of the entire mesenteric small intestine remains difficult at present. Enteroscopy can be used to evaluate patients with diffuse small bowel disease, especially if biopsy is needed, and those with unexplained gastrointestinal bleeding.

Colonoscopy is both a diagnostic and therapeutic modality. Inflammatory and neoplastic diseases of the colon are evaluated accurately. Biopsies can be obtained when needed. Using various techniques, the majority of colonic polyps can be removed through the colonoscope. When compared with the barium enema, colonoscopy is associated with more complications, including colonic perforation, and a higher mortality.

CT IMAGING

CT imaging of the chest and abdomen can portray the various organs of the gastrointestinal tract. Mucosal disease, such as ulcers, and small neoplasms will not be shown with this imaging modality. Larger gastrointestinal neoplasms, thickening of the walls of the hollow organs, and extrinsic processes can be detected with CT imaging. A major role of CT scanning, especially in the esophagus and colon, is the staging of malignancy of these organs. In the colon, for example, CT examination is used for initial staging, especially of distant metastases, and for evaluation of recurrence following surgery. Recurrent masses appearing after surgery also may be biopsied percutaneously.

ABDOMINAL ULTRASOUND

Abdominal ultrasound has not had a major impact on evaluation of the hollow organs of the gastrointestinal tract because of their location and the problem with gas interfering with the transmission of sound. However, ultrasound can be used to assess for acute appendicitis. Endoluminal ultrasound using blind probes or those attached to an endoscope has been used in the upper gastrointestinal tract and rectum to stage malignancy.

MR IMAGING

MR imaging is the newest modality developed for cross-sectional imaging of the body, and nearly all organ systems can be evaluated with this technique. MR imaging of the hollow organs of the gastrointestinal tract is being used mainly to evaluate and stage malignancies, especially of the esophagus and rectum.

TECHNIQUE SELECTION

Patient Preparation

Preparation of the patient is needed for contrast examinations of the gastrointestinal tract and varies with the organ system being evaluated. The upper gastrointestinal tract and small bowel require minimal preparation when compared with the colon. No preparation is needed if only the pharynx and esophagus are being examined. For an upper gastrointestinal or small bowel examination, the patient should have nothing orally after midnight nor the next morning preceding the radiographic study. Fluid and food in the stomach and small intestine degrade the examination by interfering with good mucosal visualization and causing artifactual defects that may mimic disease. Also, if patients are to have other imaging examinations that may introduce fluid into the upper gastrointestinal tract, such as an abdominal CT study in which oral contrast material is used, the examinations must be scheduled on separate days.

Preparation for the barium enema examination is much more complicated and more strenuous for the patient, but it must be performed properly to obtain an accurate evaluation of the colon by this method. The presence of even small amounts of residual stool in the large bowel may mimic colonic disease, or a filling defect in the colon may be passed off as stool but be a neoplasm. Various colonic preparations have been recommended and usually combine the use of dietary changes, oral fluids, and several cathartics the day preceding the barium enema examination. At our institution, the standard preparation includes (1) a 24-h clear liquid diet, (2) oral hydration, (3) a saline cathartic (e.g., magnesium citrate) in the afternoon, (4) an irritant cathartic (e.g., castor oil) in the early evening, and (5) a tap water cleansing enema the morning of the radiographic examination 30 to 60 min before the barium enema is performed. Other cleansing options for the colon can be used if indicated clinically; for example, magnesium-containing cathartics are avoided in patients with renal failure.

Specific Contrast Examinations

A number of radiographic techniques are available to examine the gastrointestinal tract. Selection of an appropriate technique will depend on the clinical indications for the examination, the efficacy of the various techniques, and the age and physical condition of the patient being examined. Indications and efficacy of the specific contrast examinations will be emphasized. However, the age and physical condition of the patient also will affect the quality of the study performed and the types of examinations that can be done optimally.

UPPER GASTROINTESTINAL TRACT

The main indications for radiographic examination of the upper gastrointestinal tract include dysphagia, odynophagia, chest pain, pyrosis, suspicion of esophageal varices, dyspepsia, upper gastrointestinal bleeding, and evaluation of obstruction. Dysphagia may be of oropharyngeal or esophageal origin; a modified examination of the oral cavity and pharynx may be required in some patients. The most common diseases causing these symptoms that may be diagnosed by radiographic evaluation are esophageal and gastric malignancies, reflux esophagitis and peptic stricture, infectious esophagitis, lower esophageal mucosal ring, and peptic ulcers and erosions of the stomach and duodenum. Many of these diseases will be illustrated and discussed in the chapter exercises.

The efficacy of the radiographic examination of the upper gastrointestinal tract depends on the quality of the study performed and on the types of diseases being evaluated. The diseases that are detected most effectively include malignancies, peptic stricture, esophageal mucosal ring, moderate to severe reflux and infectious esophagitis, and peptic ulcers that are over 5 mm in size regardless of their location. The limitations of this examination are detection of milder inflammations, such as mild reflux esophagitis or early infectious esophagitis, small gastric and duodenal ulcers (i.e., less than 5 mm), and erosive gastritis and duodenitis.

SMALL INTESTINE

The more specific indications for small bowel examination include gastrointestinal bleeding that is not localized to the other organs of the gastrointestinal tract, diarrhea or, more specifically, steatorrhea, inflammatory bowel disease, intestinal obstruction, intraabdominal malignancy, and abdominal fistulas. The small bowel is not a common site for disease, and less specific symptoms, such as vague abdominal pain, do not warrant performance of a small bowel study. The diseases that can cause small bowel bleeding include Meckel's diverticulum, Crohn's disease, ischemic enteritis, and primary and secondary neoplasms. Small bowel obstruction is usually due to adhesions, external hernias, or intrinsic or extrinsic neoplasms. Rare diseases leading to malabsorption, such as sprue, are other considerations.

As with the upper gastrointestinal tract, the efficacy of radiographic examination of the small bowel depends on the type and quality of examination performed and the types of diseases being evaluated. The enteroclysis examination is often preferred for evaluating small bowel obstruction or potential focal lesions of the small intestine, such as Meckel's diverticulum. Most diseases of the small bowel are detected effectively by a properly performed radiographic examination. Limitations of small bowel studies, depending on the thoroughness of the examination done, include early inflammatory disease, localization of obstruction, focal structural disease, and peritoneal adhesions. Many of these diseases will be illustrated and discussed in the chapter exercises.

LARGE INTESTINE

The major indications for radiographic examination of the colon are rectal bleeding, suspicion of inflammatory bowel disease, question of neoplastic disease, and evaluation of colonic obstruction. The most common diseases causing colonic bleeding are diverticulosis, idiopathic colitis, larger colonic polyps and carcinoma, and ischemic colitis. Common causes of colonic obstruction include diverticulitis, colonic malignancy, volvulus of the large bowel, and extrinsic disorders, especially pelvic malignancy invading the rectosigmoid region of the colon. Most of these diseases will be illustrated and discussed in the chapter exercises.

As with the other studies discussed, the efficacy of the radiographic examination of the large bowel depends on the type and quality of examination performed and on the diseases being evaluated. The diseases that are detected most effectively include diverticular disease and its complications, more severe forms of idiopathic and ischemic colitis, larger colonic polyps (i.e., over 1 cm in size), and colonic carcinoma. The limitations of the barium enema include smaller colonic polyps less than 1 cm in size and mild inflammatory bowel disease, although the double-contrast examination of the colon is more effective than the single-contrast method in detecting these more subtle abnormalities. An important limitation of the barium enema in older patients is evaluation of vascular malformations. Finally, regarding active gastrointestinal bleeding, the radiographic examination can demonstrate lesions that may be bleeding but will not localize the exact site of bleeding; angiography or radionuclide studies are needed to pinpoint the bleeding site.

EXERCISE 10-1: DYSPHAGIA

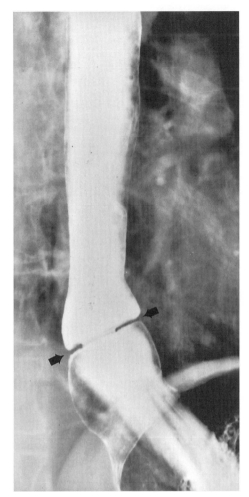

FIG. 10-E-1   *Panel A*

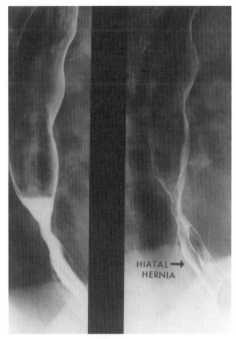

FIG. 10-E-2   *Panel A*

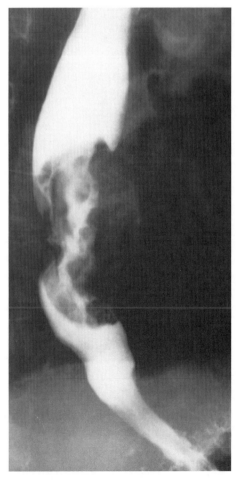

FIG. 10-E-3   *Panel A*

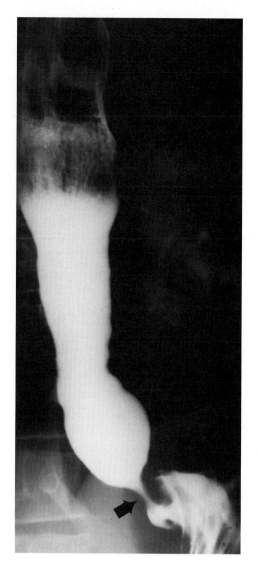

FIG. 10-E-4   *Panel A*

Clinical Histories:

CASE 10-1
A 55-year-old man presents with intermittent dysphagia for solid food (Fig. 10-E-1*A*).

CASE 10-2
A 35-year-old woman presents with gastroesophageal reflux symptoms who recently developed dysphagia (Fig. 10-E-2*A*).

CASE 10-3
A 65-year-old man presents with both dysphagia and odynophagia (Fig. 10-E-3*A*).

CASE 10-4
A 30-year-old woman presents with dysphagia and regurgitation (Fig. 10-E-4*A*).

Questions:

10-1. What is the most likely cause for the symmetric narrowing at the lower end of the esophagus (arrows) in Case 10-1?
  A. Carcinoma of the esophagus
  B. Peptic esophageal stricture
  C. Lower esophageal mucosal ring
  D. Achalasia of the esophagus
  E. None of the above

10-2. In Case 10-2, the smooth stricture above the hiatal hernia is most likely due to?
  A. *Candida* esophagitis
  B. Reflux esophagitis
  C. Herpetic esophagitis
  D. Caustic esophagitis
  E. Esophageal malignancy

10-3. The most likely cause of the focal, irregular esophageal narrowing in Case 10-3 is?
  A. Squamous cell carcinoma
  B. Adenocarcinoma
  C. Carcinoma complicating Barrett's esophagus
  D. Benign peptic stricture from reflux disease
  E. Stricture from caustic esophagitis

10-4. In Case 10-4, aperistalsis of the esophagus was present associated with smooth narrowing at the lower end of the esophagus (*arrow*) suggesting?
  A. Stricture in Barrett's esophagus
  B. Stricture in sclerodermic esophagus
  C. Peptic stricture from reflux esophagitis
  D. Achalasia of the esophagus
  E. Secondary achalasia due to gastric carcinoma

Radiologic Findings:

10-1. This case shows a smooth, symmetric, thin annular narrowing at the lower end of the esophagus that is a lower esophageal mucosal ring (*C* is the correct answer to Question 10-1).

10-2. This case demonstrates a smooth, tapered narrowing in the lower esophagus associated with a hiatal hernia that is typical for a peptic stricture (*B* is the correct answer to Question 10-2).

10-3. This case is an annular, irregular squamous cell carcinoma of the esophagus (*A* is the correct answer to Question 10-3).

10-4. This case represents idiopathic achalasia (*D* is the correct answer to Question 10-4).

Discussion:

Dysphagia is a frequent indication for radiographic examination of the esophagus. The most common esophageal causes of dysphagia are shown in the case presentations in this exercise.

The lower esophageal mucosal ring is an acquired thin, annular membrane of unknown cause that demarcates the esophagogastric junction and is a sign of hiatal hernia. More important, the mucosal ring is probably the most important cause of solid food dysphagia seen in adults. Several decades ago, Schatzki described the association of mucosal ring, which often bears his name, with dysphagia and determined that the prevalence of dysphagia related to the caliber of the ring. Rings over 20 mm in diameter cause symptoms rarely; those less than 14 mm in diameter are nearly always symptomatic,

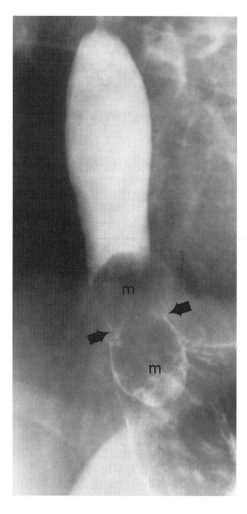

FIG. 10-E-1 (*Panel B*) Patient with solid food dysphagia and a mucosal ring measuring 16 mm in caliber. A one-half portion of a marshmallow (m) impacted at the level of the ring (*arrows*) and reproduced dysphagia.

FIG. 10-E-3 (*Panel B*) Patient with Barrett's esophagus complicated by an irregular adenocarcinoma, which may be difficult to distinguish from the accompanying changes of esophagitis and stricture. Adenocarcinoma occurs in about 5 to 10 percent of patients who have Barrett's esophagus, and periodic endoscopic surveillance is usually recommended.

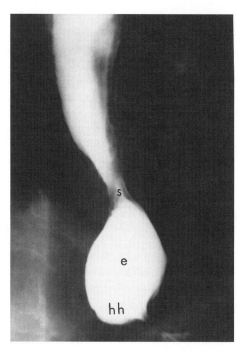

FIG. 10-E-2 (*Panel B*) Peptic stricture (s) above a normal intervening segment of esophagus (e) associated with a small hiatal hernia (hh). The esophagus between the hernia and stricture was lined by columnar epithelium at endoscopic examination.

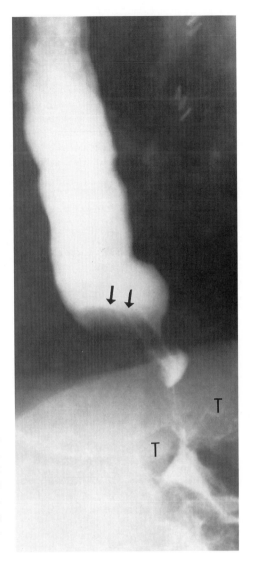

FIG. 10-E-4 (*Panel B*) An older patient with an abrupt onset of dysphagia and odynophagia. Narrowing and mass effect (*arrows*) are present at the lower end of the esophagus, which was also aperistaltic. These changes mimic idiopathic achalasia, but the tumor mass (T) in the proximal stomach proved to be a gastric adenocarcinoma causing secondary achalasia.

whereas mucosal rings 14 to 20 mm in diameter cause dysphagia in about half of patients. The mucosal ring is best detected radiographically, and use of a solid bolus, such as a portion of a marshmallow, optimizes detection of these rings and verifies the structure as a cause of dysphagia (Fig. 10-E-1*B*).

Peptic stricture of the esophagus is a complication of reflux esophagitis and is the second most common benign cause of dysphagia. Reflux strictures typically occur at the esophagogastric junction and are associated with a hiatal hernia in virtually all patients. Peptic strictures show a variety of morphologic appearances from a smooth, tapered appearance to an annular configuration that may resemble a mucosal ring. Irregularity of the stricture margin also may be seen and must be differentiated from an esophageal malignancy. Barrett's esophagus is another complication of gastroesophageal reflux disease and is suggested radiographically when a peptic stricture is located above the esophagogastric junction (Fig. 10-E-2*B*).

Squamous cell carcinoma is the most common primary malignancy of the esophagus, accounting for about 90 percent of esophageal cancers. The usual appearance of this malignancy is a focal, irregular narrowing with abrupt upper and lower margins, which rarely mimics a peptic stricture. Squamous cell carcinomas of the esophagus occur in older patients who often have a history of tobacco and alcohol abuse; this malignancy also may be multifocal and associated with similar lesions in the upper aerodigestive tract. Adenocarcinoma of the esophagus is seen less frequently but has increased in incidence in recent decades and is usually found in conjunction with Barrett's esophagus (Fig. 10-E-3*B*).

Idiopathic achalasia is a primary motility disorder of the esophagus of unknown cause that presents with dysphagia, regurgitation, and weight loss occasionally. The findings on esophageal manometry include total absence of primary esophageal peristalsis and a dysfunctional lower esophageal sphincter (i.e., failure of relaxation). The radiographic features mirror the manometric findings; aperistalsis is observed, and the lower end of the esophagus has a smooth, tapered, or "beaklike" appearance. In achalasia, hiatal hernia is an uncommon observation, which is usually seen in patients with peptic stricture or scleroderma of the esophagus. An important differential diagnosis is secondary achalasia due to an infiltrative gastric adenocarcinoma (Fig. 10-E-4*B*); patients are usually older and have a more abrupt onset of symptoms, which often include odynophagia.

EXERCISE 10-2: UPPER GASTROINTESTINAL BLEEDING

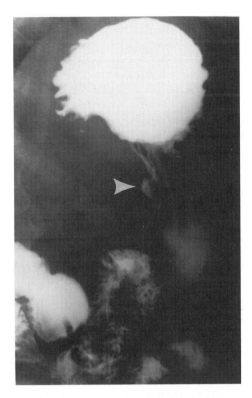

FIG. 10-E-5 *Panel A*

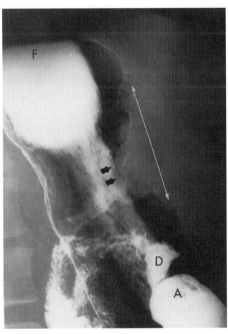

FIG. 10-E-6 *Panel A*

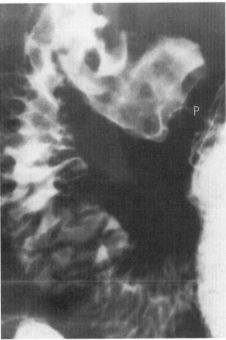

FIG. 10-E-7 *Panel A*

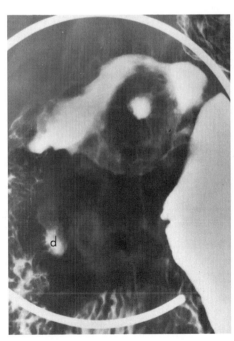

FIG. 10-E-8 *Panel A*

Clinical Histories:

CASE 10-5

A 28-year-old man presents with epigastric pain and occult blood in his stools. (Fig. 10-E-5*A*).

CASE 10-6

A 63-year-old woman presents with epigastric pain, weight loss, and anemia (Fig. 10-E-6*A*).

CASE 10-7

A 32-year-old alcoholic man presents with severe epigastric pain and hematemesis (Fig. 10-E-7*A*).

CASE 10-8

A 44-year-old woman presents with postprandial epigastric pain relieved with meals and occult blood in the stools (Fig. 10-E-8*A*).

Questions:

10-5. What is the most likely cause of the gastric lesion (*arrowhead*) shown in Case 10-5?
   A. Malignant gastric ulcer
   B. Gastric diverticulum
   C. Lymphoma of the stomach
   D. Polypoid carcinoma of the stomach
   E. Benign gastric ulcer

10-6. In Case 10-6, an irregular polypoid lesion (*arrows*) projects into the anterior body of the stomach (*F,* fundus; *A,* antrum; *D,* duodenal bulb). What is the *least* likely cause of this abnormality?
   A. Benign gastric ulcer
   B. Polypoid gastric carcinoma
   C. Gastric lymphoma
   D. Leiomyosarcoma of the stomach
   E. Secondary malignancy of the stomach

10-7. What is the best possibility for the nodular appearance of the duodenal bulb in Case 10-7 (*P,* pylorus)?
   A. Duodenal ulcer
   B. Erosive duodenitis
   C. Brunner's gland hyperplasia
   D. Duodenal carcinoma
   E. Multiple swallowed olive pits

10-8. In Case 10-8, what is the most likely cause of the barium collection seen in the duodenal bulb with the patient in the *prone* position (*d,* duodenal diverticulum)?
   A. Benign duodenal ulcer on posterior wall
   B. Malignant duodenal ulcer
   C. Benign duodenal polyp
   D. Benign duodenal ulcer on anterior wall
   E. None of the above

Radiologic Findings:

10-5. This case shows a small, smooth collection of barium projecting from the lesser curvature of the stomach associated with a lucent collar at the neck of the collection. This combination of findings indicates a benign gastric ulcer (*E* is the correct answer to Question 10-5).

10-6. This case shows an irregular, polypoid mass arising from the anterior wall of the stomach and projecting into the gastric lumen. A neoplasm of the stomach is the most likely cause, which in this patient was a primary adenocarcinoma. A benign gastric ulcer is the least likely explanation (*A* is the correct answer to Question 10-6).

10-7. This is a close-up film of the duodenal bulb and loop. Multiple nodules, some with central collections of barium, are present within the bulb and represent duodenal erosions (*B* is the correct answer to Question 10-7).

10-8. This case demonstrates a smooth collection of barium within the central portion of the duodenal bulb, which was an anterior wall duodenal ulcer (*D* is the correct answer to Question 10-8).

Discussion:

Many causes of upper gastrointestinal bleeding can be detected on a radiographic examination of this portion of the gastrointestinal tract. As illustrated in the cases of this exercise, gastric or duodenal erosions and ulcers and carcinoma of the stomach are the most important causes.

The radiographic features that suggest a benign gastric ulcer include (1) projection from the lumen of the stomach, (2) smooth lucent line (Hampton's line) or collar (as in this case) at the neck of the ulcer, (3) normal rugal folds that radiate to the edge of the ulcer collection, and (4) complete and permanent healing of the ulcer on repeat radiographic or endoscopic examination of the stomach. If at least two or more of these findings are present, a confident radiographic diagnosis of benign gastric ulcer is possible. A malignant gastric ulcer, which represents a small minority of all ulcers seen in the stomach, is suggested when the collection of barium within the ulcer is irregular and projects within the gastric lumen (i.e., within a neoplastic mass), a smooth line or collar at the ulcer margin is not present, or the rugal folds are nodular and terminate abruptly (Fig. 10-E-5*B*). Lack of healing of a gastric ulcer is not a specific sign of malignancy.

Adenocarcinoma is the most common primary malignancy of the stomach but has decreased in incidence recently in the United States. Gastric adenocarcinoma comprises about 95 percent of all primary malignancies of the stomach; lymphoma and leiomyosarcoma account for most of the remainder, although Kaposi's sarcoma is seen in patients with AIDS. The morphologic types of gastric carcinoma include ulcerative forms, polypoid or nodular lesions (Fig. 10-E-6*B*), and focal or diffuse infiltrative processes, especially if the histologic subtype is a scirrhous carcinoma (Fig. 10-E-6*C*). A properly performed radiographic examination of the stomach will detect virtually all gastric carcinomas.

Erosions in the stomach and duodenum are a common cause of upper gastrointestinal bleeding. Because these erosions may be few in number and small in size, endoscopic examination of the stomach and duodenum is more sensitive in their detection than radiologic evaluation. The radiographic features of duodenitis depend on the sever-

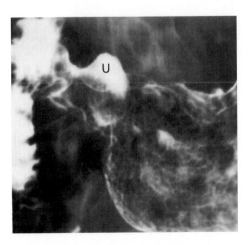

FIG. 10-E-5 (*Panel B*) An irregular ulcer (U) in the gastric antrum that does not project from the lumen nor show a smooth ulcer margin. Fixed antral narrowing was present, and the mucosal surface is distorted adjacent to the ulcer. An ulcerated adenocarcinoma of the stomach was found on biopsies from an endoscopic examination.

FIG. 10-E-6 (*Panel B*) Nodular fixed narrowing of the gastric antrum associated with a small nodule at the base of the duodenal bulb (*arrow*). Although gastric carcinoma would be a likely possibility, lymphoma of the stomach was diagnosed at surgery. (*Panel C*) Mildly irregular narrowing of the proximal half of the stomach due to scirrhous carcinoma, which may mimic benign narrowing of the stomach.

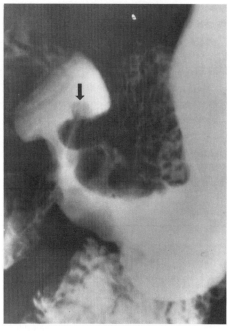

B

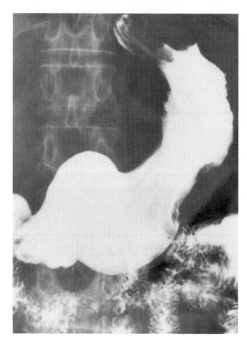

C

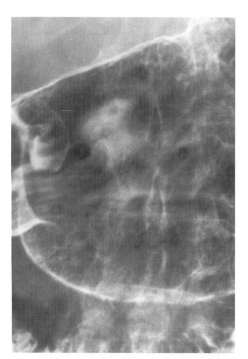

FIG. 10-E-7 (*Panel B*) Close-up double-contrast radiograph of the gastric antrum showing multiple erosions that appear as small nodular defects with a central punctate collection of barium. On endoscopic examination, erosions present as reddened nodules with a central yellow exudate at the site of mucosal disruption.

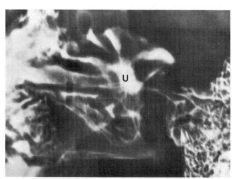

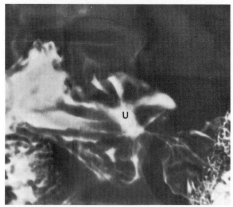

FIG. 10-E-8 (*Panel B*) Two views of the duodenal bulb with the patient in a supine position demonstrating a posterior wall ulcer (u) with radiating folds extending around the circumference of the barium collection.

ity of the disease and include thickening and nodularity of the duodenal folds or the presence of erosions that appear as punctate collections of barium centered on a nodule. Brunner's gland hyperplasia may have an appearance similar to duodenitis, but erosions are not seen and patients may not be symptomatic. Carcinoma of the duodenal bulb is extremely rare and does not typically enter the differential diagnosis of inflammatory lesions in this anatomic region. Gastric erosions also appear as nodular defects usually within the antrum of the stomach (Fig. 10-E-7B).

Approximately 95 percent of duodenal ulcers occur within the duodenal bulb and have about an equal distribution on the anterior and posterior walls of the duodenum. The remaining 5 percent of duodenal ulcers are located near the apex of the bulb. On radiographic examination, a duodenal ulcer is seen as a round or oval collection of barium that should maintain a fixed size and shape on multiple radiographs of the collection; inconsistent collections of barium, often seen in the duodenal fornices or at the apex or in the presence of bulbar deformity, may be mistaken for an active ulcer. Anterior wall duodenal ulcers are best shown with the patient in the prone position (as in this case), whereas posterior wall ulcers are seen well with the patient supine (Fig. 10-E-8B). As with duodenal carcinomas, polyps in the bulb are rare and would appear as lucent filling defects and not a collection of barium.

EXERCISE 10-3: SMALL BOWEL BLEEDING

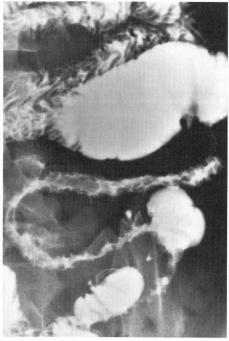

FIG. 10-E-9   *Panel A*

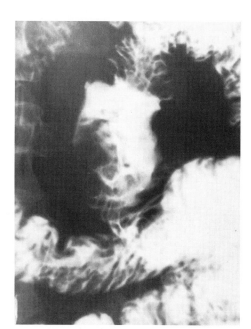

FIG. 10-E-10   *Panel A*

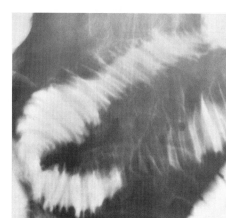

FIG. 10-E-11   *Panel A*

FIG. 10-E-12   *Panel A*

Clinical Histories:

CASE 10-9
A 24-year-old woman presents with intermittent abdominal pain, diarrhea, and anemia (Fig. 10-E-9*A*).

CASE 10-10
A 48-year-old man presents with rectal bleeding but no other symptoms (Fig. 10-E-10*A*).

CASE 10-11

A 72-year-old woman presents with sudden onset of abdominal pain and occult rectal bleeding (Fig. 10-E-11*A*).

CASE 10-12

A 58-year-old man presents with abdominal pain, anemia, and intermittent rectal bleeding (Fig. 10-E-12*A*).

Questions:

10-9. Radiographic examination of the small bowel in Case 10-9 is suggestive of which disease?
A. Crohn's disease
B. Tuberculosis
C. Whipple's disease
D. Lymphoma of small bowel
E. Small bowel metastases

10-10. Which is the most likely explanation of the saccular structure (*x*) seen in the distal small bowel?
A. Normal loop of small bowel
B. Large ulcer of small bowel
C. Meckel's diverticulum
D. Ulcerated small bowel malignancy
E. None of the above

10-11. What is the *least* likely explanation for the diffuse fold thickening in the central small bowel in Case 10-11?
A. Ischemic enteritis
B. Small bowel hemorrhage
C. Radiation enteritis
D. Small bowel edema
E. Malignancy of small bowel

10-12. In Case 10-12, select the *least* likely possibility to explain the irregular, ulcerated small bowel lesion?
A. Leiomyosarcoma
B. Ulcerated lymphoma
C. Metastatic ulcerated mass
D. Large benign small bowel ulcer
E. Ulcerated adenocarcinoma

Radiologic Findings:

10-9. This case demonstrates multifocal segments of narrowed and nodular small bowel most consistent with Crohn's disease (*A* is the correct answer to Question 10-9). Tuberculosis could appear similar but is rare, and neoplasms of the bowel typically present as focal masses.

10-10. This case shows a smooth, saccular structure of the distal small bowel that proved to be a Meckel's diverticulum (*C* is the correct answer to Question 10-10). Benign ulcers of the small bowel are rare, and ulcerated malignancies are usually irregular in appearance.

10-11. This case illustrates a long segment of small bowel of normal caliber with smooth thickening of the folds (i.e., valvulae conniventes). This appearance is usually due to submucosal infiltration of fluid (i.e., edema) or blood and can be seen in all the choices given except a small bowel malignancy (*E* is the correct answer to Question 10-11). This patient had ischemic enteritis.

10-12. This case shows an expansible ulcerated mass of the small bowel that usually occurs in an ulcerated malignancy of various histologic types, including metastatic neoplasms. In this case, the cause was lymphoma. As stated previously, benign small bowel ulcers are extremely rare (*D* is the correct answer to Question 10-12).

Discussion:

Small bowel bleeding and obstruction can be caused by a wide assortment of diseases, some of which may present with both signs. Crohn's disease and ischemia of the small bowel are likely the two most common causes in younger and older patients, respectively.

Crohn's disease is an inflammatory disorder of the gastrointestinal tract of unknown etiology. The small bowel and the ileocecal region are the most common sites of involvement. Crohn's disease may affect a single segment, often the terminal ileum, or multiple areas of the small bowel with normal intervening loops (i.e., skip segments). The involved bowel is usually narrowed with a nodular mucosal surface due to crisscrossing transverse and longitudinal ulcerations. Deeper ulcerations can progress to sinus tracts and fistulas with adjacent organs. Marked narrowing of the bowel lumen from inflammation and spasm may mimic stricture and cause partial small bowel obstruction (Fig. 10-E-9*B*).

Meckel's diverticulum is one of the most common anomalies of the gastrointestinal tract and occurs in about 2 to 3 percent of the general population. The diverticulum is usually asymptomatic and is found incidentally, but it may be a cause of intestinal bleeding if the structure contains ulcerated ectopic gastric mucosa. When shown on radiographic examination of the small bowel, especially using the enteroclysis technique, Meckel's diverticulum appears as a changeable saccular outpouching along the antimesenteric border of the bowel within a short distance from the terminal ileum. A rarer complication of a Meckel's diverticulum is inversion into the lumen of the small bowel with subsequent obstruction (Figs. 10-E-10*B,C*).

Ischemic disease of the small intestine can be caused by nonobstructive hypoperfusion of the organ or result from thrombotic or embolic vascular disease. The radiographic findings are variable depending on the extent and severity of the underlying process and

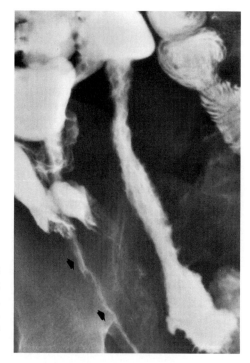

FIG. 10-E-9 (*Panel B*) Another patient with Crohn's disease of the distal small bowel with narrowing and irregularity of several segments. The terminal ileum (arrows) is severely narrowed, an appearance called the "string sign," which is often due to spasm.

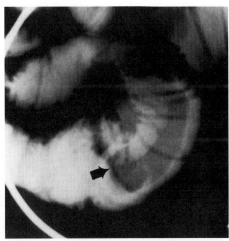

B

FIG. 10-E-10 (*Panel B*) Inverted Meckel's diverticulum (*arrow*) appearing as a luminal filling defect in the ileum and simulating a polypoid neoplasm. (*Panel C*) CT of inverted Meckel's diverticulum showing a central fat density (*arrow*). (*Used with permission from Chen YM et al: Inverted Meckel's diverticulum. Comput Med Imaging Graph 13:477, 1989.*)

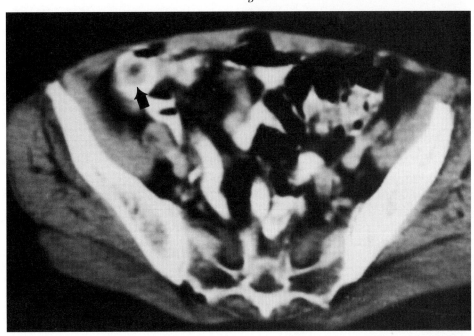

C

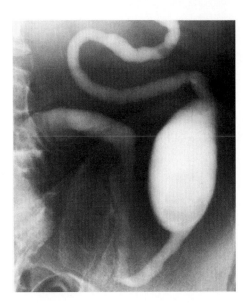

FIG. 10-E-11 (*Panel B*) Another patient with small bowel ischemia that progressed to diffuse multifocal stricture.

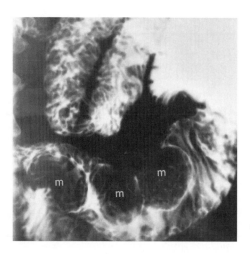

FIG. 10-E-12 (*Panel B*) Multiple polypoid metastases (m) to the small bowel from a malignant melanoma. (*Used with permission from Chen MYM et al: Radiology of the Small Bowel. New York, Igaku-Shoin, 1992.*)

its duration and promptness of treatment. Small bowel dilatation from ileus or narrowing due to spasm and submucosal edema and hemorrhage are opposite appearances that may be seen. Submucosal infiltration of the small bowel, as seen in ischemic enteritis, may occur in other disorders and have identical appearances; small bowel hemorrhages related to anticoagulants, trauma, hemophilia, or vasculitis from many causes are other considerations. Also, edematous conditions (e.g., hypoproteinemia and heart or renal failure) are further causes. Small bowel ischemia may resolve spontaneously or progress to perforation; stricture is a late complication (Fig. 10-E-11*B*).

Primary small bowel neoplasms are rare. Benign neoplasms of the small intestine are less often symptomatic compared with malignancies. Adenomas, lipomas, and leiomyomas are the most common benign neoplasms but comprise only 60 percent of the benign total due to a large number of miscellaneous lesions. Symptomatic small bowel neoplasms are usually malignant, and nearly all are adenocarcinoma, lymphoma, carcinoid tumor, or leiomyosarcoma. These malignancies, along with metastatic neoplasm to the small bowel (Fig. 10-E-12*B*), show a wide spectrum of appearances varying from polypoid and ulcerated masses (as in this case) to multifocal and infiltrative processes.

EXERCISE 10-4: SMALL BOWEL OBSTRUCTION

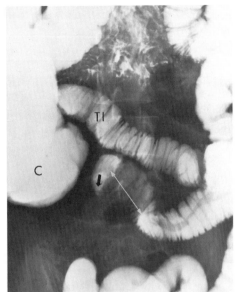

FIG. 10-E-13 *Panel A*

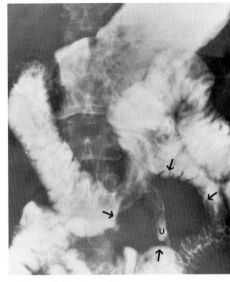

FIG. 10-E-14 *Panel A*

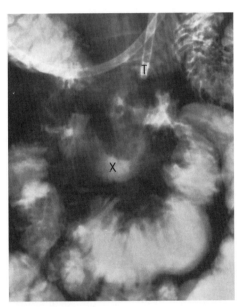

FIG. 10-E-15 *Panel A*

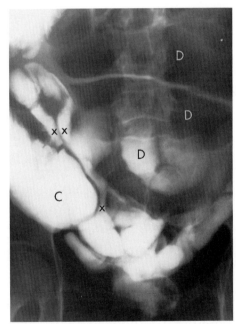

FIG. 10-E-16 *Panel A*

Clinical Histories:

CASE 10-13
A 38-year-old woman with previous abdominal surgery presents with distension of the abdomen and vomiting (Fig. 10-E-13*A*).

CASE 10-14
A 68-year-old man presents with abdominal pain, vomiting, and a mass in the abdomen on physical examination (Fig. 10-E-14*A*).

CASE 10-15

A 56-year-old man is seen who had epigastric pain and nausea (Fig. 10-E-15*A*).

CASE 10-16

A 42-year-old woman with a gynecologic malignancy presents with abdominal distension and vomiting (Fig. 10-E-16*A*).

Questions:

10-13. Barium enema (*C*, cecum) with reflux into a normal terminal ileum (TI) shows a small bowel obstruction (*arrow*) and a lucent band (*connected arrows*) most likely due to?
A. Ileocolic intussusception
B. Obstructing adhesions
C. Meckel's diverticulum
D. Small bowel volvulus
E. Polypoid malignancy

10-14. What is the *least* likely cause for the small bowel mass (*arrows*) with central ulceration (*u*) causing obstruction in Case 10-14?
A. Lymphoma of the small bowel
B. Ulcerated leiomyosarcoma
C. Leiomyoma with central ulceration
D. Metastatic mass with ulceration
E. Adenocarcinoma of small bowel

10-15. Enteroclysis (*T*, tip of tube) shows an angulated small bowel mass (*X*) in the proximal jejunum that is *least* likely to be?
A. Carcinoid tumor
B. Metastatic mass
C. Small bowel lymphoma
D. Polypoid mass with intussusception
E. Adenocarcinoma of small bowel

10-16. Barium enema (*C*, cecum) with reflux in the small bowel with multiple areas of ileal narrowing (*x*) and proximal small bowel dilatation (*D*) that is most likely due to?
A. Peritoneal adhesions
B. Primary small bowel carcinomas
C. Peritoneal metastases
D. Radiation enteritis
E. Small bowel intussusceptions

Radiologic Findings:

10-13. This case shows obstruction of the distal small bowel with a lucent band caused by adhesions (*B* is the correct answer to Questions 10-13).

10-14. This case demonstrates an ulcerated small bowel mass that is most likely a primary or metastatic malignancy. Lymphoma and leiomyosarcoma (the diagnosis in this patient) would be the most likely considerations. Adenocarcinoma usually does not present as a large mass displacing adjacent small bowel loops (*E* is the correct answer to Question 10-14).

10-15. This case displays an angulated mass in the proximal small bowel that is most likely a primary or metastatic neoplasm. Adenocarcinoma would more likely cause focal narrowing and may have this appearance, although in this patient a carcinoid tumor was found at surgery. A polypoid neoplasm with intussusception would present with focal dilatation (*D* is the correct answer to Question 10-15).

10-16. This case shows obstruction of the distal small bowel at multiple sites on a reflux examination. With a history of gynecologic malignancy, peritoneal metastasis with serosal implants causing obstruction is a common occurrence (*C* is the correct answer to Question 10-16).

Discussion:

The most common causes of small bowel obstruction are adhesions, hernias, and primary or secondary neoplasms of the small intestine. External hernias (e.g., inguinal canal) causing bowel obstruction are seen less often in recent decades, and internal hernias remain uncommon.

Peritoneal adhesions most often cause small bowel obstruction in adults. Previous abdominal surgery is the usual explanation for development of peritoneal adhesions. The patient described in Case 10-13 had previous abdominal surgery and presented with suspected small bowel obstruction on plain films of the abdomen. A nasogastric tube had been placed, and injection of contrast material into the stomach caused further vomiting; also, dilution of the contrast material in a dilated, fluid-filled jejunum degraded the examination. Consequently, a barium enema was performed with the main purpose being to reflux the distal small bowel to the level of obstruction, which was accomplished. Whether to perform an antegrade (i.e., peroral examination or enteroclysis) or retrograde study of the small bowel in suspected obstruction is not easily decided and is often based on clinical correlation and findings on plain films of the abdomen. Focal small bowel obstruction is diagnosed on contrast examination by demonstrating an area of caliber transition from dilated to normal-caliber bowel. If angulated loops are seen at a caliber transition in the absence of a mass effect, adhesions are a likely cause of the obstruction (Fig. 10-E-13*B*).

Small bowel malignancies were discussed briefly in the preceding exercise. Adenocarcinomas of the small bowel occur most often in the duodenum and jejunum and are much less common in the ileum. The morphologic appearances of adenocarcinomas of the small intestine consist of polypoid, ulcerative, stenosing, and infiltrative forms, which are similar to their counterparts in the stomach and colon. Primary lymphomas of the small bowel are a heterogeneous group of tumors, and controversy persists regarding definition of primary and secondary forms of this neoplasm. Lymphomas may involve any level of the small intestine but are most common in the ileum; the gross pathologic patterns include nodular or polypoid masses, constricting lesions that resemble carcinoma, or a more diffusely infiltrative process.

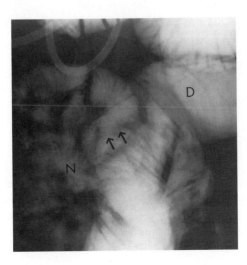

FIG. 10-E-13 (*Panel B*) Enteroclysis examination (tube in upper left corner) in a patient with suspected small bowel obstruction. Caliber transition is seen between dilated (D) and normal (N) bowel with angulated loops (*arrows*). Peritoneal adhesions were the cause of the obstruction at surgery.

Leiomyosarcoma and carcinoid tumor are the other two primary malignancies seen in the small bowel. Leiomyosarcomas (Fig. 10-E-14B) usually occur as single lesions and are most often found in the jejunum and ileum. Pathologically, this tumor typically presents as a polypoid lesion with an intraluminal and extramural component; a bulky, irregular mass is common, and ulceration with central necrosis can occur. Carcinoid tumors arise from enterochromaffin or similar-type cells, and more than 90 percent originate in the gastrointestinal tract. Most carcinoid tumors of the small bowel are located in the ileum. Their radiologic appearances reflect their broad pathologic morphology, and they may present as single or multiple polypoid lesions or as focal stenosis leading to partial obstruction; angulation and kinking of bowel loops may occur with a desmoplastic reaction and cause a mass that is best seen on cross-sectional imaging (Fig. 10-E-15B).

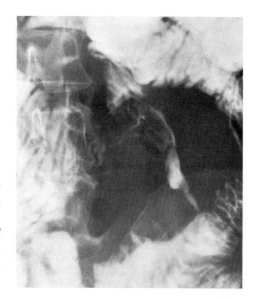

FIG. 10-E-14 (*Panel B*) Close-up view of the leiomyosarcoma of the small bowel in Case 10-14 which better demonstrates the central ulceration often seen in this malignancy. (*Used with permission from Chen MYM et al: Radiology of the Small Bowel. New York, Igaku-Shoin, 1992.*)

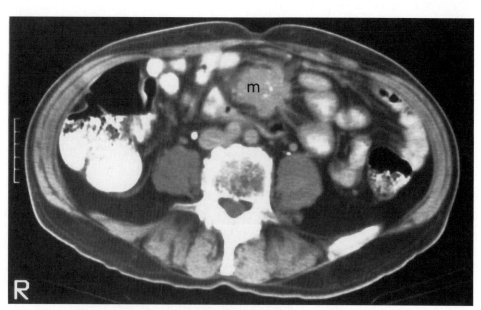

FIG. 10-E-15 (*Panel B*) CT image of the carcinoid tumor in Case 10-15 shows a mass (m) associated with the neoplasm that was not appreciated fully on the contrast examination of the small bowel. (*Used with permission from Chen MYM et al: Radiology of the Small Bowel. New York, Igaku-Shoin, 1992.*)

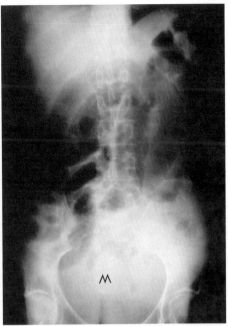

FIG. 10-E-16 (*Panel B*) A 55-year-old woman with advanced ovarian carcinoma presents with a large pelvic mass (M) and small bowel distension on plain film of the abdomen. (*Panel C*) Barium enema in this patient did not show colonic involvement, but reflux into a normal caliber terminal ileum (I) demonstrated angulated obstruction (arrows) of the small bowel due to the pelvic malignancy with more proximal dilated (D) bowel loops (C, cecum).

B

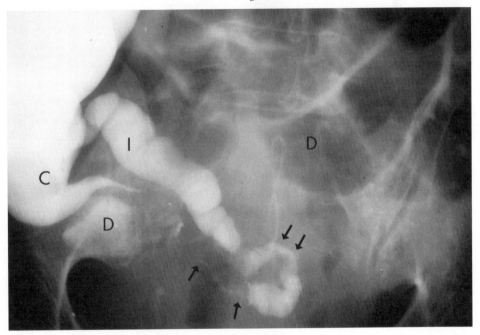

C

Secondary malignancies involving the small bowel are more common than the primary types. The three routes of secondary malignant spread to the small intestine include (1) hematogenous metastases (carcinoma of breast, lung, and melanoma most common), (2) intraperitoneal seeding of tumor from elsewhere within the abdomen, and (3) direct contiguous invasion of bowel (most often seen with pelvic malignancies). Carcinoma of the cervix, endometrium, or ovary often affects the distal small bowel by intraperitoneal seeding or direct invasion; the colon also may be involved, and radiographic evaluation of these patients may be best performed with a barium enema with one goal being reflux into the ileum (Figs. 10-E-16*B,C*).

EXERCISE 10-5: COLONIC BLEEDING

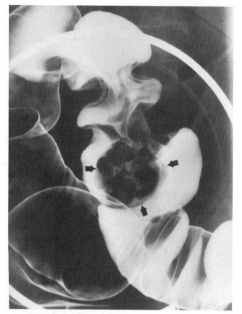

FIG. 10-E-17   *Panel A*

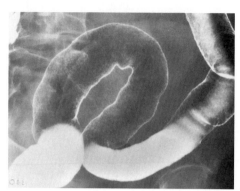

FIG. 10-E-19   *Panel A*

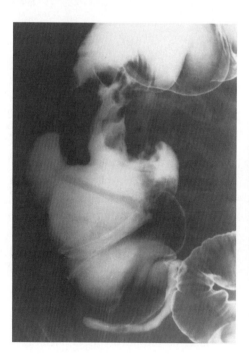

FIG. 10-E-18   *Panel A*

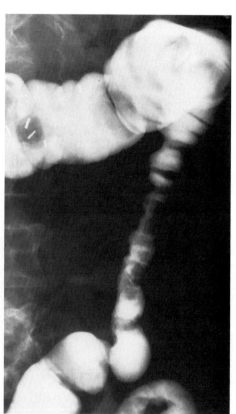

FIG. 10-E-20   *Panel A*

Clinical Histories: CASE 10-17
A 52-year-old woman presents with intermittent bright red rectal bleeding (Fig. 10-E-17A).

CASE 10-18
A 64-year-old man presents with melena and right-sided abdominal pain (Fig. 10-E-18A).

CASE 10-19
A 34-year-old woman presents with bloody diarrhea and tenesmus (Fig. 10-E-19A).

CASE 10-20
A 74-year-old man presents with cardiac disease and abrupt onset of hematochezia (Fig. 10-E-20A).

Questions:

10-17. What is the most likely cause of the large polypoid lesion (*arrows*) in the sigmoid colon of this patient?
   A. Annular carcinoma
   B. Benign lipoma
   C. Polypoid carcinoma
   D. Pedunculated benign adenoma
   E. Hyperplastic polyp

10-18. The irregular, focal narrowing in the ascending colon of this patient represents?
   A. Polypoid carcinoma
   B. Annular carcinoma
   C. Inflammatory stricture
   D. Surgical anastomosis
   E. Large lipoma

10-19. In Case 10-19, a double-contrast radiograph of the rectosigmoid region suggests what disease?
   A. Ischemic colitis
   B. Pseudomembranous colitis
   C. Lymphogranuloma venereum
   D. Crohn's colitis
   E. Ulcerative colitis

10-20. The irregular narrowing of the descending colon in Case 10-20 is most likely due to?
   A. Ischemic colitis
   B. Granulomatous colitis
   C. Ulcerative colitis
   D. Amebic colitis
   E. Pseudomembranous colitis

Radiologic Findings:

10-17. This case shows a large, lobulated (i.e., irregular surface) polypoid mass of the sigmoid colon that was a carcinoma (*C* is the correct answer to Question 10-17).

10-18. This case demonstrates an annular carcinoma of the ascending colon (*B* is the correct answer to Question 10-18).

10-19. This case shows a diffuse, irregular mucosal pattern (i.e., granularity) of the rectosigmoid colon most consistent with ulcerative colitis (*E* is the correct answer to Question 10-19).

10-20. This case represents a patient with ischemic colitis (*A* is the correct answer to Question 10-20). Granulomatous colitis (i.e., Crohn's disease) would be a second choice but unlikely at the age and with the presentation of this patient.

Discussion:

Rectal bleeding can result from a multitude of abnormalities throughout the gastrointestinal tract. This exercise illustrates the more important colonic causes of rectal bleeding. Another common cause of rectal bleeding is diverticular disease of the colon, which can be shown on barium enema examination. A further consideration, especially in older patients, is vascular malformations (e.g., angiodysplasia) of the right side of the colon, which is not seen on the barium enema study. In general, contrast studies of the gastrointestinal tract can detect many abnormalities that may be a source of bleeding but cannot determine if the lesion is bleeding actively; angiography and radionuclide studies are helpful to demonstrate bleeding.

The two most common polypoid lesions of the colon are hyperplastic and neoplastic polyps. Most hyperplastic polyps are less than 5 mm in diameter, are sessile and smooth, and may resemble small neoplastic polyps of similar size. Neoplastic polyps have a broad pathologic spectrum that includes (1) benign adenomas (tubular, tubulovillous, and villous types), (2) adenomas with focal carcinoma, and (3) polypoid carcinoma. Consequently, the radiologic appearances of neoplastic colonic polyps are varied, and benign and malignant neoplasms may appear similar. Neoplastic polyps can be sessile or pedunculated and smooth or lobulated (Fig. 10-E-17*B*). Size is an important radiologic criterion to estimate the risk of malignancy in a sessile colonic polyp; a polyp less than 1 cm in size has only a 1 percent chance of malignancy, a 1- to 2-cm polyp has about a 10 percent risk, and a polyp over 2 cm has at least a 25 percent or more chance of malignancy. The finding of a pedicle is important, regardless of the size of the head of the polyp, because even if malignancy is present, invasion down the pedicle into the adjacent colonic wall is rare. Lobulation is a less important indicator of malignancy; however, if a large colonic polyp has a smooth surface, a lipoma is a likely consideration.

Adenocarcinoma of the colon is the second most common malignancy that affects both sexes. About 95 percent of colonic carcinomas occur in patients over 40 years of age, with a peak in the late seventh decade. As with adenocarcinomas elsewhere in the gastrointestinal tract, a number of morphologic forms are seen, which include polypoid carcinoma (malignant potential discussed previously), ulcerative and infiltrative types, and the annular carcinoma (as in Case 10-18); the latter is also called the "apple-core" lesion. In the colon of an adult patient, an irregular constricting lesion having an abrupt transition with the normal colonic wall is nearly always an adenocarcinoma (Fig. 10-E-

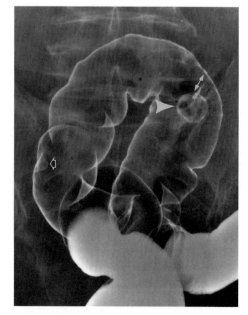

FIG. 10-E-17 (*Panel B*) Double-contrast radiograph of the rectosigmoid region shows a small, smooth, sessile adenoma (*arrow*) and a larger, pedunculated (*interconnected arrows*) adenoma (*arrowhead*) more proximally.

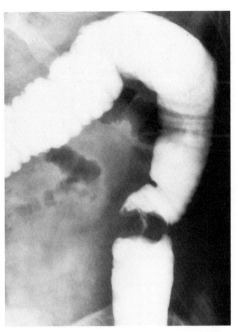

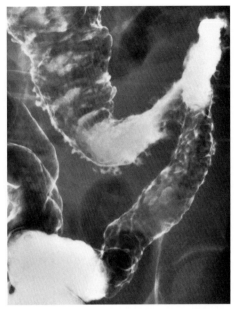

FIG. 10-E-18 (*Panel B*) Radiograph from a single-contrast barium enema showing an annular carcinoma of the descending colon.

FIG. 10-E-19 (*Panel B*) Segmental Crohn's disease of the transverse and descending portions of the colon showing multiple deep ulcers projecting from the margins of the affected colon and small "aphthoid" ulcers appearing like erosions seen in the upper gastrointestinal tract.

18*B*). Inflammatory strictures and surgical anastomoses typically have a smooth and often tapered appearance.

Ulcerative colitis and Crohn's colitis are the two common idiopathic inflammatory diseases of the colon. Other causes of colitis include infections of various types, drug-related types (i.e., antibiotic colitis), radiation-induced colitis (usually proctitis), ischemic colitis, and miscellaneous disorders. A number of these disorders may mimic the idiopathic types, and clinical correlation and exclusion of colonic infection are important. Radiographic differentiation between ulcerative and Crohn's colitis is usually possible in most patients. The features most suggestive of ulcerative colitis are continuous disease with rectal involvement, ahaustral shortening of the colon, and a finely ulcerated or granular mucosal surface (as seen in Case 10-19). The more specific findings of Crohn's colitis include discontinuous disease (i.e., skip areas) with ileitis, eccentric wall involvement, discrete (i.e., aphthoid ulcers) or deep ulceration, intramural fissuring, and formation of fistulas to adjacent organs (Fig. 10-E-19*B*). Complications that may occur in idiopathic colitis include toxic megacolon, carcinoma, sclerosing cholangitis, and abnormalities of the eyes, skin, and joints. Toxic megacolon and complicating carcinoma are more common in ulcerative colitis.

Ischemic colitis usually affects older patients and, like ischemic disease of the small bowel, may result from nonobstructive causes or from thrombotic or embolic disease. The most common location for ischemic involvement of the colon is the region of the splenic flexure and descending colon, which is the vascular "watershed" area for the superior and inferior mesenteric arteries. Other regions of the colon can be affected, although ischemic disease of the rectum is rare. The radiologic features of ischemic disease of the colon depend on the location of involvement, severity and duration of its

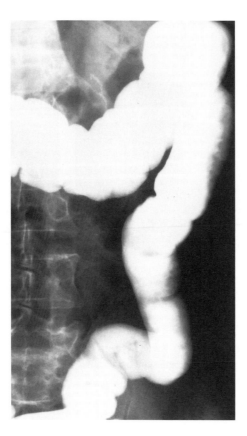

FIG. 10-E-20 (*Panel B*) Same patient 6 weeks following the acute onset of ischemic colitis in which the previously affected colon has returned to normal.

cause, and temporal changes during recovery of the colon. In the severest form, colonic infarction and perforation may occur, often with dire consequences for the patient. The most common appearances relate to submucosal hemorrhage that causes narrowing of the affected colon associated with irregular, smooth margins, often called thumbprinting (as in Case 10-20); complete healing and return to normal may occur (Fig. 10-E-20*B*) or progression to a smooth, tapered stricture can result.

EXERCISE 10-6: COLONIC OBSTRUCTION

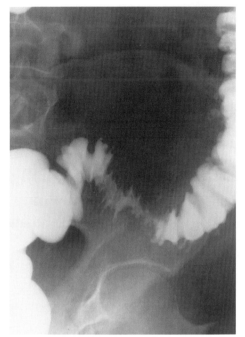

FIG. 10-E-21 *Panel A*

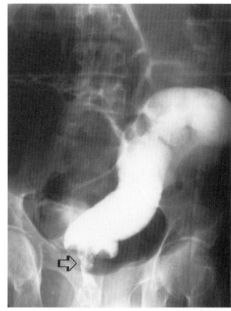

FIG. 10-E-22 *Panel A*

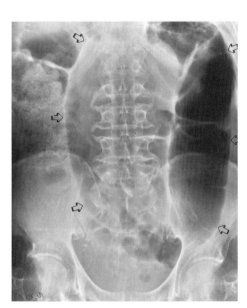

FIG. 10-E-23 *Panel A*

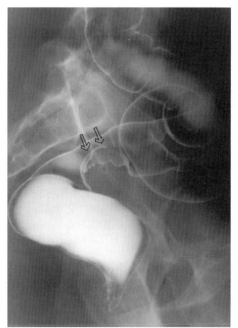

FIG. 10-E-24 *Panel A*

Clinical Histories:

CASE 10-21
A 47-year-old man presents with left lower abdominal pain and change in bowel habits (Fig. 10-E-21*A*).

CASE 10-22
A 69-year-old woman presents with rectal bleeding and obstipation (Fig. 10-E-22*A*).

CASE 10-23

A 57-year-old man presents with acute abdominal distension and obstipation (Fig. 10-E-23*A*).

CASE 10-24

A 33-year-old woman presents with cyclic lower abdominal pain, change in bowel habits, and rectal bleeding (Fig. 10-E-24*A*).

Questions:

10-21. A radiograph of the sigmoid-descending colon affected by diverticula and showing an area of long narrowing most likely caused by?

    A.   Annular carcinoma

    B.   Ischemic colitis

    C.   Ulcerative colitis

    D.   Sigmoid diverticulitis

    E.   Peritoneal metastases

10-22. Limited single-contrast barium enema of an obstructing rectal process (*arrow*) causing colonic obstruction and likely due to?

    A.   Rectal carcinoma

    B.   Lymphoma of the rectum

    C.   Crohn's proctitis

    D.   Infectious proctitis

    E.   Invasive carcinoma of cervix

10-23. What is the most likely explanation for the two adjacent loops of distended colon (*arrows*) in Case 10-23?

    A.   Right colon volvulus

    B.   Sigmoid volvulus

    C.   Ileocecal intussusception

    D.   Functional colonic ileus

    E.   Internal colonic hernia

10-24. In Case 10-24, a smooth mass (*arrows*) partially obstructing the anterior rectosigmoid region is likely due to?

    A.   Polypoid colon carcinoma

    B.   Rectosigmoid diverticulitis

    C.   Pelvic endometriosis

    D.   Invasive endometrial carcinoma

    E.   Posterior cul-de-sac metastases

Radiologic Findings:

10-21. This case shows an area of long narrowing in the sigmoid colon associated with diverticula that was caused by an acute diverticulitis (D is the correct answer to Question 10-21). Crohn's disease of the sigmoid colon may simulate diverticulitis. An annular carcinoma would not involve such a long segment and also would demonstrate mucosal destruction.

10-22. This case involves an annular rectal carcinoma causing distal colonic obstruction (A is the correct answer to Question 10-22). Rectal lymphoma is rare, and the other possibilities listed do not typically cause circumferential narrowing of the rectum.

10-23. This is a patient with sigmoid volvulus (*B* is the correct answer to Question 10-23). Sigmoid involvement is most likely because the involved loops are pointing inferiorly into the pelvis.

10-24. This is a woman with pelvic endometriosis that has invaded the rectosigmoid junction anteriorly (C is the correct answer to Question 10-24). The location is rare for diverticulitis, and the patient is rather young for the other options offered.

Discussion:

Colonic obstruction, when seen in adults, is usually caused by diverticulitis or carcinoma of the colon. Volvulus of the colon is much less common. However, extrinsic involvement of the rectum or sigmoid colon from pelvic malignancies is an important consideration in the middle-aged or older patient.

Diverticulitis is always a differential consideration in the adult patient with a suspected obstruction of the distal colon. Diverticulitis is usually due to perforation of a single diverticulum with subsequent formation of a paracolic abscess and typically is located in the sigmoid colon (as in Case 10-21). The radiographic findings suggesting diverticulitis on contrast enema of the colon include (1) extravasation into an abscess (most definitive finding), (2) eccentric or circumferential narrowing of the colon, and (3) transverse or longitudinal sinus tracts (also seen in Crohn's disease). Complications of sigmoid diverticulitis are obstruction (Fig. 10-E-21*B*), fistula formation (especially to the bladder), and development of a stricture. Free communication with the peritoneal cavity is rare. CT examination of the pelvis is useful in the evaluation of diverticulitis; also, percutaneous drainage of a diverticular abscess can be performed using CT guidance.

Adenocarcinoma of the colon was discussed in the preceding exercise as a common source of rectal bleeding but is also an important cause of colonic obstruction. The location and morphologic type of colonic carcinoma will have an impact on the clinical presentation of the patient. Carcinomas of the right side of the colon are often polypoid, may grow to a large size, and more often present clinically with localized pain, palpable mass, and melena. In the left side of the colon, carcinomas usually present at an earlier stage because obstructive symptoms are more common, often due to an annular carcinoma (Fig. 10-E-22*B*). Although carcinomas of the colon have shown a rightward shift in location in recent decades, about half these malignancies still originate in the rectum or sigmoid colon.

Sigmoid volvulus is a closed-loop colonic obstruction due to twisting along the mesenteric or long axis of the bowel. Although colonic volvulus is not common, about 90 percent occur in the sigmoid colon. On plain abdominal films, the sigmoid volvulus forms an inverted U-shaped structure with the twisted sigmoid loops lying adjacent and having an oval appearance called the "coffee bean" sign (as in Case 10-23). On barium enema examination, tapered obstruction of the sigmoid colon is found (Fig. 10-E-23*B*). Cecal volvulus results from a twisting obstruction of the right side of the colon and

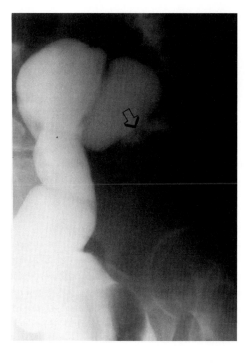

FIG. 10-E-21 (*Panel B*) Another patient with sigmoid diverticulitis causing near-complete colonic obstruction (*arrow*).

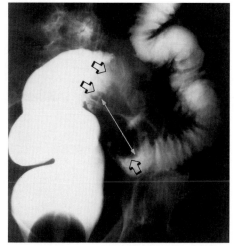

FIG. 10-E-22 (*Panel B*) Obstructing sigmoid carcinoma (*interconnected arrows*) near the rectosigmoid junction. Diverticulitis would be the main differential diagnosis; however, the abrupt, irregular areas of transition (*arrows*) favor a malignancy.

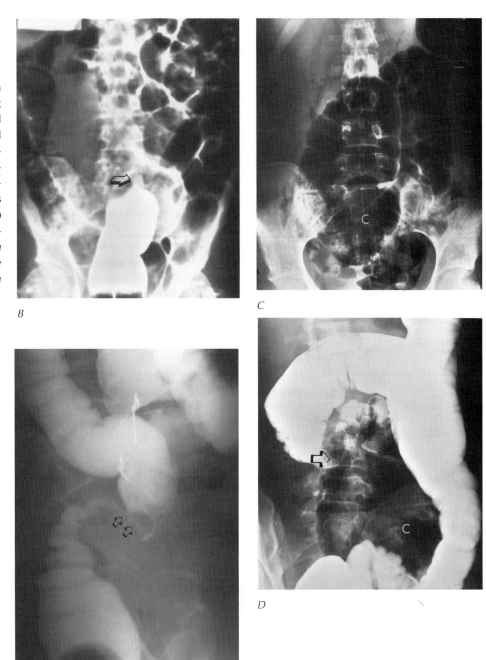

FIG. 10-E-23 (*Panel B*) Barium enema in same patient showing obstruction at the rectosigmoid junction (*arrow*) due to sigmoid volvulus. (*Panel C*) Plain abdominal radiograph of right colon volvulus (C, cecum). (*Panel D*) Barium enema in same patient shows near-complete obstruction (*arrow*) in the ascending colon (C, cecum). (*Used with permission from Ott DJ, Chen MYM: Specific acute colonic disorders. Radiol Clin North Am 32:871, 1994.*)

FIG. 10-E-24 (*Panel B*) A 54-year-old woman with advanced carcinoma of the uterine cervix that has invaded posteriorly causing obstruction at the rectosigmoid junction (*arrows*).

rarely involves the cecum only. The dilated proximal colon may be seen as an oval structure in the midabdomen or in the left upper quadrant but rarely points into the pelvis (Fig. 10-E-23*C*). Barium enema examination will locate the obstruction to the right side of the colon (Fig. 10-E-23*D*).

The anterior wall of the rectosigmoid colon is a common site for involvement of the colon by extrinsic inflammatory or neoplastic diseases. Inflammatory processes may spread into the posterior cul-de-sac and secondarily involve the colon; endometriosis can arise in this same area, implant on the colonic serosa, and invade into the colonic wall as occurred in Case 10-24. However, pelvic malignancies related to the uterine cervix, endometrium, ovary, bladder, and prostate are the most common neoplastic processes that can affect the rectosigmoid colon. Circumferential narrowing may occur with these extrinsic malignancies and mimic a primary carcinoma of the colon (Fig. 10-E-24*B*).

BIBLIOGRAPHY

Chen MYM et al: *Radiology of the Small Bowel.* New York, Igaku-Shoin, 1992.

Gelfand DW: *Gastrointestinal Radiology.* New York, Churchill-Livingstone, 1984.

Gore RM et al (eds): *Textbook of Gastrointestinal Radiology.* Philadelphia, Saunders, 1994.

Halpert RD, Goodman P: *Gastrointestinal Radiology: The Requisites.* St. Louis, Mosby, 1993.

Laufer I, Levine MS: *Double Contrast Gastrointestinal Radiology,* 2d ed. Philadelphia, Saunders, 1992.

Ott DJ: Radiology of the oropharynx and esophagus, in *The Esophagus,* edited by DO Castell. Boston, Little, Brown, 1992.

11

LIVER, BILIARY TRACT, AND PANCREAS

Robert E. Bechtold

The diagnosis of diseases of the liver, biliary tract, and pancreas optimally depends on using both clinical and radiographic data. Understanding the proper use of these data and ordering radiographic studies in the optimal sequence are very helpful for making the diagnosis most efficiently. Frequently, the clinical presentation and associated laboratory work provide most of the clues for diagnosis. Physical examination, history, and pertinent laboratory values are often helpful in making the diagnosis or at least in providing clues for selecting the optimal radiographic studies. If clinical information is insufficient, or if radiographic confirmation is necessary, plain films and contrast studies may be performed. Upright and supine plain radiographs are helpful for the detection of free air, calcifications, and other abnormalities. Contrast studies such as endoscopic retrograde cholangiopancreatography (ERCP) and percutaneous transhepatic cholangiography (PTC) are often helpful in analyzing diseases of the liver, biliary tree, and pancreas. For instance, pancreatic or biliary ductal systems, fistulas from these ductal systems, and associated abnormalities such as encasing tumors can be diagnosed cholangiographically.

Digital cross-sectional imaging, nuclear medicine (NM), and angiography have provided considerable information in analyzing diseases of these organs, which cannot be visualized directly with plain radiography, even using traditional contrast material, i.e., barium. Cross-sectional techniques consist of ultrasound (US), computed tomography (CT), and magnetic resonance (MR) imaging. This chapter reviews the use of cross-sectional imaging and, where pertinent, nuclear medicine and angiography to evaluate abnormalities of the liver, biliary tract, and pancreas.

TECHNIQUES

Ultrasound

Ultrasound utilizes a high-frequency sound wave transmission through the body. A transducer is used both to emit and to receive a very high frequency sound (2 to 10 MHz). The technique employs a radarlike detection of objects within the beam, in which the high-frequency sound waves are bounced off the objects and detected by the transducer. These signals are relayed to a computer, which displays a two-dimensional image in whatever plane is defined by the orientation of the transducer. The term for different shades within a US image is *echogenicity*. Vascular flow may be represented with colored images, in which color shade and color intensity reflect blood flow direction and velocity, respectively, or as a sine-wave form in which peaks represent increasing velocity and valleys represent decreasing velocity of flow.

Nuclear Medicine

Nuclear medicine techniques use the administration of radioactively labeled substances chemically bonded to physiologic agents. These combined substances are administered to the patient and travel to the organs that concentrate the physiologic agents. The radioactivity within the labeled substances is then detected with a camera sensitive to the presence of radioactive emissions. The term for different shades within a nuclear medicine image is *activity*.

Computed Tomography

Computed tomography (CT) uses x-rays and a ring-shaped structure called a *gantry*. The gantry contains an x-ray tube, which is directed toward a row of detectors on the other side of the gantry. The patient is placed on a table that is incrementally shifted through the opening of the gantry. The x-ray tube rotates around the patient, emitting a focused beam that passes through the patient. The attenuated beam is received by the detectors. These signals are transmitted to a computer, which reconstructs a series of two-dimensional images in a transverse plane through the body, much like cutting a loaf of bread. Blood vessels can be demonstrated by using intravenously injected contrast material, and the bowel can be demonstrated by means of an orally administered contrast agent. These images can be reconstructed in other planes or in a three-dimensional image. The term for different shades with a CT image is *attenuation,* or *density*.

Angiography

In angiography, contrast agents are administered intravascularly, and complex radiographic machines trace the injected contrast material through the blood vessels by a rapid sequence of x-ray films or with digital imaging techniques. The term for different shades within an angiographic image is *density*.

Magnetic Resonance Imaging

Magnetic resonance (MR) imaging is a very complex technique that evaluates magnetism within the patient. The device is outwardly similar to a CT unit. The patient is placed on a table that carries the patient into a cylinder that contains a magnet. The magnet emits a radiofrequency pulse that causes the protons of the atoms within the body to line up together. The magnet then emits another radiofrequency pulse, which perturbs the orientation of the protons so that as a group they are flipped to the side. The protons then return to their original orientation, and their return is accompanied by a release of energy. The rate at which the protons return to normal orientation and release energy is defined by the characteristics of the tissue, which in turn are defined by the relaxation times, T1 and T2, of the protons. Blood flow and proton density also affect the image. Signals from this process are sent to a computer, which reconstructs either a two-dimensional image in any plane or a three-dimensional image. The term for different shades within an MR image is *signal intensity*. Flow is identified by signal-intensity changes in the blood vessels.

Normal Anatomy

With US, normal organs are displayed as structures of different echogenicity. In general, fluid is anechoic (has no echoes). Soft tissue has echoes of mild to moderate intensity. Bone has extremely strong echoes. Abnormal organs are displayed as areas of diffuse inhomogeneity or as focal regions of decreased or increased echogenicity within the organ. The normal appearances of the liver, biliary system, and pancreas have been well established. The liver is second to the pancreas in echogenicity among organs in the upper abdomen. The liver typically has homogenous parenchymal detail (Fig. 11-1). Numerous intrahepatic vessels, including protal veins and hepatic veins, are easily seen within the liver. The gallbladder appears as an anechoic pear-shaped structure along the inferior aspect of the liver (Fig. 11-2). It normally has a thin, homogeneous wall less than 3 mm in thickness. The degree of distension of the gallbladder varies with postprandial intervals. The biliary ducts are thin tubes, the walls of which are 1.5 mm or less. The ducts increase in caliber as they extend from the liver to the sphincter of Oddi (Fig. 11-3). The upper limit in caliber of the extrahepatic biliary ducts increases with age. The pancreas is the most echogenic organ in the abdomen (Fig. 11-4). It is homogeneous, comma-shaped, and parallel to splenic vein and extends from the left upper quadrant caudally and to the right. In anteroposterior dimension, the pancreatic head is 3 cm, the body 2.5 cm, and the tail 2 cm.

With NM studies, normal organs are displayed as regions of homogeneous activity conforming to the general shape of the organ. Abnormal organs are displayed as diffuse inhomogeneity or as focal areas of reduced or increased activity. In the past, the liver was most commonly studied with NM with technetium-labeled sulfur colloid. However, this technique has largely been replaced by CT, US, and MR imaging. The most common NM study of the liver today uses technetium-labeled red blood cells to detect cavernous hemangioma. Evaluation of the biliary system is a very common application for NM studies. Technetium-labeled hepatobiliary imaging iminodiacetic acid derivatives, especially disophenin and mebrophenin, are taken up by the liver, excreted into the bile, carried to the biliary tree and gallbladder, and from there travel to the bowel through the extrahepatic ducts (Fig. 11-5). Currently, no practical imaging of the pancreas is done by means of NM techniques.

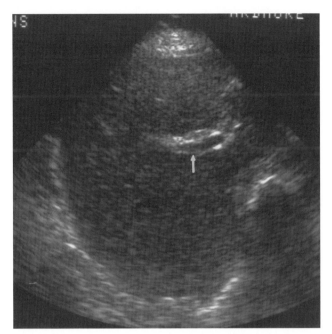

FIG. 11-1 Transverse US image of the normal liver showing homogeneous parenchymal detail, the hyperechoic hemidiaphragmatic surface, the linear protal vein, and the parallel biliary duct (*arrow*).

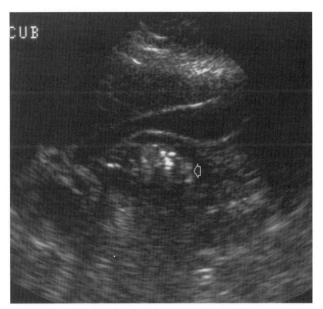

FIG. 11-2 Longitudinal US image of the normal gallbladder showing the anechoic lumen and smooth, thin walls of the gallbladder. Air-filled, echogenic duodenum is immediately behind the gallbladder (*open arrow*).

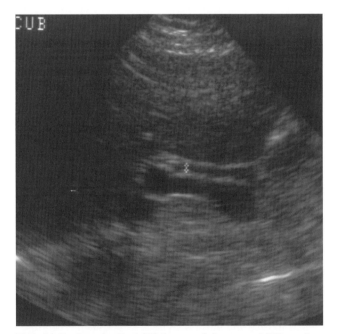

FIG. 11-3 Longitudinal US image of the normal biliary duct showing the narrow caliber and the thin, uniform ductal walls (cursors denote the internal walls of the duct).

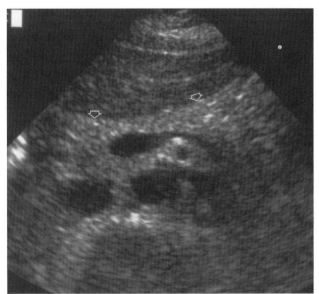

FIG. 11-4 Transverse US image of the normal pancreas showing the homogeneous, echogenic pancreatic head, body, and tail (*open arrows*) lying in front of the splenic and superior mesenteric veins.

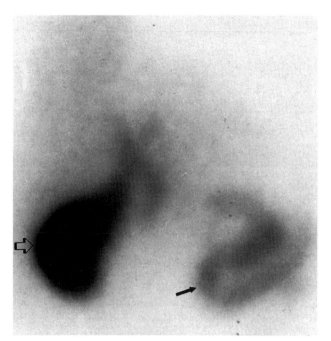

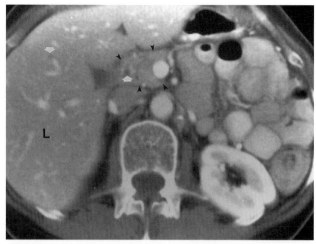

FIG. 11-6 CT showing liver (L), pancreas (*arrowheads*), and biliary tree in both the liver and pancreas (*arrows*).

FIG. 11-5 Hepatobiliary NM scan showing the presence of radiopharmaceutical within the gallbladder lumen (*open arrow*) and duodenum (*closed arrow*), demonstrating the patency of both cystic and common bile duct. (*Courtesy of Robert Cowan, M.D., Winston-Salem, N.C.*)

With CT, normal organs are displayed as regions of differing attenuation. Abnormal organs are displayed as diffuse inhomogeneity or as focal areas of decreased or increased attenuation. The liver, biliary system, and pancreas are well demonstrated by CT (Fig. 11-6). The liver is the most dense organ in the abdomen. The normal liver parenchyma appears homogeneous, just as with US. The portal

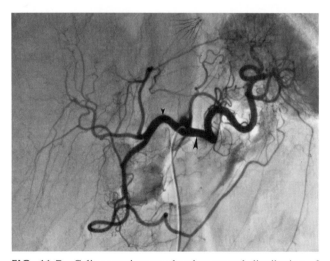

FIG. 11-7 Celiac arteriogram showing normal distribution of the splenic (*large black arrowhead*) and hepatic (*small black arrowhead*) arteries and the normal homogeneous stain of the spleen in the left upper quadrant.

and hepatic vessels and the biliary ductal system are likewise easy to identify. Overall measurements of wall thickness and biliary duct caliber are the same as with US. The pancreas is easily identified on CT, and the pancreatic duct is frequently well seen.

At angiography, normal organs enhance to variable extents. Abnormal organs either enhance inhomogeneously or have focal areas of decreased or increased enhancement. Although the parenchyma of the normal organs is rarely demonstrated, the blood vessels of these organs are seen in exquisite detail (Fig. 11-7). In the liver, both the hepatic artery and all its branches can be seen. Delayed studies through the liver in the venous phase demonstrate the portal vein. The cystic artery and any collateral vessels can be demonstrated angiographically. Angiographic studies of the pancreas can demonstrate major pancreatic branches, as well as encasement, displacement, stenosis, or occlusion.

With MR imaging, normal organs have homogeneous signal intensity or well-recognized variations in signal intensity. Abnormal organs have inhomogeneous signal intensity or areas of increased or decreased signal intensity. The normal liver, biliary system, and pancreas are well demonstrated on MR imaging (Fig. 11-8). The liver has a homogeneous signal intensity that is usually higher than that of muscle and lower than that of the spleen. The biliary system is normally demonstrated as an area of low signal intensity on T1-weighted images and high signal intensity on T2-weighted images. This appearance reflects the fluid bile within the gallbladder and biliary tree. The pancreas is of intermediate signal on both T1- and T2-weighted images and may be hard to differentiate from bowel if no oral contrast agent is administered to the patient. As with CT and US, the normal fatty change within the pancreas that occurs with age is visible with MR imaging.

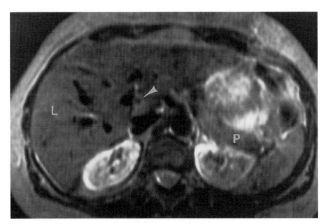

FIG. 11-8 T2-weighted MR imaging scan showing normal liver (L), pancreas (P), and biliary tree (*arrowhead*).

TECHNIQUE SELECTION

Diseases of the liver, biliary system, and pancreas can be conveniently, if arbitrarily, separated into the following categories to help illustrate the optimal sequences of imaging techniques: diffuse hepatocellular disease, focal hepatic diseases, abdominal trauma, inflammatory disease of the biliary tract, and pancreatic inflammation or neoplasm.

Diffuse Hepatocellular Disease

In diffuse hepatocellular disease, CT is probably the first study used to survey the liver because it is moderately sensitive to liver lesions and is also helpful for evaluating surrounding organs. US may have application unless fatty liver is present, since fat attenuates the US beam. NM has only infrequent applications. Angiography may be used to study collateral formation in cirrhosis. MR imaging is very sensitive for many diffuse liver diseases, including cirrhosis and hemochromatosis.

Focal Hepatic Diseases

In focal diseases of the liver, US is often used first, since it is inexpensive, widely available, and moderately sensitive to localized lesions. It is, however, of limited value in obese patients and whenever air is present, e.g., when air-filled bowel obscures the liver. CT is a pivotal examination, often employed after US. It is used as a survey of the entire body, is easy to compare in serial studies, and is sensitive to disease. Air and bone do not interfere with CT examinations. CT can be used in conjunction with angiography to perform CT angioportography, which is considered the most sensitive current means of evaluating liver metastases. NM techniques may be used to analyze a focal lesion within the liver for possible cavernous hemangioma. MR imaging is used frequently to characterize focal lesions

within the liver, especially after survey techniques that use US or CT. In fact, NM and MR imaging are considered the optimal means for evaluating the liver for cavernous hemangioma, and both are highly accurate (approximately 95 percent) in evaluating the liver for cavernous hemangioma. In the opinion of some authorities, MR imaging is the optimal means for both detection and characterization of focal liver lesions of all types. Angiography is used primarily to provide a vascular road map in planning surgery for focal liver lesions.

Abdominal Trauma

The only commonly accepted means for analyzing abdominal trauma, particularly of the liver, is CT. CT is reasonably accurate in the detection of trauma-related abnormalities of the liver, biliary system, and pancreas. US may be useful if CT is not available or to quickly identify intraperitoneal hemorrhage in patients who are in the emergency department and are going directly to the operating room. Angiography may be useful to embolize persistently bleeding arteries in the liver or spleen when surgery is not possible. Currently, NM and MR imaging have no application in studying the liver, biliary tract, or pancreas in trauma.

Pancreatic Inflammation or Neoplasm

US is often the primary means to study pancreatic inflammation or neoplasm. It is very effective in evaluating the pancreas if not interrupted by surrounding bowel gas. If ileus is present, or if a lesion has already been detected by US and additional confirmation is required, CT is the method of choice. NM has no major current application in studying the pancreas. MR imaging may be useful to study endocrine tumors of the pancreas. Angiography is useful to identify bleeding arteries as a source of hemorrhagic pancreatitis but is occasionally used to identify encasement of arteries in a pancreatic neoplasm.

Patient Preparation for Radiographic Techniques

Generally, these radiographic techniques require very little patient preparation. This is convenient, especially in evaluation of trauma. Ideally, a patient should fast after midnight before US examination. As a minimum, the patient should fast for 6 hours. Patients ideally should fast before CT examinations as well. Dilute oral contrast medium is administered at least 2 hours in advance and again just before the examination begins. Intravenous contrast material is often given as a bolus by a power injector immediately prior to the study. Proper laboratory evaluation of renal function, including a serum creatinine level below 1.5 mg/dL, is usually required before administering intravenous contrast material. Ideally, NM is also performed after fasting. Preparation for angiography again requires fasting and laboratory evaluation of renal function. Proper preparation of patients for MR imaging is controversial. However, some authorities advise administering an iron-containing oral contrast agent and an agent to relax the bowel, such as glucagon, before scanning. No assessment of renal function is necessary.

Conflicts among Examinations

These examinations may interfere with each other. No barium should be administered before US or CT. Oral contrast agents may generate bowel gas, decompress the gallbladder, and hinder US. The oral contrast agent administered prior to a CT examination interferes with angiography by obscuring the abdomen. Intravenous contrast material interferes with any subsequent NM tests studying iodine metabolism because intravenous contrast agents contain iodine. Previous angiography usually requires that a CT examination be postponed for a day or two so that residual contrast material within the kidneys may be excreted. Usually, there are no conflicts between these examinations and NM or MR imaging.

EXERCISE 11-1: DIFFUSE LIVER DISEASE

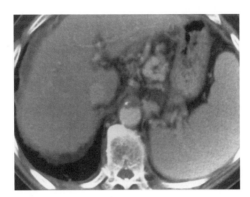

FIG. 11-E-1 *Panel A*

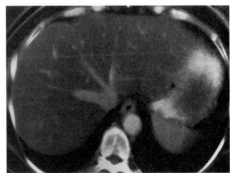

FIG. 11-E-2 *Panel A*

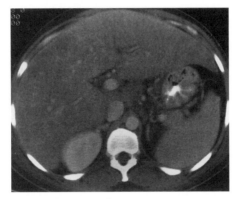

FIG. 11-E-3 *Panel A*

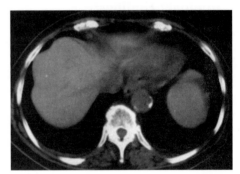

FIG. 11-E-4

Clinical Histories:

CASE 11-1
A 55-year-old American patient presents with abdominal swelling (Fig. 11-E-1*A*).

CASE 11-2
A 33-year old long-time diabetic patient presents with right upper quadrant "mass" (Fig. 11-E-2*A*).

CASE 11-3
A 65-year-old patient presents with fever and increased liver function tests (Fig. 11-E-3*A*).

CASE 11-4
An 80-year-old patient presents without symptoms referable to the abdomen (Fig. 11-E-4).

Questions:

11-1. Most likely diagnosis in Case 11-1?
   A. Cirrhosis
   B. Diffuse liver tumor
   C. Budd-Chiari syndrome
   D. Schistosomiasis

11-2. Most likely diagnosis in Case 11-2?
- A. Cirrhosis
- B. Fatty liver
- C. Hepatic iron overload
- D. Old granulomatous disease

11-3. Most likely diagnosis in Case 11-3?
- A. Cirrhosis
- B. Thorotrast-induced liver disease
- C. Hepatitis
- D. Hepatic iron overload

11-4. Most likely diagnosis in Case 11-4?
- A. Cirrhosis
- B. Old granulomatous disease
- C. Fatty liver
- D. Osler-Weber-Rendu disease

Radiologic Findings:

11-1. In this case, the overall liver size is small, especially the right lobe, with disproportionate enlargement of the left and caudate lobes, multiple collaterals are present around stomach and in central upper abdomen, and ascites is present, all findings of cirrhosis (*A* is the correct answer to Question 11-1).

11-2. In this case, the overall liver size is large, a predominant finding is marked low density throughout the entire liver, and no mass effect is present on any vessel, all findings of fatty liver (*B* is the correct answer to Question 11-2).

11-3. In this case, the overall liver size is enlarged, attenuation is inhomogeneous and mildly reduced, and no focal mass is present, all findings of hepatitis (*C* is the correct answer to Question 11-3).

11-4. In this case, multiple small, highly attenuating, punctate lesions are scattered throughout liver and spleen, characteristic of calcifications from old granulomatous disease, without any other predominant finding (*B* is the correct answer to Question 11-4).

Discussion:

Differentiation of liver disease into diffuse or focal disease is an artificial but convenient way to analyze liver disorders radiographically. Diffuse hepatocellular diseases are a common diagnostic problem. Although historical, physical examination, and laboratory testing are the first means for identifying these diseases, imaging may be required as a part of the overall assessment of the patient.

Cirrhosis is a chronic disease of the liver. It is characterized by injury and regeneration of hepatic parenchymal cells and is accompanied by formation of connective tissue within the liver. In the United States, the most common cause of cirrhosis is alcoholism. The process results in disproportionate diminution of the right lobe compared with the left lobe and caudate lobe of the liver (Fig. 11-E-1*B*). Nodular regeneration of the liver results in a nodular edge of the liver and inhomogeneity of the parenchyma. The process is accompanied by, first, increased resistance to normal hepatopedal (toward the liver) flow and, finally, the development of hepatofugal (away from the liver) flow. The increased resistance in the portal vein secondarily enlarges the spleen. This process also creates enlarged collateral venous channels to reroute blood around the liver (Fig. 11-E-1*A*). These portosystemic collaterals are visible frequently on cross-sectional imaging studies, most commonly in paraumbilical veins, coronary veins, and even spontaneous splenorenal shunts. Ascites is nearly always present.

Diffuse tumor in the liver can occur in patients with certain primary malignancies (Fig. 11-E-1*C*), particularly breast carcinoma. It is usually distributed uniformly rather than nonuniformly within the left and caudate lobes. Collateral veins normally are not

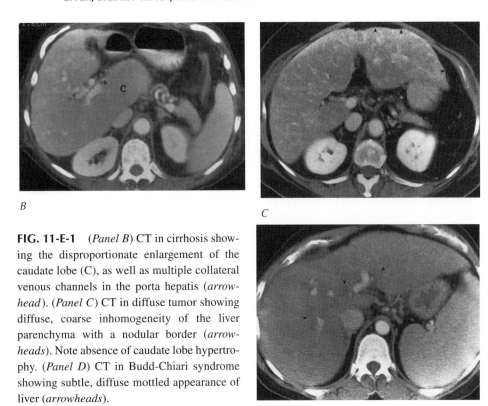

FIG. 11-E-1 (*Panel B*) CT in cirrhosis showing the disproportionate enlargement of the caudate lobe (C), as well as multiple collateral venous channels in the porta hepatis (*arrowhead*). (*Panel C*) CT in diffuse tumor showing diffuse, coarse inhomogeneity of the liver parenchyma with a nodular border (*arrowheads*). Note absence of caudate lobe hypertrophy. (*Panel D*) CT in Budd-Chiari syndrome showing subtle, diffuse mottled appearance of liver (*arrowheads*).

found. Portal venous or intrahepatic biliary radicles may be compromised or displaced, although portal vein thrombosis is uncommon.

Budd-Chiari syndrome is a condition involving obstruction of the hepatic veins or the intrahepatic inferior vena cava. It is due to hypercoagulable states that produce thrombosis; tumors of the liver, kidneys, adrenal glands, or inferior vena cava (IVC); trauma (the three *T*s, i.e., thrombosis, tumors, trauma); pregnancy; and even webs or membranes in the lumen of the inferior vena cava. This syndrome produces a marked congestion of the liver resulting from resistance to flow out of the liver, and the liver consequently enlarges and becomes edematous. The liver has a mottled appearance on CT that is due to the interstitial edema, especially after administration of intravenous contrast material (Fig. 11-E-1*D*).

Schistosomiasis is one of the world's most common parasitic diseases. This disease process is rarely seen in persons living outside the endemic areas of China, Japan, the Middle East, and Africa, but it does occur in immigrants to this country. The larvae are hosts that enter the human body, pass into lymphatic channels, migrate into mesenteric veins and portal veins, and, as adult worms, deposit ova that embolize to the portal system. This process leads to a granulomatous inflammation, periportal fibrosis, portal vein occlusion, varices, and splenomegaly. Imaging studies demonstrate periportal fibrosis. The fibrosis enhances on CT after contrast material administration and appears on US as increased echogenicity of the periportal sheath surrounding the portal veins.

Fatty liver is a common disorder. It is found in up to 50 percent of diabetic and alcoholic patients, as well as in up to 25 percent of nonalcoholic, healthy adults who die accidentally. The many causes of fatty liver, besides diabetes and alcoholism, include (1) obesity, (2) chronic illness, (3) corticosteroid excess, (4) parenteral nutrition, and (5) hepatotoxins, including chemotherapy. Fatty liver may be distributed evenly or focally. When distributed uniformly, fatty liver is recognizable as a pattern of homogeneous increased echogenicity on US, decreased attenuation on CT (Fig. 11-E-2*A*), or increased signal intensity on T1-weighted MR images. When distributed nonuniformly, it resem-

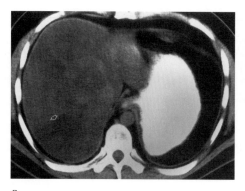

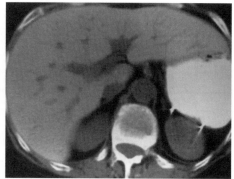

FIG. 11-E-2 (*Panel B*) CT in geographic fatty infiltration of the liver showing well-marginated, focal, low-density portion of the liver posteriorly (*white arrow*). (*Panel C*) CT in iron overload showing dense liver in relationship to the lower-density intrahepatic portal vessels.

B

C

bles focal disease of the liver in that normal islands of liver tissue are seen against the background of lower-density fatty liver (Fig. 11-E-2*B*). Specialized MR scans, NM studies, or biopsy may be required to differentiate among the possibilities.

Hepatic iron overload can be due to deposition in hepatocytes or reticuloendothelium. Parenchymal iron deposition occurs in primary idiopathic hemochromatosis, secondary hemochromatosis, cirrhosis, or intravascular hemolysis; the iron overload in these conditions is generally referred to as *hemochromatosis.* Reticuloendothelial iron deposition occurs in transfusional iron overload or rhabdomyolysis; the iron overload in these conditions is referred to as *hemosiderosis.* The liver, including the right lobe, is enlarged greatly unless cirrhosis is present. On CT, the density of the liver is very high (Fig. 11-E-2*C*) and on MR imaging, the liver has extremely low signal on both T1- and T2-weighted images. Patients with hepatic iron overload are predisposed to develop hepatocellular carcinoma.

Old granulomatous disease is a disorder in which prior granulomatous inflammation, usually caused by *Histoplasma capsulatum,* involves the liver. Other granulomatous inflammatory conditions that could be involved include sarcoidosis, Wegener's granulomatosis, and certain toxins. The granuloma tends to undergo necrosis, and dystrophic calcification forms within the lesion. This gives the lesion its most characteristic form, multiple small calcifications. The granuloma is visible on US as focal, extremely hyperechoic, shadowing lesions and on CT as extremely high density punctate lesions (Fig. 11-E-4).

Thorotrast, a thorium-containing contrast agent, was used in the 1920s for angiography and other purposes. Unfortunately, Thorotrast emits alpha and beta radiation, has a biologic half-life of 400 years because it is not excreted, and therefore has been responsible for the development of several malignancies of the liver and spleen, including angiosarcoma and hepatoma. The particles are taken up by liver, spleen, lymphatics, and bone marrow. They appear on CT studies as large, dense particles in the liver, spleen, and peripancreatic and periportal lymph nodes (Fig. 11-E-3*B*). US shows typical calcifications.

Hepatitis is a diffuse inflammation of the liver occurring as either acute or chronic disease. Patients with acute hepatitis have hepatocellular necrosis. In chronic cases, periportal inflammation and even fibrosis may occur. In acute hepatitis, the echogenicity of the parenchyma is decreased as a result of the edema, and the portal radicles are more evident; this has been termed the 'starry sky' appearance. In chronic hepatitis, the texture of the liver is coarsened as a result of the fibrotic change in the periportal space, and this may decrease the visibility of the portal vein radicles. Findings on CT include hepatomegaly and decreased density (Fig. 11-E-3*A*). Most commonly, no important findings except hepatomegaly occur on CT in hepatitis. On MR imaging, the liver has low signal intensity on T1-weighted images and high signal intensity on T2-weighted images because of the edema of inflammation.

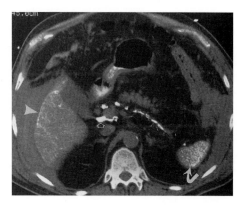

FIG. 11-E-3 (*Panel B*) CT in Thorotrast administration showing the presence of high-density Thorotrast in the liver (*white arrowhead*), lymph nodes (*open white arrow*), and spleen (*curved white arrow*).

Osler-Weber-Rendu disease, or hereditary hemorrhagic telangiectasia, affects many organs and is seen predominantly, but not exclusively, in skin and the gastrointestinal tract. In the liver it produces either telangiectasias, cirrhosis, or both. Multiple small aneurysms may be present, and hematomas may occur if the aneurysms bleed. These aneurysms and any consequent hematomas are visible on both US and CT. Angiography can demonstrate enlarged hepatic arteries and early but not immediate hepatic vein opacification.

EXERCISE 11-2: FOCAL LIVER DISEASES

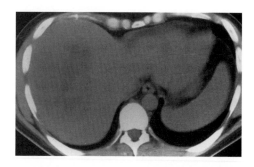

FIG. 11-E-5   *Panel A*

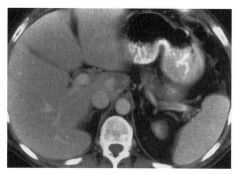

FIG. 11-E-6   *Panels A and B*

A

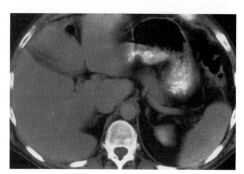

B

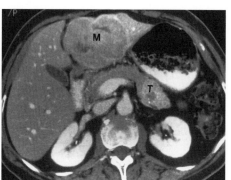

FIG. 11-E-7   *Panel A*

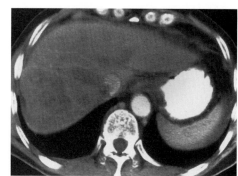

FIG. 11-E-8

Clinical Histories:

CASE 11-5
A 44-year-old patient presents with right upper quadrant pain and fever (Fig. 11-E-5*A*).

CASE 11-6
A 45-year-old woman presents with an incidentally discovered liver lesion (Fig. 11-E-6*A,B*).

CASE 11-7
A 65-year-old woman presents with a long history of a pancreatic mass (Fig. 11-E-7*A*).

CASE 11-8
A 61-year-old man presents with upper abdominal pain (Fig. 11-E-8).

Questions:

11-5. Most likely diagnosis in Case 11-5?
A. Pyogenic liver abscess
B. Echinococcal disease
C. Candidiasis
D. Amebic abscess

11-6. Most likely diagnosis in Case 11-6?
A. Hemangioma
B. Metastatic disease
C. Angiosarcoma
D. Focal nodular hyperplasia

11-7. Most likely diagnosis in Case 11-7?
A. Hemangioma
B. Hepatocellular carcinoma
C. Metastatic disease
D. Liver cell adenoma

11-8. Most likely diagnosis in Case 11-8?
A. Metastatic disease
B. Hepatocellular carcinoma
C. Liver cell adenoma
D. Abscess

Radiologic Findings:

11-5. In this case, there is an inhomogeneous liver lesion with central necrosis and a peripheral rim of edema. Although this could conceivably represent an echinococcal or amebic abscess in this patient with fever, since the patient is from the United States rather than from a foreign country, the most likely diagnosis is a pyogenic abscess (*A* is the correct answer). As more individuals from other countries, especially third world nations, immigrate to this nation, however, more echinococcal or amebic abscesses will be seen.

11-6. In this case, there is a focal lesion in the caudate lobe of the liver, which enhances early and fills in later with contrast material. This early peripheral and nodular-appearing distribution of intravenous contrast material within the lesion and eventual centripetal accumulation of contrast material to fill in the lesion are characteristic of cavernous hemangioma (*A* is the correct answer).

11-7. In this case, there is a focal lesion occupying the left lobe of the liver (M), and there is a focal enhancing mass in the pancreatic tail (T), representing a pancreatic neoplasm metastatic to the liver (*C* is the correct answer).

11-8. In this case, there is a focal lesion within the right lobe of the liver that is associated with a clot entering the hepatic vein and even the inferior vena cava, findings typical for hepatocellular carcinoma (*B* is the correct answer).

Discussion:

Recognition of the focal or diffuse nature of liver disease is helpful for sorting out the possible causes. The two can overlap, especially since one may lead to another, e.g., cirrhosis can cause hepatoma.

Pyogenic liver abscesses are relatively common focal inflammatory lesions of the liver caused by bacteria. These lesions have high morbidity and mortality rates if undiscovered. They are multiple in many cases, involving the right and left lobes. These abscesses create a severe leukocytosis. Pyogenic abscesses occur when collections of leukocytes undergo necrosis and become walled off. The imaging studies, while not definitive, have helpful findings. On US, these lesions often are well demarcated, may be multiloculated, and have fluid centers and irregular walls. Gas within an abscess creates an echogenic structure with shadowing. On CT, the abscess appears as a low-density lesion. Intraabscess gas occurs in approximately 50 percent of abscesses (Fig. 11-E-5*B*), and enhancement of the border of the lesion after intravenous contrast material infusion also occurs in approximately 50 percent of abscesses. Low-density edema may surround the abscess (Fig. 11-E-5*A*). Rapid enhancement of the edge of an abscess after bolus injection of contrast material may be helpful. On technetium-99m sulphur colloid scans, the abscess appears as a defect within the liver. MR images demonstrate signs of an irregular, fluid-containing lesion, i.e., low signal intensity on T1-weighted examinations and high signal intensity on T2-weighted examinations. Edema may be visible surrounding the lesion on T2-weighted images.

Echinococcal disease is a parasitic infestation that involves multiple organs, most commonly the liver. It is endemic in several regions around the world. The most common form is due to *Echinococcus granulosis,* which, after being ingested by humans, is carried into the gut, transmitted to the portal circulation, and eventually deposited in the liver, where it develops into large, occasionally multiloculated cysts. These cysts may calcify. On US, these lesions appear as well-defined cysts with regular borders, which may contain swirling debris and multiple septae. Smaller "daughter" cysts often surround them. Small calcifications are present. CT shows similar morphologic findings, as well as enhancement of the wall after intravenous contrast material infusion. Calcifications are crescentic, corresponding to the membranes. MR imaging shows a cystic mass with a rimlike periphery of low signal intensity on both T1- and T2-weighted images and a central matrix of high signal intensity.

Candidiasis is a fungal disease. It affects the liver primarily in renal transplant patients and patients who are immunocompromised by malignancy or chemotherapy for the malignancy. The organism forms multiple microabscesses, which create the characteristic appearance on imaging studies. US shows several patterns, the most common being multiple small hypoechoic structures containing a hyperechoic central spot, the

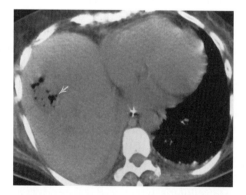

B

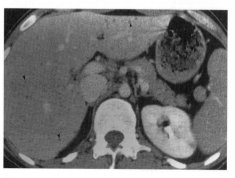

C

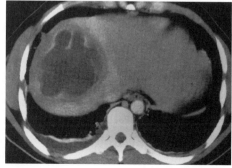

D

FIG. 11-E-5   (*Panel B*) CT in pyogenic abscess showing the presence of gas within the lesion (*arrow*). (*Panel C*) CT in candidiasis showing multiple small, low-density lesions scattered throughout the liver (*arrowheads*), representing multifocal fungal abscesses. (*Panel D*) CT in amebic abscess showing the presence of an irregular peripherally enhancing lesion within the liver. This is indistinguishable from a pyogenic abscess.

"bull's-eye" lesion. Other patterns may occur. CT shows similar multiple small abscesses (Fig. 11-E-5*C*), including the bull's-eye lesion.

Amebic abscesses are caused by a parasite, *Entamoeba histolytica,* and the liver is the most commonly involved organ. The leukocytosis is much less severe than with a pyogenic abscess. Unlike pyogenic abscesses, which require drainage, amebic abscesses often can be cured by medical treatment. Like echinococcal abscesses, amebic abscesses start when organisms reach the liver through the portal circulation from the bowel. The abscesses may rupture into the peritoneal cavity or even into the thorax. Imaging studies, including NM, US, and CT, are usually nonspecific and demonstrate focal defects within the liver (Fig. 11-E-5*D*). The lesions can resemble echinococcal abscesses. One helpful finding is intraperitoneal or intrathoracic fluid, if rupture has occurred.

Hemangioma is the most common benign tumor of the liver and is second only to metastases as the most common tumor overall within the liver. Symptomatic tumors are more often found in women, probably because of bleeding. Hemangiomas are often peripherally located in the liver, less than 2 cm in diameter, and not associated with abnormalities in liver function tests. They are most commonly single. On US, they are usually homogeneous and hyperechoic (Fig. 11-E-6*C*). They are often peripheral, with posterior acoustic enhancement. Some large lesions have central scars. CT shows homogeneous, low-attenuation lesions that enhance after intravenous contrast material administration, have nodular peripheral enhancement, and accumulate contrast material centripetally over a period of several minutes (Fig. 11-E-6*A,B*). This finding is most useful when the patient has no known primary tumor; otherwise, this pattern is more likely due to a metastasis. Technetium-99m–labeled red blood cell scans are diagnostic for hemangioma when early vascular-phase images show decreased activity and delayed blood pool scans demonstrate increased activity at the lesion site (Fig. 11-E-6*D*). MR imaging

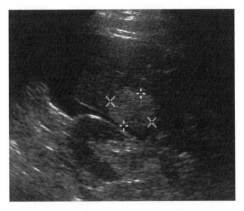

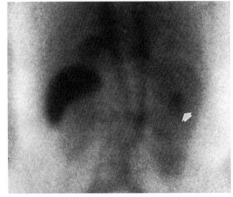

C   *D*

FIG. 11-E-6   (*Panel C*) Transverse US in cavernous hemangioma showing a hyperechoic, well-defined, homogeneous lesion at the posterior edge of the liver (*cursors*). (*Panel D*) Tagged red blood cell NM scan showing the presence of a region of increased activity within the liver (*white arrow*). Note image obtained over the posterior aspect of the patient so that liver is on left side of image. (*Courtesy of Nat Watson, M.D., Winston-Salem, N.C.*) (*Panel E*) T2-weighted transverse MR image in cavernous hemangioma showing extremely high signal intensity lesion (H) in posterior aspect of the right lobe of the liver (compare the signal intensity of this lesion with that of the lesion in part *J*). Capillary (*Panel F*) and venous (*Panel G*) phase hepatic arteriograms in cavernous hemangioma showing the dense and persistent stain of the lesions (*arrowhead*). (*Panel H*) Longitudinal US in liver metastasis showing a lesion in the posterior aspect of the liver, including a peripheral halo of decreased echogenicity (*arrows*). (*Panel I*) CT in liver metastasis showing multiple, poorly defined liver lesions scattered throughout the liver (*arrowheads*). (*Panel J*) T2-weighted transverse MR image in liver metastasis showing the presence of intermediately high-signal-intensity liver lesions (compare the signal intensity of this lesion with that of the lesion in part *E*). (*Panel K*) CT in angiosarcoma showing a low-density lesion in the right lobe of the liver (*arrowheads*). This is indistinguishable from any other liver neoplasm. (*Panel L*) CT in FNH showing a low-density lesion occupying the majority of the right lobe of the liver and demonstrating a central scar (*arrowhead*). MR images in FNH in the left lobe showing a nonspecific appearance of low signal intensity (*arrowheads*) on T1-weighted (*Panel M*) and mildly high signal intensity (*arrowheads*) on T2-weighted images (*Panel N*).

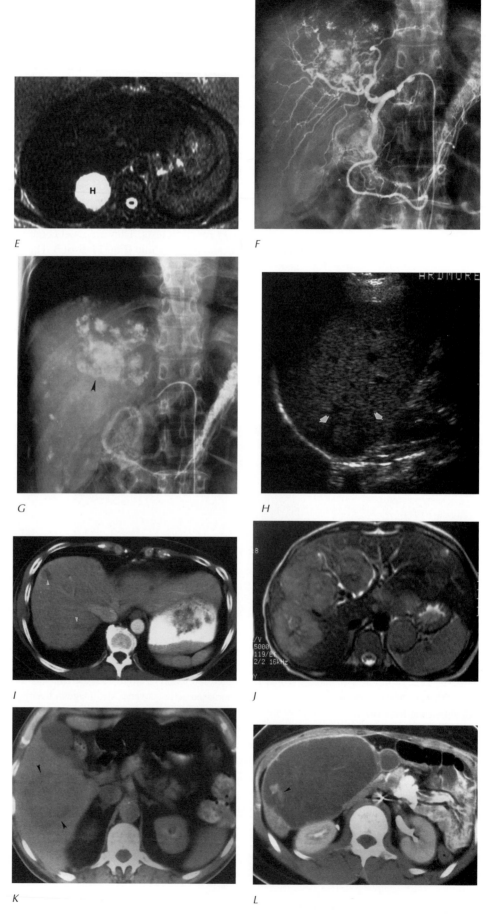

E

F

G

H

I

J

K

L

FIG. 11-E-6   (*Continued*)

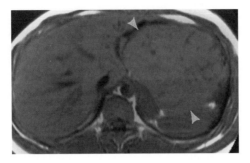 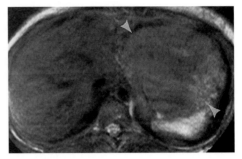

FIG. 11-E-6 (*Continued*)

M

N

demonstrates lesions with low signal intensity on T1-weighted scans, which is typical for most lesions. However, T2-weighted MR images demonstrate very high signal intensity similar to that of fluid, which is considered diagnostic of hemangioma or cyst (Fig. 11-E-6*E*). Angiography can be very helpful, since it shows punctate collections of contrast material shortly after injection (Fig. 11-E-6*F*). These collections become denser, usually within a minute, because contrast puddles in the vascular spaces of the tumor (Fig. 11-E-6*G*).

The liver is a very common and important site for metastatic disease. As many as 25 to 50 percent of cancer patients have liver metastases at autopsy. Most tumors metastasize to the liver, and metastases to the liver strongly affect stage of the tumor and prognosis of the patient. Most metastases are multiple, diffusely distributed, variable in size, and solid. They may be necrotic and appear more cystic. Liver metastases may be present even when both general and specific serum markers for tumor, e.g., liver function tests and carcinoembryonic antigen, are normal. Metastases may be poorly vascularized or highly vascular, a difference that affects their appearance after intravenous contrast material administration. Mucin-producing carcinomas, e.g., breast and colon carcinomas, frequently produce calcification, which can be detected with imaging studies. Metastases are almost always evaluated with cross-sectional imaging studies. Although US can be useful in evaluating liver metastases when used by skilled operators, it is limited by ileus. On US, metastases are usually hypoechoic, poorly defined, and hypovascular, and they may have a peripheral halo (Fig. 11-E-6*H*). Some types, such as breast cancer, may be diffusely distributed in minute form. In most institutions, CT is used to survey and monitor patients for liver metastases, since CT can detect metastases and is probably the most useful technique for evaluating extrahepatic disease. On CT, metastases are usually multifocal, of low attenuation, and often (but not always) better shown with administration of intravenous contrast material when compared with preinfusion scans (Fig. 11-E-6*I*). Again, some forms present as diffuse inhomogeneity. Because of its sensitivity and potential for characterizing some lesions specifically, MR imaging may become the technique of choice in the future for detecting and characterizing liver metastases. Lesions have low signal intensity on T1-weighted images and higher signal intensity (but never as high as in cavernous hemangioma) on T2-weighted studies (Fig. 11-E-6*J*). Certain lesions, e.g., melanoma, carcinoid, and endocrine tumors of the pancreas, have very high signal with strongly T2-weighted scans.

Angiosarcoma is a rare, highly vascular tumor of the liver. It is seen in patients who have had an occupational exposure to certain chemicals, particularly polyvinyl chloride or Thorotrast. If lesions rupture, they may produce serious hemorrhagic sequelae. On US, angiosarcoma is usually hypoechoic. Sometimes the attendant fibrosis so obscures the tumor that it is impossible to identify. On CT, the lesions have low attenuation (Fig. 11-E-6*K*), may enhance markedly, and if arising in the presence of Thorotrast, can displace and distort the Thorotrast collections.

Focal nodular hyperplasia (FNH) and liver cell adenoma are easily confused. Both are histologically benign liver disorders that produce focal (or multifocal) lesions. Both processes can occur in young adults. On imaging studies, both can resemble either primary or metastatic liver tumors. Finally, both can be single or multiple. However, some important differences pertain. FNH is probably a hamartoma of the liver, i.e., a localized overgrowth of mature cells that are identical to the types constituting the liver and contain fibrous tissue, blood vessels, bile ducts, and occasional well-differentiated hepatocytes. Adenoma is a true benign tumor composed of one tissue element of the liver, the hepatocyte. FNH often contains a central fibrotic scar. Adenoma is associated with the use of oral contraceptives, whereas FNH probably is not. Adenoma, unlike FNH, tends to undergo hemorrhage and thus to present acutely. US is nonspecific in studying FNH. Adenoma is usually hyperechoic but heterogeneous. On CT, FNH is transiently but markedly hypervascular, and the central scar may be seen (Fig. 11-E-6*L*). Adenoma usually shows low density, may hemorrhage as high-density collections on preinfusion scans, and enhances variably. On NM, FNH can show either increased, decreased, or normal activity compared with that of liver. Adenoma usually shows no increased uptake in NM studies, but this varies. FNH has low signal intensity on T1-weighted MR images and slightly high signal intensity on T2-weighted images (Fig. 11-E-6*M,N*). If the central scar is present, it may exhibit high signal intensity on T2-weighted images. Adenoma, like many lesions, has a nonspecific appearance of low signal intensity on T1-weighted examinations and slightly high signal intensity on T2-weighted examinations. Hemorrhage is recognizable as high signal intensity on T1-weighted images. Angiographically, FNH is hypervascular with radiating branches that produce a "spoked-wheel" appearance. Adenoma has a variable appearance but is generally less vascular than FNH.

Hepatocellular carcinoma, or hepatoma, is a primary malignancy of the liver. It is found in older cirrhotics in the United States but in younger patients in areas of the Far East and Africa where it is endemic. Chronic hepatitis B infection and exposure to aflatoxin predispose to the formation of hepatoma. On imaging studies, hepatoma appears as (1) a single predominant lesion (most common form), (2) a predominant lesion with multiple, smaller, surrounding daughter lesions, or (3) diffuse tumor. Portal vein invasion by the tumor in any form is relatively common and can aid in distinguishing hepatoma from other lesions. On US, hepatoma is most commonly a discrete lesion with increased, similar, or decreased echogenicity in comparison with that of liver. Hepatoma may be multiple or single, and portal vein invasion can be detected. On CT, lesions are most commonly of low density and may enhance if fast scans are performed after contrast material administration (Fig. 11-E-7*B*). Portal venous thrombosis can be seen, and preexisting cirrhosis or Thorotrast can be demonstrated. MR imaging findings are similar to those of CT, but as with CT, the lesion is inhomogeneous.

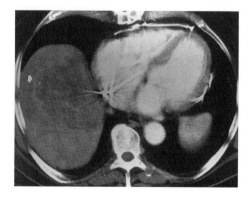

FIG. 11-E-7 (*Panel B*) CT in hepatoma showing the presence of an inhomogeneous lesion that enhances mildly in its periphery (*arrow*).

EXERCISE 11-3: UPPER ABDOMINAL TRAUMA

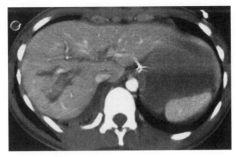

FIG. 11-E-9   *Panel A*

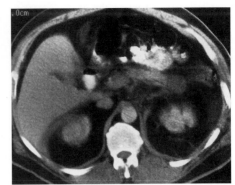

FIG. 11-E-10   *Panel A*

Clinical Histories:

CASE 11-9
A 45-year-old motor vehicle accident victim presents with upper abdominal pain (Fig. 11-E-9*A*).

CASE 11-10
A 57-year-old man presents who was beaten in the abdomen with a baseball bat (Fig. 11-E-10*A*).

Questions:

11-9. Most likely diagnosis in Case 11-9?
   A.   Hepatic contusion
   B.   Hepatic laceration
   C.   Uncomplicated ascites

11-10. Most likely diagnosis in Case 11-10?
   A.   Pancreatic trauma
   B.   Bowel injury
   C.   Mesenteric injury

Radiographic Findings:

   11-9. In this case, the liver has an irregularly linear lesion in its central aspect, representing a liver laceration (*B* is the correct answer).
   11-10. In this case, there is a low-density bulbous enlargement of the pancreatic tail, representing a pancreatic injury (*A* is the correct answer).

Discussion:

Hepatic injury is common after blunt trauma. Hepatic injuries may be life-threatening as a result of exsanguination and shock, but more often operative management is not even required. Observation and systemic support may be the only treatment necessary. Like trauma to any other organ, injury to the liver occurs within a spectrum from mild to severe. A mild injury of the liver produces a localized collection of traumatized liver tissue and an interstitial hematoma, like a bruise, which is termed a *contusion*. More severe injuries that involve complete disruption of the tissue into fracture planes, perhaps involving the hepatic veins, inferior vena cava, or portal veins, are called *lacerations*.
   Most blunt abdominal trauma in the United States is radiographically evaluated with CT. Angiography is used to a lesser extent. US, NM, and MR imaging are of little or no value in a general survey of abdominal trauma. On CT, hepatic contusion is seen as a

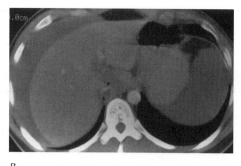

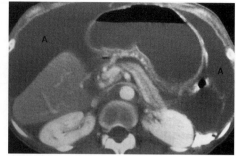

FIG. 11-E-9 (*Panel B*) CT in liver laceration showing the extension of the laceration into the IVC (*arrowheads*). (*Panel C*) CT in ascites showing fluid diffusely distributed throughout the abdomen (A).

B

C

low-attenuation lesion, perhaps with mass effect on surrounding hepatic vessels. Associated hemoperitoneum is not usually seen. On CT, hepatic laceration appears as an irregular, stellate, or linear lesion through the liver parenchyma (Fig. 11-E-9*A*), sometimes extending to porta, liver capsule, or IVC (Fig. 11-E-9*B*). A hallmark of severe trauma to upper abdominal organs is accompanying hemoperitoneum, which appears as a collection of high-density material at the site of bleeding and is termed the *sentinel clot*. Acute blood that has migrated away from the site of active bleeding or old hemoperitoneum at any site often is the attenuation of simple or near-simple fluid and can resemble intraperitoneal fluid, or ascites, from a number of causes.

Ascites is a nonspecific reaction of the peritoneal space to a variety of causes, including tumor, inflammation, trauma, increased systemic venous resistance (e.g., congestive heart failure), renal or hepatic insufficiency, and many other conditions. It is characterized by the production of intraperitoneal fluid. This fluid can be simple, a transudate, in which case it has fluid density (Fig. 11-E-9*C*) and is free to move to the dependent portion of the abdominal or pelvic cavity with patient movement. Alternatively, it can be complex, an exudate, in which case it is denser than simple fluid, is accompanied by solid tissue (e.g., tumor deposits in peritoneal metastases) or layered material (e.g., blood from trauma or inflammatory cellular debris in peritonitis), and often is loculated, or unable to move freely throughout the intraperitoneal cavity (e.g., abscess).

Pancreatic injury is an uncommon problem but is potentially extremely important. Mortality from pancreatic injuries is nearly 20 percent. Being crushed against the spine probably accounts for the frequency of injury to the body of the pancreas. Pancreatic trauma may or may not be associated with increased amylase. Usually caused by blunt trauma, these injuries are often associated with injuries to various other organs, such as liver and bowel. These injuries produce intraperitoneal blood and fluid and interstitial mesenteric edema, which can be confusing. As with hepatic trauma, CT is usually the modality of choice to evaluate pancreatic trauma, but even on CT, the diagnosis can be difficult to make. On CT, the pancreas may be ill-defined, enlarged, or even disrupted, i.e., fractured.

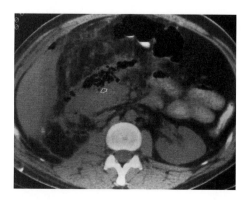

FIG. 11-E-10 (*Panel B*) CT in bowel injury showing the presence of extraluminal gas (*arrow*) due to bowel perforation.

Bowel and mesenteric injuries are found in approximately 5 percent of all patients undergoing laparotomy after motor vehicle accidents. Injuries of the bowel and mesentery frequently accompany injury to the liver or pancreas. These injuries can result in massive intraperitoneal bleeding from disruption of mesenteric vessels or peritonitis from bowel perforation. As elsewhere, CT is the modality of choice to evaluate patients for possible bowel or mesenteric injuries, but these injuries, like injuries to the pancreas, can be difficult to detect. On CT, injuries of the bowel and mesentery include free air within the intraperitoneal or retroperitoneal spaces (Fig. 11-E-10*B*), free intraabdominal fluid, circumferential or eccentric bowel wall thickening, enhancement of the bowel wall, streaky soft-tissue infiltration of the mesenteric fat, free mesenteric hematoma, and especially sentinel clot. Angiography may demonstrate free extravasation of contrast material in injuries of the mesenteric vessel, and percutaneous embolization may help deter bleeding when operative management is not possible.

EXERCISE 11-4: BILIARY INFLAMMATION

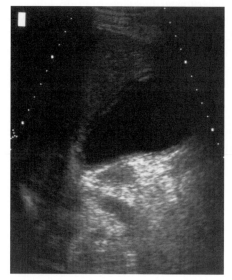

FIG. 11-E-11   *Panel A*

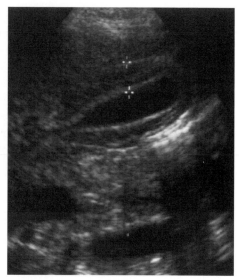

FIG. 11-E-12   *Panel A*

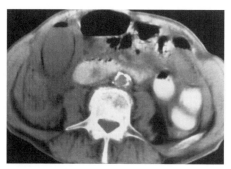

FIG. 11-E-13   *Panel A*

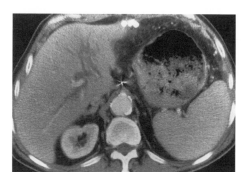

FIG. 11-E-14

Clinical Histories:

CASE 11-11
A 53-year-old man presents with acute right upper quadrant pain, fever, pain on palpation over the gallbladder, and elevated liver function tests (Fig. 11-E-11*A*).

CASE 11-12
A 22-year-old HIV-positive woman presents with debilitating and chronic illness with vague right upper quadrant pain but no tenderness on palpation over the gallbladder (Fig. 11-E-12*A*).

CASE 11-13
An 84-year-old man presents with right upper quadrant pain, marked fever, and suspicion of sepsis (Fig. 11-E-13*A*).

CASE 11-14
A 53-year-old man presents with a history of cholecystectomy, upper abdominal pain, jaundice, and fever (Fig. 11-E-14).

Questions:

11-11. Most likely diagnosis in Case 11-11?
A. Acute cholecystitis
B. Uncomplicated cholelithiasis
C. Chronic cholecystitis
D. Porcelain gallbladder

11-12. Most likely diagnosis in Case 11-12?
A. Oriental cholangiohepatitis
B. AIDS-associated cholangiopathy
C. Choledocholithiasis

11-13. Most likely diagnosis in Case 11-13?
A. Acute cholecystitis
B. Emphysematous cholecystitis
C. Porcelain gallbladder
D. Hydrops of gallbladder

11-14. Most likely diagnosis in Case 11-14?
A. Choledocholithiasis
B. Ascending cholangitis
C. Acute cholecystitis

Radiographic Findings:

11-11. In this case, the gallbladder is distended, and the wall is thickened, measuring more than 5 mm, and has multiple lamina, indicating gallbladder wall inflammation from acute cholecystitis (*A* is the correct answer).

11-12. In this case, the gallbladder wall is markedly thickened, measuring over 1 cm, with multiple lamina, but was not tender to palpation, findings seen often with AIDS-associated cholangiopathy (*B* is the correct answer).

11-13. In this case, the primary abnormality is that the gallbladder wall and lumen contain gas, indicating emphysematous cholecystitis (*B* is the correct answer).

11-14. In this case, the biliary ducts are distended and irregular, which in the clinical presentation of fever and jaundice most strongly suggest cholangitis (*B* is the correct answer).

Discussion:

Calculi are a common problem in the gallbladder and biliary ducts. Cholelithiasis is one of the most common abdominal disorders overall and is the most common cause of cholecystitis, as well as the most common indication for abdominal surgery. Gallstones develop when the composition of bile, which includes bile salts, lecithin, and cholesterol, varies from normal and creates supersaturation of cholesterol, which then precipitates. Historically, patients thought to be harboring gallstones on the basis of clinical criteria were examined by oral cholecystography, which shows filling defects in the gallbladder lumen opacified by orally ingested cholangiographic contrast material. However, this evaluation method has been largely replaced by sonography, occasionally supported by other imaging information. On US, gallstones usually appear as mobile, intraluminal, echogenic foci that cast a well-defined acoustic shadow (Fig. 11-E-11*B*). Two other possible appearances are echogenic foci in the gallbladder fossa without visible surrounding bile when the gallbladder is contracted and small, mobile, echogenic foci that do not cast a shadow. On CT, gallstones appear as dense, well-defined, intraluminal structures (Fig. 11-E-11*C*), but their density can vary from fat density to near bone density depending on the relative concentration of calcium and cholesterol. NM, MRI, and angiography have no major role at this time in the assessment of gallstones.

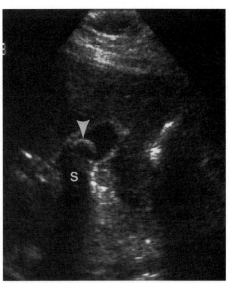

FIG. 11-E-11 (*Panel B*) Transverse US in cholelithiasis showing an echogenic structure (*arrowhead*) casting an acoustic shadow (S). (*Panel C*) CT in cholelithiasis using both soft-tissue windows (S) and bone windows (B) showing an extremely dense structure lying in the gallbladder. Note the laminated architecture of the gallstone on the bone windows (*arrowhead*).

B

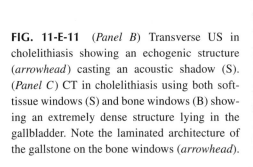

C

Choledocholithiasis occurs when calculi pass from the gallbladder into the biliary ducts or when calculi develop originally within the ductal system. Regardless of origin, they may obstruct the biliary ducts, cause biliary colic, and lead to cholangitis. Common duct stones are usually evaluated with US and CT and by direct visualization with endoscopic retrograde cholangiopancreatography (ERCP). On US, choledocholithiasis appears as echogenic foci within the lumen of the biliary duct. Sonographically, common duct stones are detected less readily than gallbladder stones, and meticulous technique is required. Choledocholithiasis can cause acoustic shadows, but for technical reasons, they are detected less frequently than those of cholelithiasis (Fig. 11-E-12*B*). On CT, choledocholithiasis appears as intraluminal biliary ductal foci, which, like gallbladder stones, may vary in density from hypodense to isodense to hyperdense to bile, depending on composition (Fig. 11-E-12*C*).

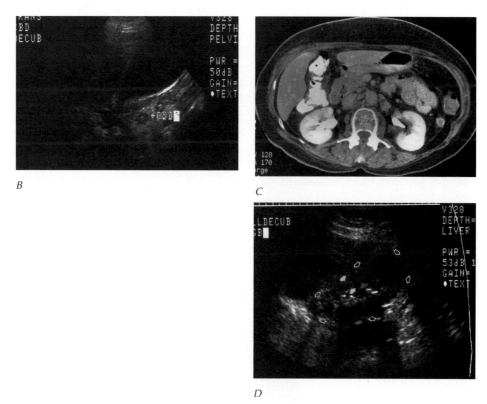

FIG. 11-E-12 (*Panel B*) Transverse US in choledocholithiasis showing the presence of an intra-ductal stone (*CBD*). Note that it does not cast an acoustic shadow, which, unlike gallbladder stones, is typical of intraductal stones. (*Panel C*) CT in choledocholithiasis showing the presence of a stone within the common bile duct (*arrowheads*). Note that it is soft-tissue density, which is often, though not always, the case with intraductal stones. (*Panel D*) Longitudinal US in acute cholecystitis showing thickened gallbladder wall (*white arrows*), gallstones, casting an acoustic shadow. Open arrows are gallbladder boundary. The patient was extremely tender to palpation by the transducer right over the gallbladder (sonographic Murphy's sign). (*Panel E*) NM hepatobiliary scan in acute cholecystitis showing the absence of gallbladder activity in the gallbladder fossa (*white arrow*) 60 min following administration of the agent and even after administration of morphine. (*Courtesy of James Ball, M.D., Winston-Salem, N.C.*)

Cholecystitis is inflammation of the gallbladder that is almost always caused by ob-struction of the cystic duct, usually by an impacted calculus. The inflammation may be acute or chronic, uncomplicated or complicated, calculous or acalculous. As the gall-bladder continues to accumulate bile, intraluminal pressure increases, and vascular in-sufficiency of the wall occurs, causing ischemia, necrosis, and often supervening inflam-mation. The gallbladder distends, the gallbladder wall thickens from edema, and the patient is tender to palpation over the gallbladder (positive Murphy's sign).

Both US and hepatobiliary NM studies are the modalities of choice to evaluate pos-sible cholecystitis. Sonographic signs of acute cholecystitis include cholelithiasis, gall-bladder wall thickening (greater than 3 mm), irregular or linear hypoechoic structures within the gallbladder wall, a positive Murphy's sign, and marked gallbladder distension (Fig. 11-E-12*D*). A combination of these signs is a good positive predictor of acute cholecystitis. In marked chronic cholecystitis, US shows persistent gallbladder wall thickening or sludge, stones, and contraction of the gallbladder. However, in the presence of cholelithiasis, the gallbladder almost always shows signs of chronic inflammation his-tologically, even without symptoms or sonographic findings.

The primary hepatobiliary sign of acute cholecystitis is the absence of activity in the gallbladder despite good hepatic uptake, given sufficient time after injection of the agent

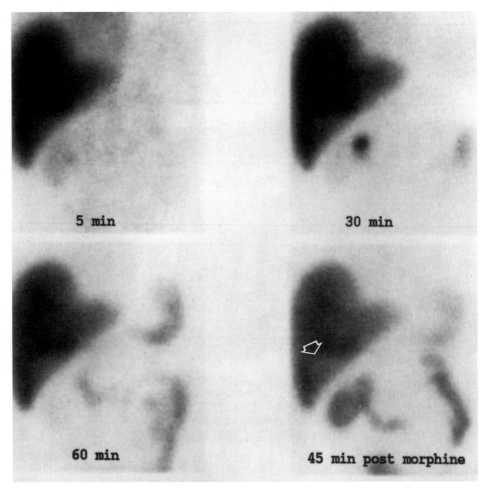

5 min

30 min

60 min

45 min post morphine

FIG. 11-E-12 (*Continued*)

E

(Fig. 11-E-12*E*). This time depends on whether or not morphine is administered. Morphine increases the tone of the sphincter of Oddi and increases intraluminal common bile duct pressure to overcome the resistance to bile flow into the gallbladder in chronic cholecystitis but not in acute cholecystitis when a stone obstructs the duct. Acute cholecystitis is diagnosed when absence of activity is noted either 45 min after morphine augmentation or after 4 h without morphine augmentation. Delayed gallbladder visualization after 1 h usually reflects chronic cholecystitis. On CT, the morphologic findings in patients with acute cholecystitis are similar to the US findings, including gallstones and a thickened and inhomogeneous gallbladder wall. However, CT is not as sensitive as US or NM. MR imaging and angiography have no established role as yet in the diagnosis of cholecystitis.

Many potential complications and conditions are associated with cholecystitis. These include hydrops, porcelain gallbladder, milk-of-calcium bile, and emphysematous cholecystitis.

Hydrops refers to the marked distension of the gallbladder by clear, sterile mucus, usually under conditions of chronic, complete cystic duct obstruction. On imaging studies, the primary finding is enlargement of the gallbladder (Fig. 11-E-13*B*).

Porcelain gallbladder refers to calcification of the gallbladder wall as a result of chronic inflammation causing dystrophic calcification and often associated with recurrent acute cholecystitis. Gallbladder stones are usually present, and there is a higher incidence (approximately 10 to 20 percent) of gallbladder carcinoma. On imaging studies, complete or incomplete circular wall calcification is present and is seen as a curvilinear, highly echogenic wall on US or as a curvilinear, high-attenuation wall on CT (Fig. 11-E-13*C*).

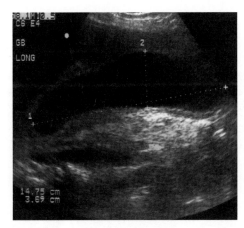

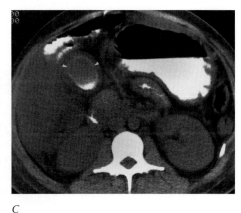

C

B

FIG. 11-E-13 (*Panel B*) Longitudinal US in hydrops showing a massively enlarged gallbladder due to complete obstruction of the cystic duct and accumulation of clear mucus. (*Panel C*) CT in porcelain gallbladder showing the calcification of the gallbladder wall (*arrowheads*) and the dependent accumulation of calcified material in the gallbladder lumen.

Milk-of-calcium bile refers to a precipitation of calcified material within the lumen of the gallbladder, usually associated with chronic cholecystitis. US shows echogenic sludgelike material, possibly with gallstones. CT demonstrates the distinctive appearance of a horizontal bile-calcium level.

Emphysematous cholecystitis is a distinctive condition. Like acute cholecystitis, it is marked by intense gallbladder wall inflammation, but unlike acute cholecystitis, it is not necessarily associated with gallstones. It may be related to ischemia of the gallbladder wall from small-vessel disease, and it affects an older age group than does acute cholecystitis. Gas is released by bacterial invasion and accumulates in the gallbladder wall, lumen, or both. On US, gas is seen as an echogenic focus producing poorly defined or "dirty" shadowing behind it. The wall is thickened, perhaps focally, with gas. On CT, air-density gas is seen within the lumen or wall (Fig. 11-E-13*A*). MR imaging and angiography have no current role in evaluation of these complications.

Like inflammation of the gallbladder, inflammation of the biliary ducts, or *cholangitis,* is an important clinical condition. It is less common than cholecystitis. AIDS-associated cholangiopathy, ascending cholangitis, and oriental cholangiohepatitis are three important forms of cholangitis.

AIDS-associated cholangiopathy is marked by the frequent isolation of opportunistic organisms, including *Cryptosporidium* and cytomegalovirus from the bile, and by considerable inflammation of the bile duct wall. On US or CT, the gallbladder or biliary duct walls may be markedly thickened (greater than 4 mm) (Fig. 11-E-12*A*) and may contain irregular lamina. Inflammation is present, but stones may or may not be present. Cholangiography shows irregular strictures, papillary stenosis, or both.

Ascending cholangitis is a bacterial inflammation of both walls and lumina of the biliary system, including the gallbladder. It is almost always due to obstruction of the biliary tract, especially when caused by choledocholithiasis and distal bile duct stenosis. The presence of grossly purulent material within the duct indicates suppurative cholangitis. Cross-sectional imaging studies are used to define the level and cause of obstruction. Cholangiography can show the abnormal biliary ducts directly. The purulent material of suppurative cholangitis may be seen as echogenic material on US, high-density material on CT, or filling defects on cholangiography.

Oriental cholangiohepatitis is a common illness endemic to some areas of Asia and can be seen in Asian immigrants in this country. It may be caused by bile duct wall injury from the parasitic infestation. Ductal stones commonly form, and the ducts are dilated. A characteristic finding is the presence of intraductal (especially intrahepatic ductal) calculi. These findings are readily demonstrated with US, CT, and cholangiography.

EXERCISE 11-5: PANCREATIC INFLAMMATION

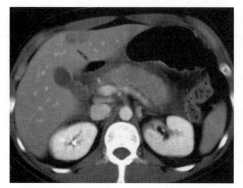

FIG. 11-E-15 *Panel A*

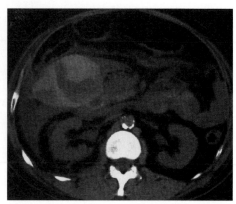

FIG. 11-E-16 *Panel A*

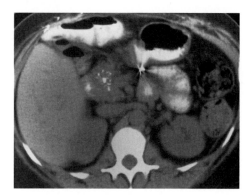

FIG. 11-E-17 *Panel A*

Clinical Histories:

CASE 11-15
A 54-year-old alcoholic man presents with marked epigastric pain and increased amylase (Fig. 11-E-15*A*).

CASE 11-16
A 45-year-old man presents with marked epigastric pain and falling hematocrit and is "crashing" (Fig. 11-E-16*A*).

CASE 11-17
A 65-year-old man presents with epigastric pain (Fig. 11-E-17*A*).

Questions:

11-15. Most likely diagnosis in Case 11-15?
    A.   Acute edematous pancreatitis
    B.   Pancreatic abscess
    C.   Pancreatic phlegmon

11-16. Most likely diagnosis in Case 11-16?
    A.   Acute edematous pancreatitis
    B.   Hemorrhagic pancreatitis
    C.   Gastroduodenal artery pseudoaneurysm

11-17. Most likely diagnosis in Case 11-17?
- A. Acute edematous pancreatitis
- B. Chronic pancreatitis
- C. Pancreatic phlegmon
- D. Hemorrhagic pancreatitis

Radiographic Findings:

11-15. In this case, the overall size of the pancreas is enlarged, the tissue around the pancreas is edematous, and the fat planes between the pancreas and the stomach are blurred, findings of acute edematous pancreatitis (*A* is the correct answer).

11-16. In this case, peripancreatic inflammatory changes and a high-density collection are seen adjacent to the pancreatic head, representing a collection of blood created by hemorrhagic pancreatitis (*B* is the correct answer).

11-17. In this case, multiple high-density calcifications are distributed throughout the pancreatic head, and the pancreatic head is mildly enlarged, findings of chronic calcific pancreatitis (*B* is the correct answer).

Discussion:

Pancreatitis, an inflammatory condition of the pancreas, has a number of causes, including alcohol abuse, trauma, cholelithiasis, peptic ulcer, hyperlipoproteinemia, hypercalcemia, and infection. Pancreatic inflammation may be acute or chronic. Acute pancreatitis and chronic pancreatitis may not represent different stages of the same disease.

Acute pancreatitis can occur once or repetitively and usually has the potential for healing. It can be associated with mild to severe inflammatory edema (edematous or interstitial pancreatitis) or with hemorrhage (hemorrhagic or necrotizing pancreatitis). These two forms of acute pancreatitis may be distinguishable only by the severity and time course of the disease. Edematous pancreatitis resolves within 2 to 3 days with appropriate therapy, whereas hemorrhagic pancreatitis requires much longer to resolve. The diagnosis of simple pancreatitis is usually based on medical history, physical examination, and laboratory results. With this information, imaging studies are usually unnecessary, and scans show the pancreas to be normal or only slightly enlarged. The surrounding fat is edematous. The pancreas appears hypoechoic on US (Fig. 11-E-15*B*). On CT, the surrounding fat appears as areas of streaky interstitial soft-tissue density in the transverse mesocolon around the pancreas (Fig. 11-E-15*C*).

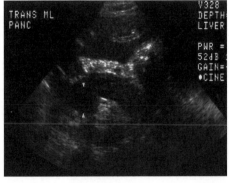
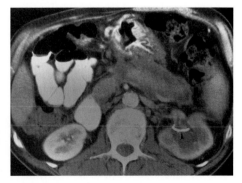

B   *C*

FIG. 11-E-15 (*Panel B*) Transverse US in acute pancreatitis showing a diffusely hypoechoic pancreas with more pronounced hypoechogenicity in the pancreatic head (*arrowheads*). (*Panel C*) CT in pancreatitis showing the presence of poorly defined soft-tissue planes around the pancreas obscuring the boundary between the pancreas and the stomach and colon. Note the stent in the renal pelvis (*black arrowhead*) of the left kidney, placed to relieve urinary obstruction.

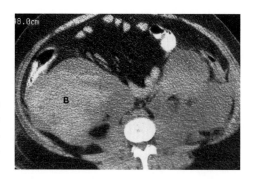

FIG. 11-E-17 (*Panel B*) CT in hemorrhagic pancreatitis showing diffusely distributed pancreatic inflammatory exudate containing high-density blood (B) in the right side of the abdomen.

Clinical criteria to predict the severity or likelihood of complications of pancreatitis correlate well with the presence and extent of extrapancreatic abnormalities on imaging studies. Imaging is useful in acute pancreatitis when assessing potential complications. These complications include hemorrhagic pancreatitis, vascular complications, phlegmon, and abscess.

Hemorrhagic pancreatitis is usually due to erosion of small vessels. Hemorrhagic pancreatitis is often a very serious problem and indicates that the patient is acutely and critically ill. It appears as a collection of echogenic material on US. On CT, it appears as a collection of high-density material and can be extremely extensive, since it is an aggressive process (Fig. 11-E-17*B*). This material represents blood.

Large vessels are at risk for developing pseudoaneurysms when the histiolytic enzymes released by the inflamed pancreas erode their walls, leading to a focal, highly vascular structure within the region of the pancreas. The splenic, gastroduodenal, and hepatic arteries are particularly prone to this complication. On US and CT, flow within an enlarged, rounded vessel can be seen. Angiography is the standard means of establishing the diagnosis by showing a focally enlarged vessel, sometimes with extravasation.

Phlegmon is an inflammatory, boggy, edematous soft-tissue mass, distinct from fluid, arising from the pancreas and diffusely spreading away from it. Phlegmon appears as a diffuse soft-tissue echogenicity or density process surrounding the pancreas and contains neither blood of hemorrhagic pancreatitis nor the fluid of abscess (Fig. 11-E-16*B*).

Abscesses are a potentially life-threatening complication of pancreatitis. Infection associated with pancreatitis can be thought of as representing infected necrosis (diffuse infection without pus collection) or pancreatic abscess (collection of pus surrounded by a capsule). Infected necrosis is harder to identify on imaging studies than is pancreatic abscess, since it is less distinct and blends into the surrounding edema. On US, abscess appears as a poorly defined anechoic or hypoechoic lesion. It enhances sound posteriorly and may contain debris. Gas appears as a poorly defined echogenic focus within the nondependent aspect of the lesion and casts a "dirty" shadow. On CT, the lesion is poorly defined and may contain gas collections (Fig. 11-E-16*C*). After contrast material infusion,

FIG. 11-E-16 (*Panel B*) CT in pancreatic phlegmon showing the presence of poorly defined phlegmonous exudate (P) surrounding the entire pancreas and extending from the pancreas toward the anterior abdominal wall. (*Panel C*) CT in pancreatic abscess showing the presence of gas in the pancreatic tail (G) from a gas-forming organism.

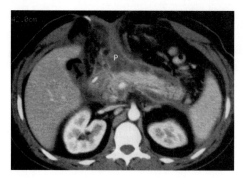

B

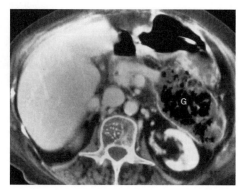

C

the border enhances. If gas is absent, abscess cannot be differentiated from phlegmon or pseudocyst. In general, NM, MR imaging and angiography do not have a major role in the evaluation of acute pancreatitis.

Unlike acute pancreatitis, chronic pancreatitis is considered to indicate permanent pancreatic damage. Chronic pancreatitis may or may not be preceded by prior attacks of acute pancreatitis. The pancreas will develop calcifications within the ductal system (Fig. 11-E-17A). Masslike enlargement of the pancreas can occur periodically, but often the gland eventually atrophies. The pancreatic duct may dilate. These findings are visible on both US and CT. NM, MR imaging and angiography do not have a current major role in the evaluation of chronic pancreatitis.

EXERCISE 11-6: PANCREATIC NEOPLASM

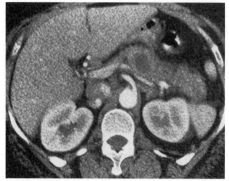

FIG. 11-E-18 *Panel A*

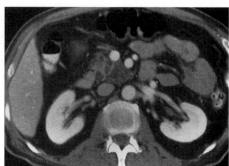

FIG. 11-E-19

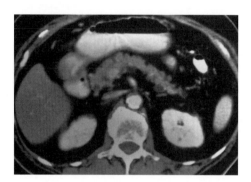

FIG. 11-E-20

Clinical Histories:

CASE 11-18
A 62-year-old woman presents with vague, deep, and persistent abdominal pain (Fig. 11-E-18*A*).

CASE 11-19
A 65-year-old man presents with midepigastric pain over a long period of time (Fig. 11-E-19).

CASE 11-20
A 32-year-old healthy, asymptomatic woman (Fig. 11-E-20).

Questions:

11-18. Most likely diagnosis in Case 11-18?
  A. Pancreatic cyst
  B. Ductal pancreatic carcinoma
  C. Pancreatic metastasis
  D. Peripancreatic lymphadenopathy

11-19. Most likely diagnosis in Case 11-19?
  A. Cholangiocarcinoma
  B. Cystic pancreatic neoplasm
  C. Ductal pancreatic carcinoma

11-20. Most likely diagnosis in Case 11-20?
A. Acute edematous pancreatitis
B. Pancreatic pseudocyst
C. Pancreatic cyst
D. Cystic pancreatic neoplasm

Radiographic Findings:

11-18. In this case, there is a low-density, but not fluid, lesion in the pancreatic body, expanding the contour of the pancreas, and not associated with any inflammatory changes in the peripancreatic fat, findings most consistent with a ductal adenocarcinoma (*B* is the correct answer).

11-19. In this case, there is a fluid-density lesion within the pancreatic head and uncinate process of the pancreas, not associated with inflammatory changes in the peripancreatic fat, findings most compatible with a cystic neoplasm of the pancreas (*B* is the correct answer).

11-20. In this case, several small, simple, unilocular cysts are seen in the pancreatic parenchyma, without inflammatory changes or signs of peripancreatic extension of any disease process (*C* is the correct answer).

Discussion:

Pancreatic masses include tumors, tumorlike masses such as cysts and developmental anomalies, and inflammatory lesions. These can overlap in appearance, such as when an inflammatory mass simulates a neoplastic mass on imaging studies. They can be causally related, such as when a neoplastic mass secondarily causes an inflammatory mass. Therefore, differentiation among them is not entirely possible, either clinically or radiographically. However, the prognostic and management implications of the lesions that create pancreatic masses differ considerably and therefore require extensive and often invasive investigation. Although contrast studies of the gastrointestinal tract can be used to infer the presence of a mass, usually cross-sectional imaging studies are employed to establish the diagnosis.

Tumors of the pancreas are important clinical entities; some have an extremely poor prognosis, and some produce serious clinical symptoms. They can be classified according to origin as epithelial tumors, endocrine tumors, and miscellaneous lesions. Epithelial tumors can be solid or cystic. Solid ductal adenocarcinoma is the most common overall and carries the worst prognosis (mean survival 4 months). Cystic tumors, such as cystadenocarcinoma, have a less serious prognosis. Endocrine, or islet cell, tumors elaborate hormonal substances and can create serious symptoms. The two most common of these are insulinoma, which releases insulin and produces hypoglycemia, and gastrinoma, which releases gastrin and produces Zollinger-Ellison syndrome. There are many other important kinds of hormonally active pancreatic endocrine tumors, and each is designated by the hormone it secretes (e.g., glucagonoma, somatostatinoma). Miscellaneous lesions arise from pancreatic parenchymal tissue (e.g., metastases, especially from melanoma, and lung or breast cancer) or from tissue other than pancreas (e.g., intrapancreatic cholangiocarcinoma or peripancreatic lymph node). These miscellaneous lesions are important because they sometimes strongly simulate true pancreatic neoplasms on imaging studies.

Ductal adenocarcinoma has a variety of appearances on imaging studies. On US, it usually is seen as a focal, hypoechoic, irregular, solid mass. Rarely, it is isoechoic or involves the entire gland. In some pancreatic head masses, the only finding may be that the uncinate process is rounded. The pancreatic or biliary duct may be dilated by the obstructing tumor. Pseudocysts, cystic collections in or around the pancreas, may form because of pancreatic duct dilatation and perforation. On CT, the tumor presents as a solid, low-density, irregular mass, perhaps with ductal dilatation, pseudocyst formation, or both (Fig. 11-E-18*A*). Occasionally, the tumors will enhance brightly (Fig. 11-E-18*B*). Angiography may be used to demonstrate the vascular anatomy and establish defini-

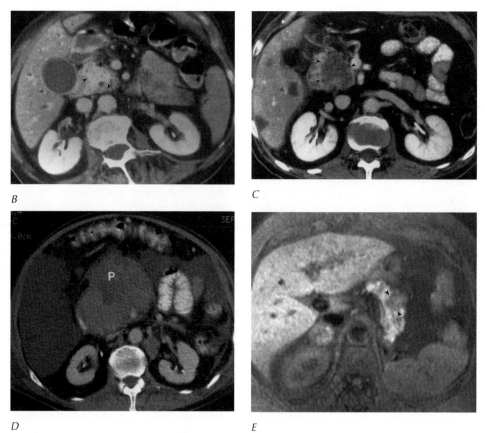

B   *C*

D   *E*

FIG. 11-E-18 (*Panel B*) CT in pancreatic ductal adenocarcinoma showing an enhancing tumor in the pancreatic head (*arrowheads*). (*Panel C*) CT in metastatic pancreatic carcinoma showing a pancreatic mass (*arrowheads*) and numerous liver metastases. (*Panel D*) CT in parapancreatic lymphadenopathy showing the presence of a large soft-tissue mass (P) simulating a pancreatic carcinoma but without the biliary duct obstruction that is normally caused by a lesion this size (normal biliary tree not shown). (*Panel E*) Transverse MRI image of a pancreatic metastasis from lung carcinoma (*arrowheads*).

tively whether certain key vessels (e.g., the superior mesenteric artery or vein) are encased. If so, the lesion is unresectable. NM and MR imaging currently have no established role in evaluation of pancreatic tumors. Associated metastases in the liver establish the fact that a pancreatic mass cannot be simply inflammatory (Fig. 11-E-18*C*). General pertinent negatives on cross-sectional imaging may help to differentiate adenocarcinoma from other nontumorous masses. Calcification is rarely, if ever, seen in ductal adenocarcinoma, and it is almost never hypervascular.

Ductal adenocarcinoma is simulated by a number of other entities. These include peripancreatic lymphadenopathy, intrapancreatic cholangiocarcinoma, and pancreatic metastases. Peripancreatic lymphadenopathy from lymphoma, leukemia, or any other primary malignancy can closely resemble a pancreatic mass. On imaging studies, it may appear as solid soft tissue in the pancreatic region (Fig. 11-E-18*D*). Keys to differentiating lymphadenopathy from a primary solid mass include smooth lobulation and pseudoseptations caused by incomplete coalescence of the lymph nodes. Also, peripancreatic lymphadenopathy is much less likely to obstruct the pancreatic duct, although suprapancreatic lymph nodes obstruct the biliary duct as it passes through the porta hepatis.

Two uncommon neoplastic processes that occur in the pancreas are cholangiocarcinoma and metastases. Cholangiocarcinoma usually does not occur within the pancreas, but when it does, it can exactly mimic a pancreatic head mass to the extent of producing biductal dilatation. Metastases appear as solid intrapancreatic lesions. If they necrose, they appear as fluid masses. Since they may be completely indistinguishable from primary tumors, the diagnosis may be inferred only from the clinical history. Pancreatic metastases are quite uncommon, usually arise from melanoma or lung primary lesions, and mimic a focal mass lesion of any neoplastic origin (Fig. 11-E-18*E*).

Pancreatic endocrine tumors also may simulate ductal adenocarcinoma, and in fact, no specific features consistently distinguish the two. Occasionally, however, certain imaging features can be helpful, especially when combined with the history. Many islet cell tumors appear simply as solid masses within the pancreas. However, some (especially in insulinoma) may appear hypervascular when studied with fast bolus, or dynamic, CT, and they may appear as extremely dense lesions immediately after enhancement with intravenous contrast material. Calcifications, which sometimes are very dense, are more commonly seen with islet cell tumors. MR imaging may have a role in the evaluation of islet cell tumors, since these tumors have a characteristic appearance on MR imaging studies. Islet cell tumors and their metastases have extremely high signal intensity on T2-weighted MR images, which can be used to characterize the origin of the lesion.

Primary cystic pancreatic malignancies and pancreatic cysts are not readily confused with typical ductal adenocarcinoma. Currently, cystic malignancies are classified as either microsystic adenomas or mucinous cystic neoplasms. This classification is helpful, since the two lesions are distinguishable from each other and from solid lesions on imaging studies. Microcystic adenomas are composed of innumerable very small cysts (1 mm to 2 cm) and contain highly vascularized fibrous septa and a central stellate fibrotic scar, which may calcify. They are not thought to be malignant or premalignant. Mucinous cystic neoplasms are composed of unilocular or multilocular cysts larger than 5 cm and may have large papillary excrescences. They are considered malignant or premalignant lesions. Both microcystic adenomas and mucinous cystic neoplasms are cystic, but differences in the sizes of the cysts can be recognized on US or CT. Pancreatic cysts can occur as isolated congenital cysts or as part of a more generalized multiorgan process that includes adult polycystic disease or von Hippel–Lindau disease. Regardless, their appearance is similar to that of a cyst in any other organ (Fig. 11-E-20). US and CT depict a uniloculated or multiloculated cyst. A pancreatic cyst may be difficult to differentiate from a mucinous cystic neoplasm.

BIBLIOGRAPHY

Friedman AC, Dachman AH: *Radiology of the Liver, Biliary Tract, and Pancreas,* 1st ed. St. Louis, Mosby, 1994.

Jeffrey RB Jr et al: Computed tomography of pancreatic trauma. *Radiology* 147:491, 1983.

Moss AA et al: *Computed Tomography of the Body with Magnetic Resonance Imaging,* 2d ed. Philadelphia, Saunders, 1993.

Nghiem HV et al: CT of blunt trauma to the bowel and mesentery. *AJR* 160:53, 1993.

PART 5

HEAD AND SPINE

12

BRAIN AND ITS COVERINGS

Daniel W. Williams III

Technologic advances in radiology during the past 20 years have vastly improved our ability to diagnose neurologic diseases. Prior to the introduction of computed tomography in 1974, neuroradiologic examinations of the brain consisted primarily of plain films of the skull, cerebral arteriography, pneumoencephalography, and conventional nuclear medicine studies. Unfortunately, these techniques for the most part provided only indirect information about suspected intracranial processes, were insensitive in detecting subtle or early brain lesions, or were potentially harmful to the patient. Computed tomography revolutionized the radiologic workup of central nervous system abnormalities because for the first time normal and abnormal structures could be visualized directly with minimal risk to the patient. With the recent development of other neuroimaging techniques (magnetic resonance imaging, ultrasonography, single photon emission computed tomography, and positron emission tomography) and with improvements in older techniques such as arteriography, the neuroradiologist today has a variety of sophisticated ways in which to evaluate the brain and brain function.

The main purpose of this chapter is to acquaint the reader with the major radiologic techniques used currently to evaluate the brain and its coverings. The strengths and weaknesses of these techniques are discussed. Imaging the

anatomy of the brain and its coverings is briefly reviewed. Basic guidelines for technique selection for evaluating common neurologic conditions are provided. Finally, examples of common brain abnormalities are presented. It is assumed that readers have a basic understanding of neuroanatomy and neuropathology.

Although this chapter may give some insight into neuroradiologic study interpretation, that is not its primary goal. Rather, readers should expect to become reasonably familiar with the various techniques employed to examine the brain and should gain some idea about the appropriate ordering of examinations in specific clinical situations.

TECHNIQUES

Radiologic modalities useful in evaluating the brain and its coverings can be divided into two major groups: anatomic modalities and functional modalities. Anatomic modalities, which provide information mostly of a structural nature, include plain films of the skull, computed tomography (CT), magnetic resonance (MR) imaging, cerebral arteriography (CA), and ultrasonography (US). On the other hand, single photon emission computed tomography (SPECT), positron emission tomography (PET), and magnetic resonance spectroscopy are primarily functional modalities, which give information about brain perfusion or metabolism. Some techniques provide both anatomic and functional information. For example, cerebral arteriography depicts blood vessels supplying the brain but also allows us to estimate brain circulation time. Ultrasound of the carotid bifurcation is another modality that provides both anatomic and functional information. A routine sonogram of the carotid bifurcation gives anatomic data that can be combined with Doppler data to provide information about blood flow.

The following discussion of current neuroradiologic techniques emphasizes relative examination cost and patient risk, along with the advantages and disadvantages of each technique. The normal imaging appearance of the brain and its coverings is also illustrated.

Anatomic Modalities

PLAIN FILMS

Plain films are obtained by placing a patient between an x-ray source and a recording device (i.e., x-ray film). The resulting x-ray "picture" is actually a record of x-ray beam attenuation produced by the different tissues within the structure being filmed, in this case, the skull (Fig. 12-1).

Bones of the skull can block a large number of x-rays and, therefore, cast a white "shadow" on the x-ray film. On the other hand, soft tissues such as scalp or brain cast little, if any, shadow on the film. The resulting skull film gives some information about the bony calvarium but no direct information about the intracranial contents. Indirect information about intracranial abnormalities can sometimes be obtained from the skull plain film, although this information can be quite subtle, even in the setting of advanced disease.

Another difficulty with plain-film interpretation is that the skull is a spherical structure, and therefore, bones are superimposed on one another. As a result, it is necessary to obtain multiple views of the skull to adequately assess the calvarium and to accurately localize a lesion. Routine views of the skull include the lateral view, various frontal views, and several axial views (see Fig. 12-1).

Plain films of the skull are relatively inexpensive, easy to obtain, and safe. However, they give information primarily about the bones of the skull. Since the intracranial contents are invisible on plain films, they give no direct information about most neurologic abnormalities. They can occasionally be tricky to interpret because of the large number of superimposed structures. Skull plain films have been largely replaced today by more sensitive techniques such as CT or MR imaging. Even in the setting of suspected skull fracture, plain films are rarely indicated, because CT scans also show the fracture, as well as any intracranial abnormality that might require treatment.

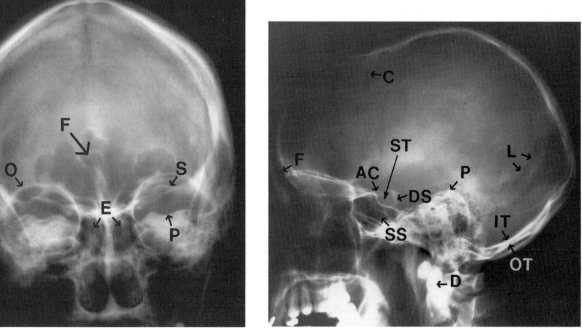

A   *B*

FIG. 12-1 Frontal (*A*) and lateral (*B*) plain films of the normal skull. Anatomic landmarks include ethmoid sinuses (E), frontal sinus (F), orbital roof (O), superior surface of the petrous portion of the temporal bone (P), sphenoid ridge (S), coronal suture (C), dens (D), anterior clinoid process (AC), dorsum sella (DS), sella turcica (ST), lambdoid suture (L), inner table of calvarium (IT), outer table of calvarium (OT), sphenoid sinus (SS).

COMPUTED TOMOGRAPHY

CT scans consist of computer-generated cross-sectional images obtained from a rotating x-ray beam and detector system. Patients typically lie on a table that incrementally moves them into the donut-shaped CT gantry. The resulting images give information about x-ray attenuation by the tissues traversed by the x-ray beam, much like that provided by plain films. However, unlike plain films, CT scans exquisitely depict and differentiate between soft tissues, thus allowing direct visualization of intracranial contents and abnormalities associated with neurologic diseases.

CT images are computer-generated and, therefore, can be viewed directly on a TV monitor. A viewer can adjust the image contrast or brightness ("window" or "level," respectively) to highlight particular tissues. In practice, images on the TV monitor are transferred to radiographic film for interpretation. Typically, a head CT consists of images adjusted to emphasize soft-tissue detail (soft-tissue windows) as well as images adjusted to visualize bony detail (bone windows) (Fig. 12-2). The CT technologist can change the slice thickness and angulation, among other technical factors, to change the way an image appears. Ax-

ial images are obtained most commonly, but coronal images can be obtained with hyperextension of the patient's neck. Since CT images are computer-generated, data making up the axial images can be reformatted in the coronal, sagittal, or oblique planes, although some resolution is lost.

CT examinations are often performed after intravenous administration of an iodinated contrast agent. These agents "light up," or enhance," normal blood vessels and dural sinuses, as well as intracranial structures that lack a blood-brain barrier (BBB), such as the pituitary gland, choroid plexus, or pineal gland. Pathologic conditions that interrupt the BBB also demonstrate enhancement after contrast material administration. For this reason, lesions that may be invisible on a noncontrast study are often obvious on a contrast-enhanced scan.

Structures seen on a normal head CT examination have variable intensity levels depending on their composition. These range from cortical bone, which appears white (has a high attenuation value), to air within the paranasal sinuses, which is black (has a low attenuation value) (see

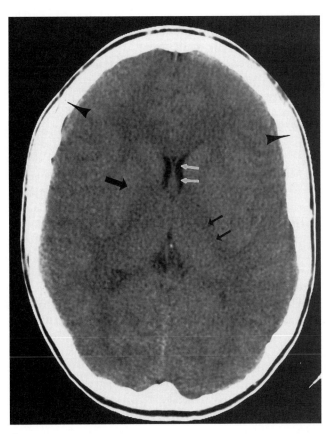
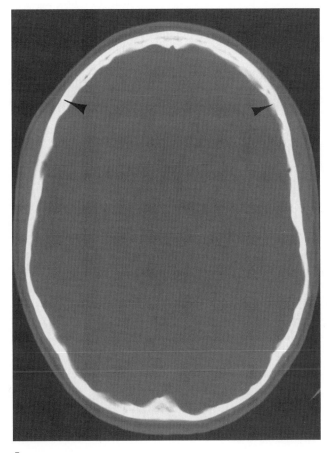

A   *B*

FIG. 12-2 Normal axial head CT images. Appropriate window selection allows visualization of both intracranial contents (*A*) and bony calvarium (*B*). Note the differences in attenuation between gray matter (right basal ganglia, *large arrow*), white matter (left internal capsule, *small black arrows*), CSF (frontal horn of the left lateral ventricle, *white arrows*), and bone (skull, *arrowheads*).

Fig. 12-2). Attenuation values are measured in CT numbers or Hounsfield units. Water has an arbitrarily assigned number of 0. Air has a negative number, as does fat, whereas soft-tissue structures have positive numbers slightly higher than that of water. Cerebral white matter has a slightly lower Hounsfield number than does cerebral gray matter and consequently appears slightly darker than gray matter on a head CT scan (Fig. 12-2*A*). Of course, bony structures have the highest CT numbers. Intracranial pathologic conditions can be either dark (low attenuation) or bright (high attenuation) depending on the particular abnormality. For example, acute intracranial hemorrhage is typically very bright, whereas an acute cerebral infarction demonstrates low attenuation when compared with the surrounding normal brain because of the presence of edema.

CT scans are moderately expensive (more than plain films but less than MR imaging) and are associated with a low level of risk to the patient. Certain patients are allergic to iodinated contrast material, and mild, moderate, or even severe reactions can occur when it is administered. The recent development of low-osmolality contrast agents has decreased the frequency of these reactions (although these agents are much more expensive than the older agents). The major advantage of CT scanning is that it allows a relatively quick assessment of intracranial contents in the setting of a neurologic deficit. Individual 1-cm slices of the

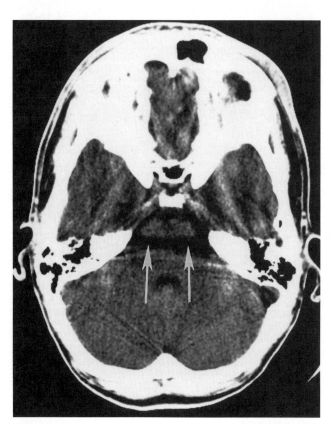

FIG. 12-3   Streak artifacts (*arrows*) commonly obscure portions of the brain stem, posterior fossa, and temporal lobes on routine head CT scans.

brain are typically obtained in 2 s, and an entire head scan can be performed in 10 to 15 min. CT scanners are also more widely available than are MR scanners. Images obtained are very sensitive to the presence of acute hemorrhage and calcifications and give excellent pictures of bone detail of the skull and skull base. Because of the configuration of the scanner, patients are reasonably accessible for monitoring during the examination.

CT scanners do have a number of disadvantages, however. Multiplanar imaging is difficult and sometimes impossible, and patients are exposed to ionizing radiation. Imaging artifacts can interfere with accurate interpretation. In particular, images of the brain stem and posterior fossa are often degraded by "streak" artifacts from dense bone (Fig. 12-3). Streak artifacts from metallic objects (e.g., fillings, braces, surgical clips) also can obscure abnormalities. Images can be severely degraded by patient motion. Fortunately, unlike MR scans, individual CT images degraded by motion can be redone rapidly.

MR IMAGING

One of the most exciting developments in radiology during the past 15 years has been the application of the nuclear magnetic resonance phenomenon, used for decades by physicists in spectroscopic chemical analysis, to imaging. The product of this application, MR imaging, has profoundly affected the radiologic evaluation of most neurologic disorders. MR examinations, like CT scans, consist of computer-reconstructed cross-sectional images (Fig. 12-4). In MR imaging, however, unlike CT scans or plain films, the information collected is not x-ray beam attenuation. The MR image is a visual display of nuclear magnetic resonance data collected principally from nuclei within body tissues—especially hydrogen nuclei within water and fat molecules. An MR image is obtained by placing a patient inside a powerful magnetic field. Hydrogen nuclei aligned with the magnetic field are excited by a radiofrequency (rf) pulse. When the rf pulse is turned off, excited nuclei return to their original ground state (i.e., relax). During this excitation-relaxation process, these nuclei release energy that can be detected by a sensitive receiver. This energy contains information about the molecular makeup of particular tissues in the imaged volume and also spatial information necessary for proper anatomic organization of these data. This loss of excitation energy and the resulting current induced in the receiver are responsible for the MR signal and ultimately the MR image.

Obviously, the information provided by MR imaging is entirely different from that provided by CT, even though both examinations consist of computer-generated cross-sectional images. Whereas CT gives information about x-ray beam attenuation, MR imaging gives information mainly about how magnetized tissues respond (i.e., relax) after exposure to an rf pulse. Intrinsic tissue relaxation occurs by two major pathways, called *longitudinal,* or T1,

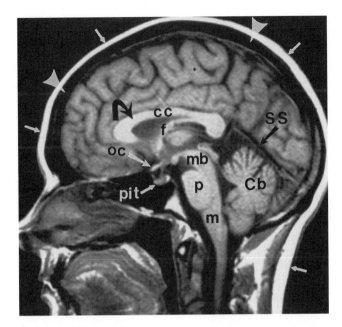

A

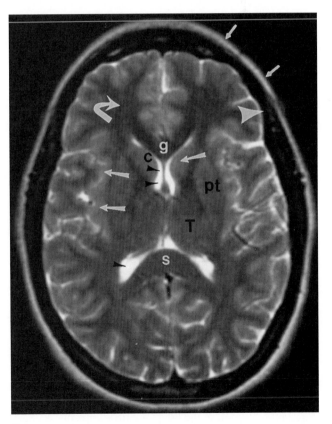

FIG. 12-4 Normal head MR images. Sagittal T1-weighted (*A*), axial T1-weighted (*B*), and axial T2-weighted (*C*) images. Note differences in signal between gray matter (*large arrows*), white matter (*curved arrows*), CFS (*small arrowheads*), fat (*small arrows*), and cortical bone (*large arrowheads*) on different pulse sequences. Normal structures include the genu (g) and splenium (s) of the corpus callosum (cc), fornix (f), optic chiasm (oc), pituitary gland (pit), midbrain (mb), pons (p), medulla (m), cerebellar vermis (Cb), straight sinus (SS), caudate head (c), putamen (pt), and thalamus (T).

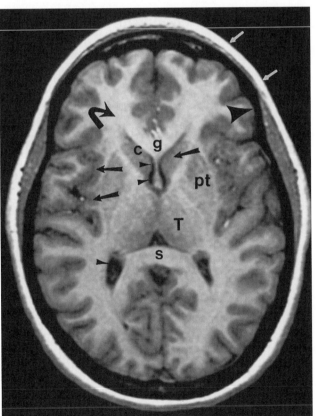

B

C

and *transverse,* or T2, *decay.* MR imaging sequences that emphasize T1 decay are commonly referred to as *T1-weighted;* sequences that bring out T2 relaxation properties are called *T2-weighted* (Fig. 12-4). Most MR scans of the brain use both these sequences, since certain abnormalities may only be obvious on one or the other. T2-weighted images are usually easy to identify because fluid (e.g., cerebrospinal, globe vitreous) is very bright; fluid on a T1-weighted scan is usually dark. Fat is bright on T1-weighted scans but darker on T2-weighted images. On the other hand, both cortical bone and air are very dark on all imaging sequences. Brain tissue has intermediate intensity; vessels can have almost any signal, depending on the velocity of flowing blood.

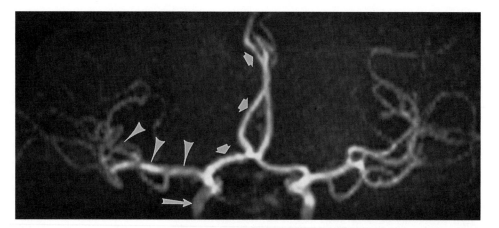

FIG. 12-5 Normal frontal view of intracranial MR angiogram at the level of the circle of Willis. Note the internal carotid artery (*large arrow*), anterior cerebral artery (*small arrows*), and middle cerebral artery (*arrowheads*).

A contrast agent is also available for MR imaging. The agent currently used is gadopentetate-dimeglumine (Gd-DTPA), which is very well tolerated and extremely safe. Its major use in the central nervous system (CNS) is to improve lesion detectability by "lighting up" pathologic conditions that either lack a BBB or have disrupted the BBB.

Since MR imaging technology has not yet matured, major advances continue to occur at a rapid pace. Recent developments include MR angiography and MR spectroscopy. MR angiography uses the MR scanner to noninvasively generate three-dimensional images of the carotid or vertebral basilar circulations (Fig. 12-5). Image quality is still not equal to that of conventional cerebral arteriograms, but it is constantly improving. Many believe that MR angiography could eventually replace much conventional arteriography, especially for evaluating carotid stenoses or for screening for intracranial aneurysms. In MR spectroscopy, the MR scanner performs in vivo tissue characterization of brain abnormalities. It is hoped that this procedure will help in the pretreatment and posttreatment evaluation of brain tumors and stroke.

A routine MR imaging study of the brain can be obtained in 30 to 60 min. It is an expensive test, typically costing about twice what a CT scan costs. MR imaging cannot be performed on everyone. There are both absolute and relative contraindications to the procedure, most of which concern implanted or foreign objects within the patient. These objects could become dislodged by the magnetic field or damaged by rf pulses used to generate an image. MR imaging is absolutely contraindicated in patients with ferromagnetic intracranial aneurysm clips, metallic foreign bodies within the orbit, cochlear implants, and cardiac pacemakers. MR imaging is avoided if possible in pregnant women, uncooperative patients, and very sick patients who require intensive monitoring.

MR imaging offers a number of advantages over CT in the workup of patients with neurologic disease. Its soft-tissue contrast resolution is superior to that of CT, and lesions that would be subtle or invisible on CT are frequently very obvious on MR imaging. MR imaging also allows acquisition of multiplanar views in the sagittal, axial, coronal, and oblique projections that may be impossible to obtain with CT. Furthermore, MR imaging gives information about blood flow without the need for a contrast agent, and bony streak artifacts that obscure lesions of the brain stem and cerebellum on CT scans are not present on MR images. Finally, MR imaging does not expose the patient to ionizing radiation.

Besides the high cost and patient contraindications previously mentioned, MR imaging has several other limitations. Fewer scanners are available for MR imaging than for CT, MR imaging is much more sensitive to motion artifacts than is CT, acutely ill patients undergoing MR imaging are difficult to monitor, and 5 percent or more of patients cannot tolerate the examination because of claustrophobia.

CEREBRAL ARTERIOGRAPHY

Cerebral arteriography (CA) involves the injection of water-soluble contrast material into a carotid or vertebral artery. Contrast material is injected into the desired vessel via a small catheter, which has been introduced into the body through the femoral or brachial artery. Information about the arterial, capillary, or venous circulation of the brain is recorded on serial plain films or digitized for viewing on a TV monitor or for storage within a computer (Fig. 12-6).

Cerebral arteriograms are expensive (two to three times as much as MR examinations) and are relatively more risky procedures than other neuroradiologic studies. The major risk of the procedure is stroke, which may occur in 1 of every 1000 patients. Stroke during CA occurs either from an embolic event (e.g., inadvertent injection of air, thrombus formation on the catheter tip, atherosclerotic plaque dislodged by catheter manipulation) or from catheter-related local vessel trauma (e.g., dissections, occlusions).

Although CA is an invasive study with well-known risks, it is invaluable in the workup of vascular diseases affecting the CNS. It is the "gold standard" for assessing vas-

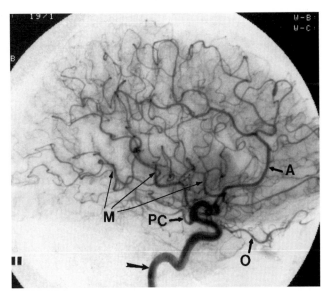

B

FIG. 12-6 Normal cerebral arteriogram. (*A*) Lateral view of the cervical carotid artery. Catheter is located within the common carotid artery, and contrast material fills internal (*arrows*) and external (*arrowheads*) carotid arteries. (*B*) Lateral view of the head after injection of the carotid artery (*arrow*). Note anterior cerebral (A), ophthalmic (O), posterior communicating (PC), and middle cerebral (M) branches.

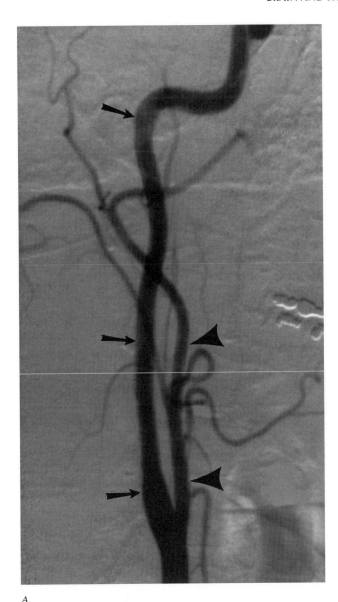

A

cular stenosis and atherosclerosis or vasculitis and is indispensable in diagnosing cerebral aneurysms and certain intracranial vascular malformations or fistulas. It is useful in assessing carotid or vertebral artery integrity after trauma to the neck. Finally, it is unsurpassed for showing vascular anatomy of the brain and is therefore useful as a preoperative road map. CT and MR scans have replaced CA in the workup of most other neurologic diseases.

One final word about CA: A new field called *interventional neuroradiology* has emerged over the past 10 years or so and has had considerable impact on the diagnosis and treatment of certain CNS diseases. Endovascular diagnostic and therapeutic procedures, based on fundamental CA principles, are becoming widely practiced and accepted. Although a full discussion of these techniques is beyond the scope of this chapter, they include balloon occlusion tests of the carotid artery, preoperative or definitive de-

vascularization of a hypervascular mass or arteriovenous malformation, carotid artery angioplasty, thrombolysis of intracranial vascular thrombosis in the setting of acute infarction, and endovascular treatment of vasospasm.

ULTRASONOGRAPHY

Ultrasonography, or sonography, is the diagnostic application of ultrasound to the human body. Ultrasonography (US) produces anatomic images from sound transmitted into and subsequently reflected from or absorbed by the organ or body part being examined. Until recently, there were two major applications of US in CNS disease: evaluation of carotid artery patency in the setting of atherosclerosis and screening evaluation of intracranial abnormalities in the newborn and young infant (Fig. 12-7). The utility of US has expanded in recent years since the addition of Doppler spectral analysis to the US examination. This addition, which allows the noninvasive measurement of blood flow, has greatly increased the usefulness and accuracy of US in evaluating carotid stenoses and has helped in the evaluation of certain intracranial processes such as vasospasm after subarachnoid hemorrhage. Ultrasound also has been used intraoperatively to demonstrate the spinal cord and surrounding structures during spine surgery and to define tumor and cyst margins during craniotomies.

US examinations, although moderately expensive, are virtually risk-free to the patient, involve no ionizing radia-

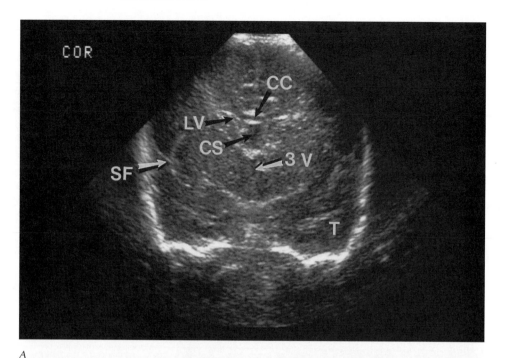

A

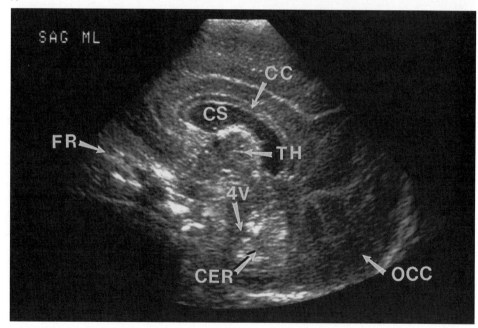

FIG. 12-7 Coronal (*A*) and sagittal (*B*) head ultrasound of a neonate. Normal structures include the corpus callosum (CC), lateral ventricle (LV), cavum septum pellucidum (CS), sylvian fissure (SF), third ventricle (3V), fourth ventricle (4V), temporal lobe (T), frontal lobe (FR), occipital lobe (OCC), cerebellum (CER), and thalamus (TH).

B

tion, and are portable (i.e., can be performed at the bedside). However, examination quality and therefore diagnostic accuracy are quite dependent on the ability of an individual sonographer to obtain truly representative information about an area being examined. Also, the heavy reliance of US on the presence of an adequate "acoustic window" through which an examination can be performed diminishes its usefulness in examining the brain after the fontanelles close in infancy. Finally, to the untrained eye, anatomic structures and pathologic processes as depicted by US are not as readily apparent as they are on CT or MR images.

Functional Modalities

Two major functional modalities are available for evaluating neurologic disease: single photon emission computed tomography (SPECT) and positron emission tomography (PET). As discussed, several of the anatomic techniques can provide functional information. For example, cerebral arteriography, ultrasonography, and MR angiography all provide information about blood flow.

MR spectroscopy gives information about brain metabolism and tissue characterization, but this technique is still primarily a research tool and is not discussed further here. SPECT and PET make up a very small portion of present neuroimaging procedures. However, since they do provide unique information about the brain and are used clinically, they are discussed briefly below.

SINGLE PHOTON EMISSION COMPUTED TOMOGRAPHY

SPECT uses a rotating gamma camera to reconstruct cross-sectional images of the distribution of a radioactive pharmaceutical that has been administered to a patient (usually intravenously). For brain imaging, radioactive iodine (^{123}I) or technetium (^{99m}Tc) is combined with a compound that rapidly crosses the BBB and localizes within brain tissue in proportion to regional blood flow. The rotating gamma camera detects gamma rays emitted by the radiopharmaceutical and produces cross-sectional images of the brain that are really a map of brain perfusion (Fig. 12-8). SPECT imaging also gives indirect information about brain metabolism, since perfusion is usually highest to parts of the brain with high metabolic activity and lowest to areas with low metabolic demand. Normal SPECT examinations demonstrate activity concentrated primarily in areas of high perfusion/metabolism, such as the cortical and deep gray matter (see Fig. 12-8).

SPECT studies are moderately expensive (as much as or more than brain MR imaging), and as expected, they provide limited anatomic information. SPECT also exposes patients to ionizing radiation. Since patients rarely have allergic reactions to the radiopharmaceuticals used, the examination is of low risk. On the other hand, SPECT does provide unique information about regional cerebral perfusion. Such information can be quite useful in the setting of stroke. SPECT also has been used with varying degrees of success in the workup of patients with epilepsy or dementia.

POSITRON EMISSION TOMOGRAPHY

PET scans consist of computer-generated cross-sectional images of the distribution and local concentration of a radiopharmaceutical. This technique is very similar to SPECT imaging. The main difference is that PET studies use radiopharmaceuticals labeled with a cyclotron-produced positron emitter. These agents are very expensive to produce and have a very short half-life (on the order of seconds to minutes). The most widely used radiotracer is ^{18}F-deoxyglucose. PET scanning with this agent gives a measurement of brain glucose metabolism. Other agents are useful in assessing regional cerebral blood flow, neuroreceptor function, and the like.

At first glance, PET scans resemble CT scans. Images can be viewed on a TV monitor or on x-ray film. Areas of high metabolic activity (i.e., cerebral cortex, deep gray nuclei) demonstrate greater radiopharmaceutical uptake than do areas of low metabolic activity, such as white matter or cerebrospinal fluid (Fig. 12-9). The bones of the skull and scalp soft tissues are, for the most part, invisible.

PET scans are very expensive, costing approximately twice as much as an MR scan. This expense is directly related to the high cost of operating the PET facility, which requires on-site physicists as well as an on-site cyclotron for radiotracer production. Therefore, PET scanning is not generally available in community hospitals. Although patients undergoing PET examinations are exposed to ionizing radiation, overall risk to the patient is low. Anatomic resolution, although not as good as with CT or MR imaging, is better than with SPECT imaging. The major advantage of PET imaging is that it provides in vivo information about brain perfusion, glucose metabolism, and ultimately, brain function.

PET scanning has been used primarily as a research tool, and its full potential is just now being realized. PET appears to provide useful information in the setting of stroke, epilepsy, dementia, and tumors. At present, the two main indications are in the workup of patients with complex partial seizures and in identifying tumor recurrence in patients who have undergone surgery, radiation therapy, or both for brain tumors.

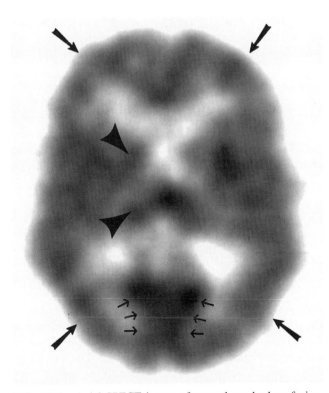

FIG. 12-8 Axial SPECT image of normal cerebral perfusion. Note that perfusion is greatest to gray matter structures, including the cerebral cortex (*large arrows*) and deep gray nuclei (*arrowheads*). White matter and ventricles are nearly invisible because of low or no perfusion. The greatest perfusion is to the visual cortex area (*small arrows*).

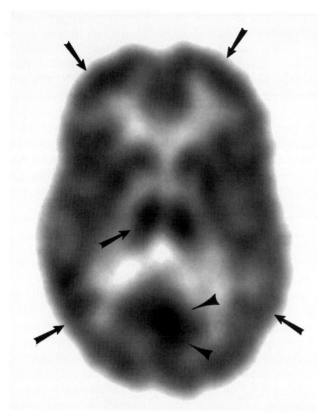

FIG. 12-9   Normal axial image of brain PET scan. As in the SPECT study (Fig. 12-8), areas of high activity correspond to metabolically active gray matter (*arrows*), especially the visual cortex (*arrowheads*).

TECHNIQUE SELECTION

The primary goal of a radiologic examination is to provide useful information for disease management. Radiologic studies can provide a diagnosis or can give information about disease extent or response to treatment. In the present medical climate, it also has become imperative that radiologic workups be performed efficiently and in a cost-effective manner. This requirement presents a problem for clinicians trying to decide which test to order in a given clinical situation.

The major strengths and weaknesses of neuroradiologic examinations have been discussed earlier in this chapter. The following brief discussion concerns the appropriate ordering of examinations in clinical situations. Several points should be emphasized. First, although a recommended modality may clearly be superior to another in evaluating a particular neurologic condition, the choice of examination is not always obvious before the diagnosis is established. For example, in patients with nonfocal headache, MR scans are more sensitive than CT scans for detecting most intracranial abnormalities. However, if the headache is produced by subarachnoid hemorrhage, CT would be a much better examination than MR imaging,

since subarachnoid hemorrhage is nearly invisible on MR images. Choice of examinations also may be limited by what is locally available. If MR imaging is unavailable, if the MR scanner is of poor quality, or if the interpreting radiologist is inadequately trained in MR image interpretation, then CT would be an excellent examination for evaluating most neurologic disorders.

Next, it is important to realize that the least expensive examination is not always the best first choice, even in this cost-conscious age. For example, most suspected skull fractures should be evaluated with CT scanning and not with plain films, despite the significant cost differential, because what is really important in management decisions is not the fracture itself but the potential underlying brain injury. Some neurologic diseases require multiple radiologic studies for accurate evaluation. Complex partial seizures refractory to medical management frequently require multiple examinations to localize the seizure focus prior to temporal lobectomy. Such a workup normally includes MR imaging and PET scanning of the brain, as well as a special cerebral arteriogram to identify cerebral dominance.

Finally, certain examinations are contraindicated in certain patients, and an alternative test must suffice. Patients with ferromagnetic cerebral aneurysm clips or pacemakers should not undergo MR imaging. Patients with a strong history of allergic reaction to iodinated contrast media should not routinely undergo contrast-enhanced CT scanning. MR imaging is frequently unsuccessful in claustrophobic or uncooperative patients unless they are sedated.

Imaging recommendations for common neurologic disorders are briefly discussed below. Please keep the preceding limitations in mind while reviewing the recommendations. The clinical situations discussed correspond to chapter subdivisions in Osborn's basic neuroradiologic text (see the Bibliography).

Congenital Anomalies

Congenital anomalies of the brain are best evaluated by MR imaging. MR imaging is the very best examination for demonstrating intracranial anatomy. It provides excellent discrimination between gray matter and white matter, superb views of the posterior fossa and craniocervical junction, and most important, the ability to view the brain in any plane. MR imaging has, for all practical purposes, completely replaced CT for this indication. The one exception is in evaluation of skull abnormalities such as suspected fusion of the sutures.

Craniocerebral Trauma

CT is the preferred modality for studying practically all acute head injuries. Examination times are short, intracranial hemorrhage is well demonstrated, and skull fractures are readily apparent. Unstable patients also can be monitored easily. Intravenous administration of contrast agents is unnecessary in this setting. Occasionally, cerebral arteriography is performed to look for carotid or vertebral artery injury when there has been penetrating trauma to the neck. Similarly, arteriography may be required to evaluate suspected carotid artery dissection associated with blunt head trauma or to assess carotid laceration in skull-base fractures.

While MR imaging is not performed routinely in the acute trauma setting, it may sometimes be helpful in patients with neurologic deficits unexplained by a head CT examination. For example, traumatic brain stem hemorrhages are often difficult to see on CT scans but are usually quite obvious on MR images. MR imaging is also useful in demonstrating tiny shear lesions within the brain in diffuse axonal injury and in assessing the brain in remote head trauma.

Intracranial Hemorrhage

The best examination to perform in most cases of suspected acute intracranial hemorrhage is a head CT scan. CT scans can be quickly obtained, allowing rapid initiation of treatment, and they are very good at demonstrating all types of intracranial hemorrhage, including subarachnoid blood. MR imaging takes much longer to perform in a potentially unstable patient, and subarachnoid hemorrhage is difficult, if not impossible, to see. MR imaging is more useful in the subacute or chronic setting, especially since it gives information about when a hemorrhagic event occurred. This information might be useful in such settings as nonaccidental head trauma (e.g., child abuse). MR imaging is also very sensitive to petechial hemorrhage, which frequently accompanies a cerebral infarction, and could potentially help to identify an underlying cause for an intracranial hemorrhage (e.g., tumor, arteriovenous malformation, occluded dural sinus). Finally, since most nontraumatic subarachnoid hemorrhage occurs secondary to a ruptured intracranial aneurysm, CA is routinely performed after detection of subarachnoid hemorrhage. MR angiography may one day replace conventional angiography to search for aneurysms.

Aneurysms

All intracranial aneurysms in which surgical intervention is planned require evaluation by CA. Cerebral arteriography not only allows aneurysm identification but also provides other critical preoperative information such as aneurysm orientation, presence of vasospasm, and location of adjacent vessels and collateral intracranial circulation. Arteriography also helps to determine which aneurysm has bled when more than one aneurysm is present. Recently, interventional neuroradiologists have treated some types of aneurysms, usually in nonsurgical patients, by placing

thrombosing material within the aneurysm itself via an endovascular approach.

Although most patients with symptomatic cerebral aneurysms present with subarachnoid hemorrhage, some aneurysms act like intracranial masses. These situations usually warrant evaluation by MR imaging as a first examination. The same is sometimes true with posterior communicating artery aneurysms (which can produce symptoms related to the adjacent third cranial nerve) or with aneurysms arising from the internal carotid artery as it courses through the cavernous sinus (which can affect any of the cranial nerves that lie within this structure, including cranial nerves III, IV, V, or VI).

Vascular Malformations

Patients with a vascular malformation (e.g., arteriovenous malformation, cavernous angioma, venous angioma, capillary telangiectasia) often seek medical attention after an intracranial hemorrhage or a seizure. In this setting, the first test that should be performed is either a CT examination (to look for intracranial hemorrhage) or MR imaging. Although an intracranial hemorrhage is usually very obvious on a CT scan, the vascular malformation itself may be difficult, if not impossible, to see unless intravenous contrast material is administered. MR imaging, on the other hand, is quite sensitive for detecting vascular malformations, whether they have bled or not. As can be seen, the choice of the initial examination for evaluation of a vascular malformation can be difficult. Usually, patients undergo noncontrast head CT scanning to look for intracranial hemorrhage when they come to the emergency department. Head CT is followed by gadolinium-enhanced MR imaging to further characterize the CT findings. If a high-flow true arteriovenous malformation is suspected, either clinically or from a cross-sectional imaging study, then CA is performed prior to initiation of treatment. MR angiography may someday replace conventional arteriography in the workup of these lesions, as with aneurysms.

Infarction

Most patients today with suspected cerebral infarction undergo CT scanning in the acute setting, even though infarctions are demonstrated earlier and are more obvious on MR imaging. So why is CT usually performed first? The answer is that clinicians who manage stroke patients are not so interested in seeing the infarct itself. Infarct location is usually suspected from the physical examination, and acute infarcts may not even be visible on CT scans for 12 to 24 h after onset of stroke symptoms. Clinicians are very interested, though, to know if a stroke is secondary to something besides an infarct (e.g., intracranial hemorrhage, brain tumor) or if an infarct is hemorrhagic, since anticoagulation agents would be contraindicated in this setting. CT can quickly answer both these questions. MR imaging is often reserved for problem cases or for suspected brain stem or posterior fossa infarcts.

The underlying cause of most cerebral infarctions is thromboembolism related to atherosclerosis. Although CT or MR scans are useful in demonstrating brain infarction, US and CA are commonly performed in the setting of stroke or transient ischemic attack to identify vascular stenoses or occlusions. These examinations are usually reserved for patients who might be candidates for carotid endarterectomy. Functional examinations (SPECT and PET) also have been used in patients with strokelike symptoms to identify regions of the brain at risk for infarction. These studies are not widely available and therefore do not enter into the imaging algorithm for most stroke patients.

Brain Tumors and Tumor-Like Conditions

The best examination to order in the setting of suspected brain tumor is a contrast-enhanced MR scan. This is true for primary neoplasms as well as for metastatic disease. MR imaging is especially useful in identifying tumors of the pituitary region, brain stem, and posterior fossa, including the cerebellar-pontine angle.

Although MR imaging is the preferred examination for intracranial neoplasms, it is occasionally supplemented by a CT scan, which can give important pretreatment information not provided by MR images. For example, CT can demonstrate tumor calcifications, occasionally a useful factor in differentiating between types of neoplasms. Also, CT is very useful in identifying bone destruction in skull base lesions.

In most medical centers, MR scans are performed to assess brain tumor response to treatment. PET scanning has shown some promise in this area and may eventually replace MR imaging in detecting recurrent or residual disease. PET scanning is currently the best examination for differentiating recurrent tumor from postradiation tissue necrosis, which can mimic tumor on an MR or a CT scan.

Cerebral arteriography is rarely performed for brain tumor evaluation today except to map the blood supply of meningiomas and other very vascular tumors prior to surgery. Such lesions also can be devascularized prior to surgery to minimize blood loss by injecting various materials into feeding vessels to occlude them.

Infection

Intracranial infections are best evaluated by contrast-enhanced MR imaging. Abscesses, cerebritis, subdural empyemas, and other infectious or inflammatory processes are all very well demonstrated. MR imaging is especially useful in assessing patients with the acquired immune deficiency syndrome (AIDS). Not only does it allow identification of secondary infections (e.g., toxoplasmosis, cryptococcosis, progressive multifocal leukoencephalopathy), but it is also exquisitely sensitive to the white matter changes produced by the human immunodeficiency virus itself. CT scanning is less sensitive than MR imaging in the detection of intracranial infections and should be reserved for patients in whom MR imaging is contraindicated. Cerebral arteriography is only useful in one particular situation—suspected vasculitis. Involvement of brain arteries and arterioles in this condition requires arteriography for diagnostic confirmation.

Inherited and Acquired Metabolic, White Matter, and Neurodegenerative Diseases

As with suspected intracranial infections, this large and diverse group of disease is best evaluated with MR imaging. It is extremely sensitive in detecting white matter abnormalities. In fact, one of the very first clear indications for MR imaging was in the workup of suspected multiple sclerosis. While brain abnormalities in these conditions may be quite obvious on MR imaging, there is one problem: Many of these conditions appear very similar, and an exact diagnosis may not be possible.

Recently, PET imaging has been used in assessing patients with dementia and suspected neurodegenerative disease. This modality is currently being evaluated to determine its role in this group of patients.

EXERCISE 12-1: CONGENITAL ANOMALIES

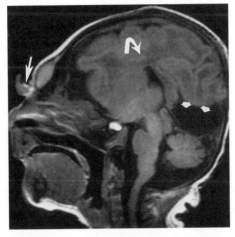 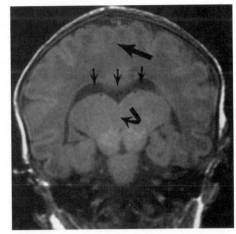

FIG. 12-E-1 *Panels A and B*

A B

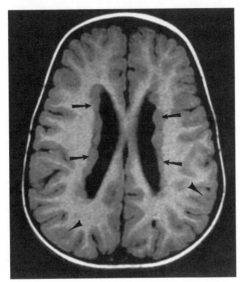 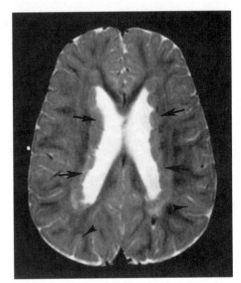

FIG. 12-E-2 *Panels A and B*

A B

Clinical Histories:

CASE 12-1
A 2-day-old male infant presents with multiple craniofacial deformities, including frontal bossing, microcephaly, and a fleshy mass on the bridge of the nose. Sagittal and coronal T1-weighted MR images of the brain are shown (Fig. 12-E-1*A,B*).

CASE 12-2
A 15-month-old female infant presents with new onset of seizures. Axial T1- and T2-weighted MR images are shown (Figs. 12-E-2*A,B*).

Questions:

12-1. In Case 12-1, what is the major abnormality?
    A. Enlarged ventricles
    B. Cyst in the posterior fossa
    C. Lack of brain cleavage into two hemispheres
    D. Herniation of intracranial contents through a skull defect
    E. Abnormal migration of gray matter

12-2. In Case 12-2, what is the cause of the patient's seizures?
   A. Brain tumor
   B. Gray matter in the wrong place (i.e., heterotopic gray matter)
   C. Congenital infection
   D. Nodules along ventricles in a patient with tuberous sclerosis
   E. Infarction of periventricular white matter

Radiologic Findings:

12-1. In this case, corpus callosum (*curved arrow*) is absent on sagittal T1-weighted MR image (Fig. 12-E-1*A*). Also note other midline abnormalities, including abnormal tissue at the bridge of the nose (*large arrow*) and a posterior cyst (*small arrows*). Coronal T1-weighted MR image (Fig. 12-E-1*B*) demonstrates monoventricle (*small arrows*) and thalamic fusion (*curved arrow*). Also note the lack of separation of the two hemispheres (*large arrow*) (*C* is the correct answer to Question 12-1).

12-2. In this case, T1-weighted (Fig. 12-E-2*A*) and T2-weighted (Fig. 12-E-2*B*) MR images show abnormal tissue lining the lateral ventricle (*arrows*). Signal of this tissue follows that of normal gray matter (*arrowheads*) on both T1- and T2-weighted images (*B* is the correct answer to Question 12-2).

Discussion:

Two common reasons for performing MR scans in young infants are illustrated by the cases in this section. Infants with craniofacial anomalies frequently have underlying congenital malformations of the central nervous system (CNS). Seizures, too, may be the first sign of an underlying brain malformation. As discussed in the section "Technique Selection," whenever a congenital brain anomaly is suspected, MR imaging is the best examination to perform.

Insults to the developing brain lead to predictable alterations in brain morphology. By analyzing patterns of altered brain morphology, we can often determine which stage of CNS development has been disrupted. This analysis, combined with a knowledge of neuroembryology, has allowed for the development of systems to classify congenital anomalies of the CNS. One simplified classification system divides congenital malformations into disorders of organogenesis (which include abnormalities of neural tube closure, diverticulation/cleavage, sulcation/cellular migration, and size, as well as destructive lesions acquired in utero), disorders of histogenesis (i.e., neurocutaneous syndromes), and disorders of cytogenesis (i.e., congenital neoplasms). Readers are referred to the Bibliography for further information on this topic.

The patient in Case 12-1 has alobar holoprosencephaly, a classic example of disordered ventral induction. In this condition, there is complete (alobar) or partial (semilobar, lobar) failure of separation of the forebrain (prosencephalon) into two hemispheres. In alobar holoprosencephaly, the most severe form of this disorder, there is no separation of the two hemispheres at all. The thalami are fused, a central monoventricle is present, and there is no corpus callosum. Infants with this form of holoprosencephaly frequently have severe facial anomalies.

In Case 12-2, the patient has heterotopic gray matter lining the lateral ventricles. This congenital anomaly is one type of disordered cellular migration. Neurons that make up the gray matter of the cerebral cortex actually develop along the edges of the lateral and third ventricles within the so-called germinal matrix zone. They then migrate outward to their final cortical location. If this normal neuronal migration is disrupted, a normal cortex may not develop, and clumps of gray matter may be present in abnormal locations along the migration route. Collections of these normal neurons in abnormal locations are called *gray matter heterotopias*. Case 12-2 demonstrates a nodular gray matter heterotopia involving the subependymal region at the edge of the lateral ventricles. Seizures frequently occur in patients with this condition, as in the patient in Case 12-2. Since MR imaging usually provides an exact diagnosis of this condition, biopsies of CNS tissue are unnecessary.

EXERCISE 12-2: STROKE

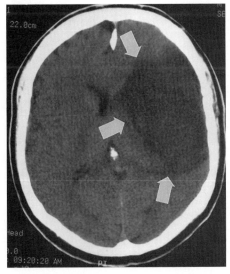

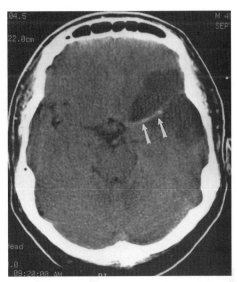

FIG. 12-E-3   *Panels A and B*

A   B

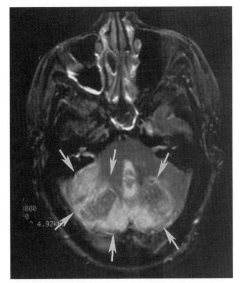

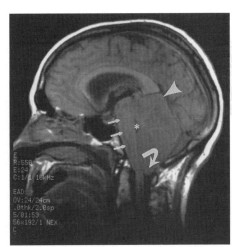

FIG. 12-E-4   *Panels A and B*

A   B

Clinical Histories:

CASE 12-3

A 45-year-old man presents with recent development of right-sided hemiplegia. Axial images from a noncontrast head CT examination are shown (Figs. 12-E-3A,B).

CASE 12-4

A 66-year-old woman presents with gradual onset of nausea, dizziness, and ataxia. The patient became comatose 24 h after the onset of symptoms. Axial T2-weighted and sagittal T1-weighted images are shown (Figs. 12-E-4A,B).

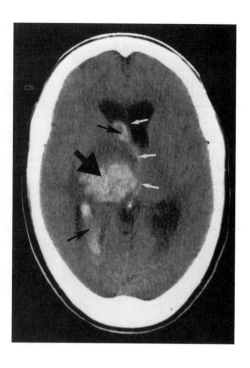

FIG. 12-E-5

CASE 12-5

A 42-year-old female hypertensive renal transplant patient presents with acute mental status changes and left hemiparesis. A single axial image from a noncontrast head CT scan is shown (Fig. 12-E-5).

Questions:

12-3. In Case 12-3, what is the most likely diagnosis?
   A.   Intracranial abscess
   B.   Arachnoid cyst
   C.   Metastatic brain tumor
   D.   Primary brain tumor
   E.   Cerebral infarction

12-4. In Case 12-4, what is the likely cause of the patient's problem?
   A.   Brain stem infarction
   B.   Brain stem compression from cerebellar infarction
   C.   Brain stem tumor
   D.   Cerebellar astrocytoma
   E.   Posterior fossa hemorrhage

12-5. In Case 12-5, what is the most likely diagnosis?
   A.   Thalamic glioma
   B.   Subarachnoid hemorrhage
   C.   Metastatic disease
   D.   Hypertensive hemorrhage in the basal ganglia
   E.   Cerebral contusion

Radiologic Findings:

12-3. In this case, the axial CT image (Fig. 12-E-3A) demonstrates a well-defined hypodensity (*arrows*) in the left middle cerebral artery (MCA) territory. In a more inferior axial image (Fig. 12-E-3B), note the bright MCA (*arrows*) corresponding to an acute thrombus in the main trunk of this vessel (E is the correct answer to Question 12-3).

12-4. In this case, an axial MR image (Fig. 12-E-4*A*) shows areas of increased T2 signal (*arrows*) corresponding to edema within the cerebellum. The sagittal T1-weighted image (Fig. 12-E-4*B*) shows a swollen cerebellum, as well as upward transtentorial (*arrowhead*) and downward tonsillar (*curved arrow*) herniation of cerebellar tissue. Also note compression of the brain stem (*small arrows*) and fourth ventricle (*asterisk*). These changes are compatible with a recent cerebellar infarction with brain stem compression caused by the swollen cerebellum (*B* is the correct answer to Question 12-4).

12-5. In this case, CT scan demonstrates a right basal ganglia hematoma (*large black arrow*) with intraventricular extension (*small black arrows*). Note the shift of midline structures (*white arrows*). This is most likely secondary to the patient's known hypertension (*D* is the correct answer to Question 12-5).

Discussion:

Stroke is a lay term for neurologic disfunction. The usual image of a stroke patient is that of an elderly individual with a hemiparesis, often associated with abnormal speech. There are actually many different causes of stroke. These include cerebral infarction, intracerebral hemorrhage, subarachnoid hemorrhage, and miscellaneous causes such as dural sinus occlusion with associated venous infarction. Although these conditions may have similar clinical presentations, they have different treatments and prognoses.

The vast majority of strokes are cerebral infarctions associated with atherosclerosis. The radiologic manifestations of cerebral infarction vary with time. The head CT scan of the patient in Case 12-3 was obtained several days after the onset of symptoms and shows typical findings of a subacute infarct in a major vascular territory, in this case the left middle cerebral artery region. By this time, the infarct is a very well defined area of low attenuation compared with normal surrounding brain. There is associated mass effect from the edematous tissue. Acute infarcts (less than 24 h since onset of symptoms) may be invisible on head CT scans, although MRI often demonstrates brain abnormalities within several hours of symptom onset. Subtle changes on head CT scans in acute infarction can sometimes be seen but may be overlooked if the examination is not closely scrutinized. Sometimes the only apparent change on CT scans is a subtle loss of gray matter–white matter differentiation in the area of infarction. CT scanning is performed in acute cerebral infarction because scans can be obtained quickly, and CT is a very good test for identifying intracranial hemorrhage, an important finding for management considerations. If the infarct is not obvious on the initial CT scan, a follow-up CT or MR scan is usually obtained within a few days to verify the clinical suspicion.

Case 12-4 illustrates an important point to consider when deciding which test to order in the setting of acute stroke. In this case, the patient's symptoms were worrisome for a brain stem process. CT scanning of the brain stem and posterior fossa is frequently degraded by streak artifacts emanating from the dense bone of the skull base. Subtle (and sometimes not so subtle) abnormalities may not be apparent. Therefore, for most neurologic conditions that involve the brain stem or posterior fossa, MR scans are much better at depicting an abnormality. Notice that the patient in Case 12-4 did not in fact have a brain stem infarct, as was suspected clinically, but rather had brain stem compression from a large cerebellar infarct.

Case 12-5 illustrates how essential an imaging examination is in managing stroke. The patient had signs and symptoms of an acute cerebral infarction. The CT scan demonstrated an obvious basal ganglia hemorrhage, probably secondary to the patient's hypertension. Management of these two conditions is considerably different. Hypertension is the main cause of nontraumatic intracranial hemorrhage. In adults, these hemorrhages typically occur in the putamen/external capsule. Other locations for hypertensive hemorrhage include the thalamus, pons, cerebellum, and rarely, subcortical white matter. Acute parenchymal hematomas, as in this case, are usually hyperdense on CT scans. With time these lesions become darker and eventually appear as round or slitlike cavities. The MR imaging appearance of a parenchymal hematoma is complex and depends largely on the presence of hemoglobin breakdown products within the clot.

EXERCISE 12-3: BRAIN TUMORS

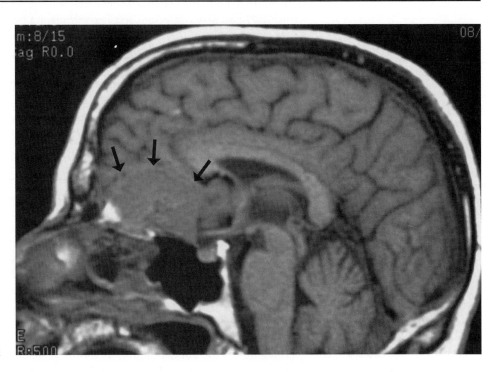

FIG. 12-E-6   *Panel A*

Clinical Histories:

CASE 12-6
A 58-year-old man presents with anosmia. Sagittal T1-weighted MR images before and after contrast administration are shown (Figs. 12-E-6*A,B*).

CASE 12-7
A 76-year-old woman presents with a 6-month history of progressive gait ataxia and frequent falling. Sagittal T2-weighted and coronal contrast-enhanced T1-weighted MR images are shown (Figs. 12-E-7*A,B*).

CASE 12-8
A 58-year-old man presents with a history of lung cancer and mental status changes. A contrast-enhanced axial CT scan and a gadolinium-enhanced axial T1-weighted MR image are shown (Figs. 12-E-8*A,B*).

Questions:

12-6. In Case 12-6, what is the most likely diagnosis?
     A.   Extraaxial brain tumor such as a meningioma
     B.   Intraaxial brain tumor such as an astrocytoma
     C.   Frontal contusion
     D.   Subdural hematoma
     E.   Encephalocele

12-7. In Case 12-7, what is the most likely cause of the patient's symptoms?
     A.   Multiple sclerosis
     B.   Inner ear abnormality
     C.   Intraventricular meningioma
     D.   Hematoma
     E.   Malignant brain tumor

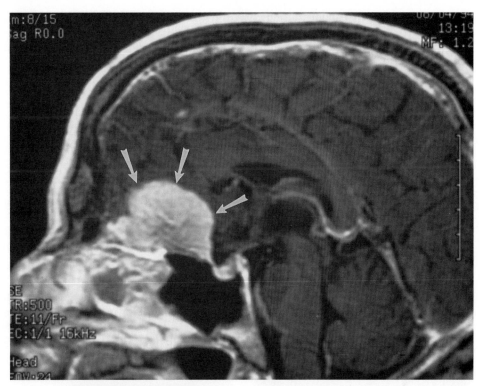

FIG. 12-E-6 *Panel B*

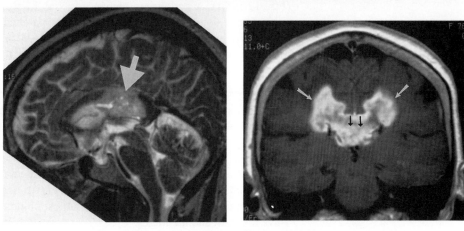

FIG. 12-E-7 *Panels A and B*

A   *B*

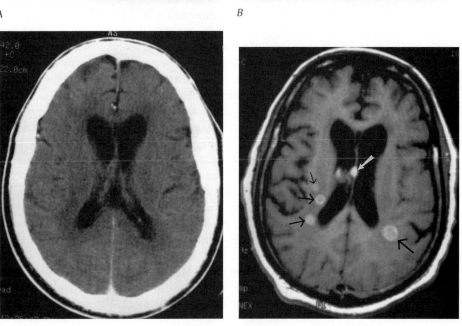

FIG. 12-E-8 *Panels A and B*

A   *B*

12-8. In Case 12-8, what is the most likely explanation for the patient's mental status changes?
  A. Metastatic disease
  B. Intracranial hemorrhage
  C. Small infarcts
  D. Sarcoidosis
  E. Arteriovenous malformation

Radiologic Findings:

12-6. In this case, sagittal T1-weighted images before and after contrast administration show an extraaxial, subfrontal mass (Figs. 12-E-6*A,B*). Subfrontal mass (*arrows*) is difficult to differentiate from normal brain tissue on an unenhanced T1-weighted MR image (Fig. 12-E-6*A*). The mass enhances after gadolinium-DTPA administration (*arrows*), allowing easy identification (Fig. 12-E-6*B*). This is fairly typical of a meningioma (*A* is the correct answer to Question 12-6).

12-7. In this case, the sagittal T2-weighted MR image (Fig. 12-E-7*A*) demonstrates a high-signal mass (*arrow*) with its epicenter in the corpus callosum. On the coronal view (Fig. 12-E-7*B*), an enhancing mass (*white arrows*) extends through the corpus callosum (*black arrows*) into both hemispheres. This is one appearance of a malignant brain tumor, in this case a glioblastoma multiforme (*E* is the correct answer to Question 12-7).

12-8. In this case, a contrast-enhanced axial CT scan shows no definite abnormality (Fig. 12-E-8*A*). A gadolinium-enhanced axial T1-weighted MR image shows multiple enhancing lesions (*arrows*) within the brain parenchyma (Fig. 12-E-8*B*). In a patient with known lung cancer, metastatic disease is the most likely explanation for multiple intracranial enhancing lesions (*A* is the correct answer to Question 12-8).

Discussion:

Brain tumors can be classified in a variety of ways. The traditional classification of intracranial neoplasms is based on histology. In this system, brain tumors are either primary (they arise from the brain and its linings) or secondary (they arise from somewhere outside the CNS, i.e., metastases). Primary tumors, which account for approximately two-thirds of all brain neoplasms, can be subdivided into glial and nonglial tumors. Secondary tumors, especially from lung and breast cancer, account for the remaining one-third of brain neoplasms. Metastases are most commonly parenchymal but also can involve the skull and meninges.

Brain tumors also can be classified according to patient age and general tumor location (i.e., adult or child, supratentorial or infratentorial). Finally, brain tumors can be classified according to the specific anatomic region involved. For example, we can generate lists of brain tumors that specifically affect the pineal or the pituitary regions.

Case 12-6 illustrates a useful principle for interpreting studies of patients with suspected brain tumors. It is very important to first decide whether a mass is within the brain parenchyma (intraaxial) or outside the brain (extraaxial). Extraaxial masses usually turn out to be meningiomas, many of which can be removed surgically with a very low incidence of recurrence. Intraaxial masses frequently turn out to be astrocytomas, and the prognosis is less favorable.

The patient in Case 12-6 has an extraaxial, subfrontal mass that markedly enhances with the MR imaging contrast agent, gadolinium-DTPA. Notice that the meningioma is isointense to normal brain tissue prior to administration of the contrast agent and could easily be overlooked if the contrast-enhanced images were not obtained. Meningiomas often demonstrate this precontrast isointensity with brain on MR images (and sometimes on CT scans).

Meningiomas are the most common nonglial primary CNS tumors. They can occur anywhere within the head but typically occur along the venous dural sinuses. The parasagittal region and cerebral convexities are the most common locations. Anterior basal or olfactory groove meningiomas, such as the one in this case, account for 5 to 10 percent of intracranial meningiomas. Anosmia results from involvement of the olfactory tracts by the tumor.

Case 12-7 demonstrates an intraaxial neoplasm in an elderly woman. This mass involves the posterior body and splenium of the corpus callosum and spreads into the deep white matter of both cerebral hemispheres. The imaging appearance resembles the wings of a butterfly, hence the commonly used name *butterfly glioma*. The intense enhancement of the mass after gadolinium-DTPA administration is quite typical of a glioblastoma multiforme. This highly malignant tumor is the most common brain neoplasm and occurs most frequently in patients over 50 years of age. Patients with glioblastoma multiforme present with neurologic deficits or with new onset of seizures. The prognosis in these patients is dismal; postoperative survival averages 8 months. Imaging studies typically demonstrate a very inhomogeneous mass with irregular margins and striking peritumoral edema.

Case 12-8 illustrates a very important point to remember when working up patients with suspected metastatic disease to the brain: MR imaging is considerably more sensitive than CT in detecting metastases. This is not a trivial point, since surgery is sometimes performed to remove single, but not multiple, brain metastases. Metastatic disease to the brain has a variety of manifestations, the most common being parenchymal involvement. Typical hematogenous brain metastases demonstrate solid or ringlike enhancement on CT or MR imaging scans, occur near gray matter–white matter junctions, and are usually surrounded by a marked amount of edema. They most commonly metastasize from lung or breast primaries.

EXERCISE 12-4: INTRACRANIAL INFECTIONS

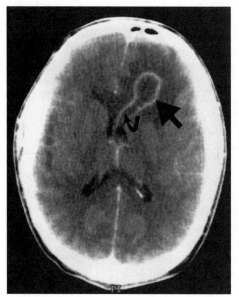

FIG. 12-E-9

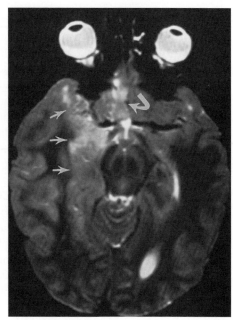

FIG. 12-E-10

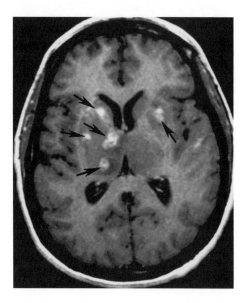

FIG. 12-E-11   *Panel A*

Clinical Histories:

CASE 12-9
A 25-year-old man with a history of atrial septal defect presents with fever and seizures after undergoing dental work. An axial image from a contrast-enhanced head CT scan is shown (Fig. 12-E-9).

CASE 12-10
A 4-year-old girl presents with lethargy and seizure activity. An axial T2-weighted MR image of the brain is shown (Fig. 12-E-10).

CASE 12-11
A 43-year-old man presents with headache and weakness. An axial contrast-enhanced T1-weighted MR image is shown (Fig. 12-E-11*A*).

Questions:

12-9. In Case 12-9, what is the most likely diagnosis?
A. Frontal contusion
B. Aneurysm with intraventricular hemorrhage
C. Frontal lobe abscess
D. Intracranial lymphoma
E. Cerebritis

12-10. In Case 12-10, the location of the abnormality is pathognomonic for which type of infection?
A. Toxoplasmosis
B. Tuberculosis
C. *Cryptococcus*
D. Herpes
E. *Staphylococcus*

12-11. In Case 12-11, the major differential diagnosis for this lesion is toxoplasmosis versus _____.
A. *Cryptococcus*
B. intracranial lymphoma
C. sarcoidosis
D. metastatic disease
E. cytomegalovirus (CMV)

Radiologic Findings:

12-9. In this case, the contrast-enhanced CT scan shows a ring-enhancing lesion (*arrow*) in the left frontal lobe. Note the involvement of the frontal horn of the left lateral ventricle (*curved arrow*) by the process. The patient's history is compatible with an intracranial infection, and the CT scan shows a classic ring-enhancing abscess (*C* is the correct answer to Question 12-9).

12-10. In this case, the T2-weighted MR image shows high signal abnormality in the medial aspect of the right temporal lobe (*arrows*) and within the inferior right frontal lobe (*curved arrow*). These changes are commonly seen in patients with herpes encephalitis (*D* is the correct answer to Question 12-10).

12-11. In this case, multiple enhancing lesions are present within the basal ganglia, especially on the right (*arrows*) on the gadolinium-enhanced T1-weighted MR image (Fig. 12-E-11*A*). The most common lesions with this appearance in an HIV-positive patient are toxoplasmosis and intracranial lymphoma (*B* is the correct answer to Question 12-11). The patient markedly improved after antitoxoplasmosis therapy, and the lesions shown on the MR image disappeared.

Discussion:

A host of infectious diseases can involve the brain and its coverings. Because the CNS has a limited number of ways of responding to an infectious agent, many intracranial infections appear identical on neuroimaging studies. It is therefore very important to closely correlate the imaging findings with the clinical presentation and other diagnostic tests, such as lumbar puncture or stereotactic brain aspiration.

For our purposes, it is useful to classify CNS infections according to the intracranial compartment involved, especially since this has treatment implications. Intracranial infections can be either parenchymal or extraparenchymal. Parenchymal manifestations include cerebritis/abscess and encephalitis. Extraparenchymal disease includes epidural abscess, subdural empyema, and leptomeningitis. Bacterial, viral, fungal, and parasitic agents can all affect the CNS. Although a few infectious agents preferentially involve a particular anatomic compartment of the CNS, most are not site-specific.

Case 12-9 demonstrates a classic ring-enhancing lesion of a pyogenic abscess. Most pyogenic abscesses result from hematogenous dissemination from a non-CNS source. Pyogenic brain abscesses also can result from direct extension of an infectious process from an adjacent area (e.g., sinusitis or mastoiditis) or from trauma (e.g., penetrating wound or surgery).

Abscesses usually occur at gray matter–white matter junctions, although they can occur anywhere in the brain. Patients frequently present with seizures or symptoms related to intracranial mass effect. If abscesses develop near the brain surface, they may rupture into the subarachnoid space, producing a meningitis; they also may produce a ventriculitis if they rupture into the ventricular system, as in this case. Most abscesses are treated surgically.

Herpes encephalitis (Case 12-10) is caused by the herpes simplex virus (HSV). Older children and adults are usually infected by HSV-1, either primarily or as a result of reactivation of a latent virus. The ensuing necrotizing encephalitis in this condition typically involves the temporal and inferior frontal lobes and insular cortex. Focal abnormalities of attenuation (on CT) or signal (on MR imaging) in these characteristic locations, often with enhancement after contrast administration, are practically pathognomonic of HSV-1 encephalitis. Early diagnosis of this condition is extremely important, since antiviral therapy can significantly affect patient outcome.

Neonatal herpes simplex infection differs from infection in the older child and adult. The offending organism is usually HSV-2, which may be acquired in utero or during birth from mothers with genital herpes. HSV-2 infection can produce severe destructive changes within the developing brain. Unlike HSV-1 infection in older children and adults, neonatal herpes encephalitis can involve any area of the brain, having no predilection for the temporal lobe.

Patients with AIDS (Case 12-11) commonly develop intracranial infections during the course of their disease. Human immunodeficiency virus (HIV) itself can infect the CNS directly, producing encephalopathy in up to 60 percent of AIDS patients. The most common neuroimaging finding in HIV encephalopathy is cerebral atrophy, often with patchy white matter hypointensity (on CT) or increased T2 signal (on MR imaging) from

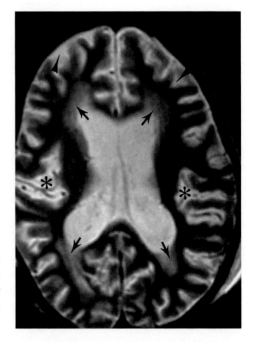

FIG. 12-E-11 (*Panel B*) An 8-year-old girl with AIDS and new onset of seizures. Axial T2-weighted image shows white matter high signal (*arrows*). Also note the diffuse prominence of gyri and sulci (*arrowheads*) and sylvian fissures (*asterisks*), compatible with cerebral atrophy.

demyelination and gliosis (Fig. 12-E-11*B*). Other common CNS infections in the immunocompromised AIDS patient include toxoplasmosis, cryptococcosis, and progressive multifocal leukoencephalopathy (from a papovavirus infection).

Toxoplasmosis lesions, usually demonstrated by ring enhancement with surrounding edema on CT or MR imaging, occur in the basal ganglia areas or at the gray matter–white matter junctions within the cerebral hemispheres. Their appearance is almost identical to that of primary intracranial lymphoma, another common intracranial condition in AIDS. Meningitis is the most frequent manifestation of cryptococcosis in AIDS, although parenchymal lesions, termed *cryptococcomas,* are encountered occasionally. In progressive multifocal leukoencephalopathy, extensive areas of white matter demyelination are shown on MR imaging. A number of other intracranial infections can occur in AIDS patients, and the reader is referred to the Bibliography for sources of further information.

EXERCISE 12-5: HEAD TRAUMA

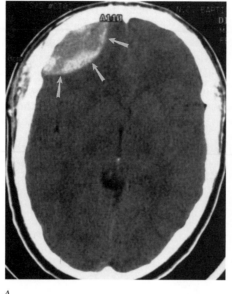 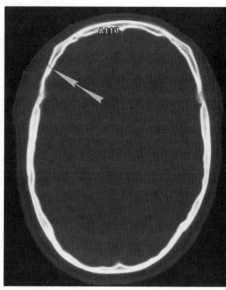

FIG. 12-E-12   *Panels A and B*

A   B

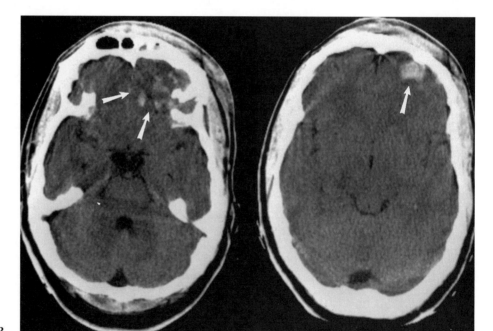

FIG. 12-E-13

Clinical Histories:

CASE 12-12

A 17-year-old boy presents with a head injury resulting from a motor vehicle accident. Soft-tissue and bone windows from axial noncontrast head CT scan are shown (Figs. 12-E-12A,B).

CASE 12-13

A 24-year-old man presents with multiple facial fractures and frontal scalp soft-tissue swelling resulting from a motor vehicle accident. Axial noncontrast head CT images are shown (Fig. 12-E-13).

Questions:

12-12. In Case 12-12, what is the diagnosis?
  A. Subdural hematoma
  B. Cerebral contusion
  C. Epidural hematoma
  D. Meningioma
  E. Subdural hygroma

12-13. In Case 12-13, what is the main radiologic finding?
  A. Subdural hematoma
  B. Epidural hematoma
  C. Duret hemorrhage
  D. Cerebral contusions
  E. Shearing injuries

Radiologic Findings:

12-12. In this case, an extraaxial hematoma (*arrows*) is producing mass effect on the right frontal lobe on an unenhanced head CT scan (Fig. 12-E-12*A*). The convex appearance of this lesion is typical of an epidural hematoma (*C* is the correct answer to Question 12-12). Also note the nondisplaced skull fracture (*arrow*) on the bone window of the CT (Fig. 12-E-12*B*).

12-13. In this case, there are multiple areas of increased attenuation within the frontal lobes, especially on the left (*arrows*) (Fig. 12-E-13). These areas correspond to multiple hemorrhagic contusions involving the brain parenchyma (*D* is the correct answer to Question 12-13).

Discussion:

Intracranial abnormalities in head trauma can be classified as either primary or secondary. Primary lesions occur at the moment of injury and include skull fractures, extracerebral hemorrhage (e.g., epidural or subdural hematomas, subarachnoid hemorrhage), and intracerebral hemorrhage (e.g., brain contusion, brain stem injury, diffuse axonal injury).

The secondary effects of head trauma are actually complications of the primary intracranial injury. Elevated intracranial pressure and cerebral herniations are responsible for most of the secondary effects of head trauma, which in many cases may be more devastating to the patients than the initial injury.

Epidural hematoma (EDH) (Case 12-12) is usually associated with skull fractures that lacerate the middle meningeal artery or a dural sinus. Up to one-half of patients with EDHs have a lucid interval after the head trauma occurs. On CT, EDHs usually appear as biconvex, high-attenuation, extraaxial masses. Most are located in the temporoparietal area. Underlying skull fractures (as in this case) are common. Intracranial brain herniation also may be a prominent feature in this condition. One important imaging feature in EDHs is that they do not cross skull sutures.

Subdural hematoma (SDH), on the other hand, is usually a crescent-shaped extraaxial collection that may cross suture lines. These lesions are more lethal than are EDHs; the SDH mortality rate is over 50 percent. CT can usually, but not always, distinguish between EDHs and SDHs.

Cerebral contusions (Case 12-13) are the second most common form of brain parenchymal injury in primary head trauma (diffuse axonal injury is the most common parenchymal injury). Cerebral contusions can be thought of as brain bruises. They result either from the brain's striking a bony ridge inside the skull during rapid acceleration/deceleration, as occurs in a motor vehicle accident, or from a depressed skull fracture. These lesions tend to occur in particular anatomic locations, especially the undersurfaces and poles of the frontal and temporal lobes. CT scans show areas of low attenuation (edema) and hemorrhage at the site of injury. Delayed hemorrhage, 1 to 2 days after a head injury, is common with contusions.

EXERCISE 12-6: INTRACRANIAL VASCULAR ABNORMALITIES

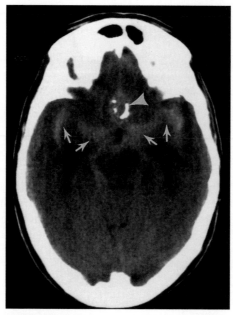

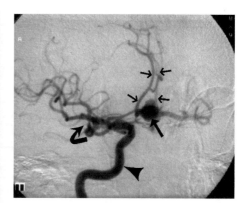

B

FIG. 12-E-14   *Panels A and B*

A

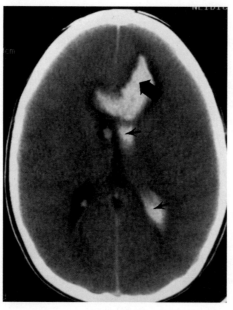

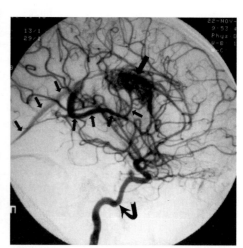

FIG. 12-E-15   *Panels A and B*

A   B

Clinical Histories: **CASE 12-14**
A 59-year-old woman presents with severe headache. An axial head CT image and a cerebral arteriogram are shown (Figs. 12-E-14*A,B*).

CASE 12-15
An 11-year-old boy presents with acute decline in mental status. Axial head CT image and cerebral arteriogram are shown (Figs. 12-E-15*A,B*).

Questions:

12-14. In Case 12-14, what is the reason for the abnormality on the CT scan?
   A. Cerebral aneurysm
   B. Arteriovenous malformation
   C. Head trauma
   D. Carotid dissection
   E. Vasculitis

12-15. In Case 12-15, what is the reason for the abnormality on the CT scan?
   A. Cerebral aneurysm
   B. Arteriovenous malformation
   C. Head trauma
   D. Carotid dissection
   E. Vasculitis

Radiologic Findings:

12-14. In this case, the CT scan (Fig. 12-E-14*A*) shows extensive subarachnoid hemorrhage filling the basal cisterns (*arrows*). Curvilinear calcifications (*arrowhead*) are present in the region of the anterior communicating artery. Oblique frontal view from a carotid arteriogram (Fig. 12-E-14*B*) demonstrates the source of this bleeding—a large aneurysm (*large arrow*) between the anterior cerebral arteries (*small arrows*). Also note the internal carotid (*arrowhead*) and middle cerebral (*curved arrow*) arteries (*A* is the correct answer to Question 12-14).

12-15. In this case, the CT scan shows intraparenchymal (*large arrow*) and intraventricular hemorrhage (*small arrows*) (Fig. 12-E-15*A*). The lateral view of a carotid arteriogram (Fig. 12-E-15*B*) demonstrates a tangle of blood vessels typical of an arteriovenous malformation (*large arrow*) with early draining veins (*small arrows*). Note the internal carotid artery (*curved arrow*) (*B* is the correct answer to Question 12-15).

Discussion:

Cerebrovascular disorders (strokes) were discussed in Exercise 12-2, which dealt mainly with cerebral infarction secondary to atherosclerosis. For information on other causes of cerebral infarction, the reader is referred to the Bibliography. This exercise addresses two other common vascular conditions affecting the CNS: aneurysms and vascular malformations.

Most cerebral aneurysms, as in Case 12-14, are saccular or "berry" aneurysms. These focal arterial dilatations tend to occur at cerebral arterial branch points. Traditionally, they have been thought to develop at congenitally weak areas of a blood vessel wall. Recent evidence, however, has questioned this view, and many now believe that saccular aneurysms are probably acquired lesions from abnormal hemodynamic stresses that damage the arterial wall.

Intracranial aneurysms are usually asymptomatic until they rupture, at which time the patient typically presents with a severe headache resulting from subarachnoid hemorrhage (SAH). The vast majority of nontraumatic SAHs occur as a result of aneurysm rupture. CT is very good at demonstrating SAH. Patients usually undergo cerebral arteriography whenever nontraumatic SAH is detected.

Common locations for intracranial aneurysms include the anterior communicating artery, the internal carotid artery at the origin of the posterior communicating artery, and the middle cerebral artery trifurcation. Posterior fossa aneurysms are less common; they make up only around 10 percent of all intracranial aneurysms.

Vascular malformations can be divided into four major types: true arteriovenous malformations (as demonstrated in Case 12-15), cavernous hemangiomas, venous angiomas, and capillary telangiectasias. Arteriovenous malformations (AVMs) are congenital lesions consisting of a tangle of abnormal blood vessels, usually within the brain parenchyma, that are fed by enlarged cerebral arteries and drained by dilated, tortuous veins. Since there is no normal intervening brain parenchyma for the blood to flow through, blood is rapidly shunted from the arterial to the venous side. This shunting is dramatically demonstrated on cerebral arteriography. Patients with AVMs usually present with intracranial hemorrhage or seizures. MRI or contrast-enhanced CT scan demonstrate the tortuous vascular channels of most AVMs, although cerebral arteriography is the definitive study in this condition.

The other intracranial vascular malformations have very characteristic appearances on MR imaging, although they are frequently invisible on cerebral arteriography. Patients with these "low-pressure" malformations can present with headaches, seizures, or rarely, intracranial hemorrhage. Many of these lesions, however, are incidentally discovered on MR scans performed for other reasons.

EXERCISE 12-7: WHITE MATTER DISEASES

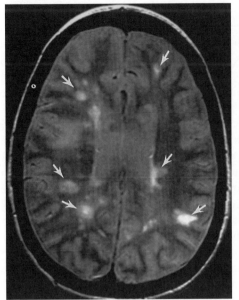

FIG. 12-E-16

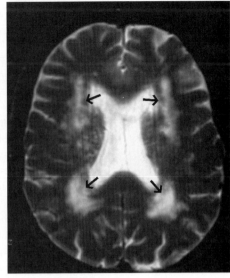

FIG. 12-E-17

Clinical Histories:

CASE 12-16
A 45-year-old woman presents with acute left-sided vision loss. An axial T2-weighted MR image of the brain is shown (Fig. 12-E-16).

CASE 12-17
A 77-year-old woman presents with a long history of hypertension and recent onset of dementia. An axial T2-weighted MR image is shown (Fig. 12-E-17).

Questions:

12-16. In Case 12-16, what is the most likely diagnosis?
   A. Pseudotumor cerebri
   B. Metastatic disease
   C. Septic emboli
   D. Radiation necrosis
   E. Multiple sclerosis

12-17. In Case 12-17, what is most likely responsible for the abnormalities seen on the MR image?
   A. Cardiac arrhythmia
   B. Chronic hypertension
   C. Remote trauma
   D. Hepatic failure
   E. Carbon monoxide poisoning

Radiologic Findings:

12-16. In this case, the axial MR image (Fig. 12-E-16) shows multiple foci of increased T2 signal within the white matter (*arrows*). These lesions are quite characteristic of multiple sclerosis (*E* is the correct answer to Question 12-16). The patient's vision loss was due to optic neuritis, a common abnormality in multiple sclerosis.

12-17. In this case, there are patchy areas of increased T2 signal (*arrows*) within the periventricular white matter (Fig. 12-E-17). Usually seen in elderly hypertensive patients, these lesions correspond to focal areas of demyelination secondary to deep white matter ischemia (*B* is the correct answer to Question 12-17).

Discussion:

Diseases that primarily affect the cerebral white matter have a host of causes. Unfortunately, very few of these conditions have specific appearances on CT or MR scans. Neuroimaging is usually performed to determine whether there are changes within the brain that are compatible with one of the white matter diseases and to rule out other conditions that might mimic white matter disease.

White matter diseases include both inherited and acquired conditions. They can be further subdivided into demyelinating conditions (destruction or injury of normally formed myelin) and dysmyelinating conditions (abnormal formation or maintenance of myelin, usually because of an enzyme deficiency). The dysmyelinating conditions are rare and, for the most part, include the leukodystrophies, such as adrenoleukodystrophy and metachromatic leukodystrophy. Although the MRI appearance can be striking in some of these diseases, it is often nonspecific. These conditions will not be discussed.

Multiple sclerosis (MS) (Case 12-16) is the most common demyelinating disease. Since there is no generally accepted etiology for MS, it is also referred to as a *primary demyelinating disease.* Secondary demyelinating conditions are those caused by a known agent or event. MS usually occurs in young adults and more often in women than in men (approximately 2:1). The disease is characterized by a relapsing and remitting course and by varying neurologic symptoms, depending on the location of the lesion within the CNS. Although the diagnosis of MS is usually based on clinical criteria, MRI can be a very helpful confirmatory test. Typical MS plaques appear as ovoid, T2 hyperintensities within the periventricular deep white matter. Lesions are also common within the corpus callosum, brain stem, cerebellar peduncles, spinal cord, and optic nerves. MS plaque enhancement on gadolinium-infused MR images suggests active disease (i.e., breakdown of the BBB). Confluent areas of T2 signal abnormality in the periventricular white matter are common in severe cases.

Ischemic demyelination (Case 12-17) is usually seen in patients with long-standing hypertension. This condition, also called *leukoaraiosis* (white matter softening), occurs because of hypertension-induced arteriolar sclerosis of penetrating medullary arteries that supply the deep white matter of the brain. This leads to a reduction in white matter blood flow with accompanying ischemic demyelination. This condition occurs most commonly in older patients and is associated with small-vessel brain infarcts (lacunar infarcts). MRI usually demonstrates patchy areas of increased T2 signal in the deep white matter. The lesions are often bilaterally symmetric and periventricular in distribution.

BIBLIOGRAPHY

Atlas SW (ed): *Magnetic Resonance Imaging of the Brain and Spine.* New York, Raven Press, 1991.

Grossman RI, Yousem DM: *Neuroradiology: The Requisites.* St. Louis, Mosby, 1994.

Osborn AG: *Diagnostic Neuroradiology.* St. Louis, Mosby, 1994.

Woodruff WW: *Fundamentals of Neuroimaging.* Philadelphia, Saunders, 1993

13

IMAGING OF THE SPINE

Lawrence E. Ginsberg

It goes without saying that the spine is critical for normal human function. The spine provides height and mobility for turning and bending and protects the spinal cord and spinal nerves. Given the wide range of pathologic conditions that may affect the spine, radiologists are frequently called on for spine imaging. Recognition of normal anatomy and variants, differentiation from abnormal anatomy, and diagnosis of different pathologic conditions are the goals of spine imaging.

It is assumed in this chapter that the reader is already familiar with basic spine anatomy learned early in medical school. With such a foundation, this presentation of the imaging appearance of the spine will serve to solidify and perhaps even enhance this knowledge base.

The purpose of this chapter is to review the different techniques employed in spine imaging and to emphasize normal anatomy as depicted with these techniques. The imaging appearance of certain common lesions also will be presented. Relative advantages and disadvantages of the various imaging modalities will be reviewed within the context of an overall imaging strategy. It is not intended that the reader will be an accomplished spine radiologist after reading this chapter. Rather, it is hoped that the reader will gain basic familiarity with normal imaging anatomy and the imaging appearance of certain types of abnormalities, as well as a sense of which test might be the best to order for a given clinical circumstance.

TECHNIQUES

Prior to the advent of computed tomography (CT) in the 1970s, spine imaging consisted primarily of plain-film radiography and an adjunct test, myelography, to be discussed below. Spine imaging was revolutionized by CT and, subsequently, magnetic resonance (MR) imaging, which for the first time allowed direct acquisition of axial and sagittal (multiplanar) images. Not until the era of CT could the spinal cord itself be visualized directly. Refinements of these cross-sectional imaging techniques are ongoing, with exciting progress undoubtedly still to come. These imaging modalities have so changed the face of spine diagnosis and treatment that virtually no neurosurgeon today would undertake spine surgery without first obtaining a CT or MR imaging study. Unfortunately, however, the widespread availability of this technology, combined with unscrupulous entrepreneurs and an adversarial legal climate, has resulted in the performance of many unnecessary scans. Perhaps health care changes, malpractice reform, or both will help to reduce the number of unnecessary examinations.

This section reviews the major modalities currently employed to image the spine. The highly specialized technique of spinal arteriography, which is used principally to detect vascular malformations, is beyond the scope of this review. Nuclear medicine scanning also will not be discussed, since seldom is it used as a primary diagnostic study in the evaluation of spine disease (though spinal metastases are frequently diagnosed with whole-body isotope bone scanning).

Plain Film

Plain films are conventional radiographs, which are commonly referred to as x-rays. They may be obtained in a frontal projection [anteroposterior (AP) or posteroanterior (PA)—the difference is insignificant in the spine], a lateral projection (side view), or an oblique projection (Figs. 13-1, 13-2, and 13-3). Plain films are most useful for the visualization of bony structures. Soft-tissue structures (everything but bone) are largely radiolucent and cannot be seen clearly on plain films unless abnormal density such as calcification is present. Although plain films depict bone anatomy quite well, certain structures may be obscured by other structures in front of or behind them. For instance, on a lateral projection, both pedicles would be superimposed on one another

(Figs. 13-1B and 13-3B). For this reason, multiple views are always obtained as part of a routine examination.

On conventional radiographs, bony structures appear white. This appearance is referred to as *radiodense* or simply *dense*. Normally mineralized bones have a recognizable radiodensity, which should always be assessed when viewing x-rays. Certain pathologic conditions (e.g., osteopenia and osteolytic metastases) can result in decreased bone density, and other conditions (e.g., osteoblastic metastases and some exotic diseases) may result in abnormally increased bone density.

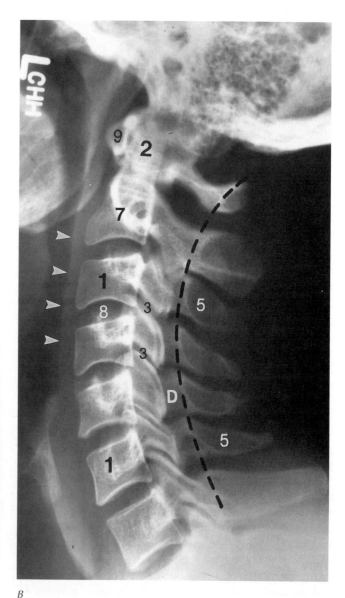

FIG. 13-1 Plain film of normal cervical spine. (*A*) Anteroposterior. (*B*) Lateral. Arrowheads indicate prevertebral soft-tissue stripe. Note normal lordosis and continuity of spinolaminar line (*dashed line*). (*C*) Oblique. (*D*) Open mouth. (*Courtesy of Stanley P. Bohrer, M.D., Bowman Gray School of Medicine.*) *Key* (for Figs. 13-1, 13-2, and 13-3): 1 = vertebral body; 2 = odontoid process (dens); 3 = articular facet joint; 4 = intervertebral (neural) foramen; 5 = spinous process; 6 = transverse process; 7 = body of axis (C2); 8 = intervertebral disk space; 9 = anterior arch of atlas (C1); A = lateral mass of atlas; B = atlantoaxial joint; C = uncinate process; D = lamina; E = pedicle; F = pars interarticularis; S = sacrum; I = sacroiliac joint.

After bone density is assessed, the next observation should be the alignment of the spine. A normal spine should show cervical and lumbar lordosis (anterior convexity) (Figs. 13-1 and 13-3) and thoracic kyphosis (posterior convexity). Abnormalities in alignment may result from incorrect positioning of the patient but often reflect an underlying problem. Such abnormalities may be minor, such as straightening or reversal of normal cervical lordosis in the case of muscle spasm. More significant misalignments, such as scoliosis, may be either idiopathic or secondary to an underlying lesion. Major alterations in alignment, such as subluxation, may result from trauma. In assessing alignment, it is important to determine whether the vertebral bodies, as well as the posterior elements (i.e., spinous processes, pedicles, and laminae), are appropriately aligned. Remember that the spinal cord rests within the spinal canal formed by the vertebral foramen of each vertebra and that the spinal cord is invisible on plain films. One must therefore evaluate where the spinal cord *should* be. The anterior margin of the spinal canal is the posterior aspect of the vertebral body. The posterior limit of the spinal canal can be approximated by locating on a lateral radiograph the junction of the spinous process and the laminae. Identification of the spinolaminar line also helps in the evaluation of alignment (Fig. 13-1*B*).

Most anatomic features of the spine are readily identifiable on plain radiographs (Figs. 13-1, 13-2, and 13-3). Vertebral bodies, facet joints, disk spaces, pedicles, laminae, transverse and spinous processes, and the neural foramen can all be visualized. Certain anatomic areas can be seen only on specialized views. For instance, the open-mouth view facilitates visualization of the atlantoaxial (C1–2) articulation and provides an additional view of the dens (Fig. 13-1*D*). This view is an essential component of a trauma workup. Oblique views allow visualization of the neural foramen in the cervical spine (lateral views are used for this purpose in the thoracolumbar spine), which transmit the paired spinal nerves (Fig. 13-1*C*). As you recall, there are 8 pairs of cervical spinal nerves, 12 pairs of thoracic spinal nerves, and 5 pairs of lumbar spinal nerves. To allow for spinal nerve exit, these neural foramina are formed by the pedicles above and below (Fig. 13-1*C* and 13-3*B*). Abnormal bony projections, known as *osteophytes,* are a common manifestation of degenerative spine disease and, if present within the neural foramen, may be a cause of nerve root compression. Spinal nerves also can be compressed by disk herniations, but this type of neural compression cannot be diagnosed by means of plain film alone.

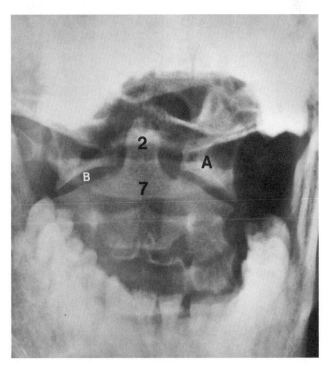

C

D

FIG. 13-1   (*Continued*)

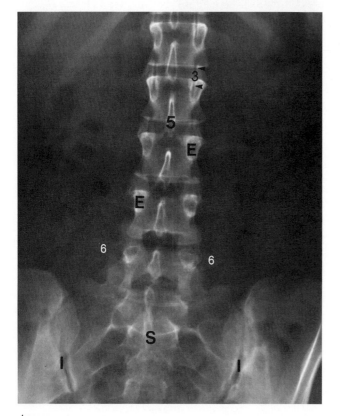

FIG. 13-2 Plain film of normal thoracic spine, anteroposterior view.

Certain small bony structures, such as the cervical transverse foramen (for the vertebral artery) and the small facets for rib articulation in the thoracic spine, are not well visualized on plain radiographs. Since soft-tissue structures also are poorly demonstrated on plain radiographs, the intervertebral disk is not well seen with x-rays unless calcified (and therefore dense). However, the soft tissues should not be ignored. In the cervical spine, for instance, one may identify calcification in the region of the carotid artery bifurcation, which may suggest atherosclerotic vascular narrowing. In the evaluation of cervical trauma, one should always include assessment of the width of the normal soft-tissue stripe that is anterior to the vertebral bodies (Fig. 13-1B). This prevertebral soft-tissue stripe may become widened in cervical spine trauma (prompting a closer search for fracture) and also in certain inflammatory conditions. When reviewing thoracic or lumbar spine films, at-

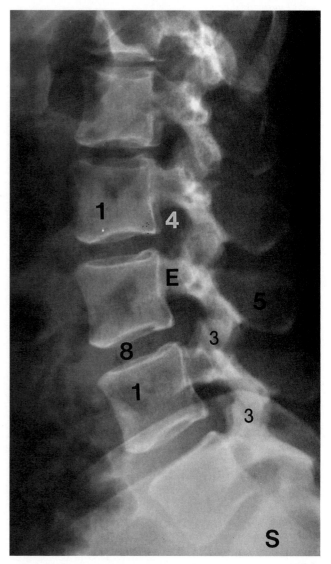

A

B

FIG. 13-3 Plain film of normal lumbar spine. (A) Anteroposterior. (B) Lateral. (C) Oblique. Notice "Scottie dog" configuration formed by facet joints and pedicle in this projection (*dashed line*).

The "neck" of the Scottie dog represents the pars interarticularis. (Part *C courtesy of Stanley P. Bohrer, M.D., Bowman Gray School of Medicine.*)

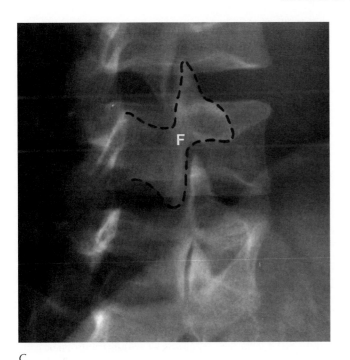

C

FIG. 13-3 (*Continued*)

tention to the soft tissues may facilitate diagnosis of a host of conditions ranging from pneumonia and lung cancer to retroperitoneal diseases and abdominal aortic aneurysms. Therefore, it is important not to focus only on the spine when interpreting spine radiographs.

Myelography

Contrast myelography has been around since its accidental discovery in 1922, when Sicard and Forestier, intending to administer extradural Lipiodol to treat sciatica, inadvertently introduced the material into the subarachnoid space. This radiopaque oil was noted to move freely, and it was immediately recognized that with the use of fluoroscopy (real-time radiography) and conventional radiography, this procedure would be useful for diagnosing intraspinal tumors. Lipiodol quickly replaced air as the medium of choice for myelography (air is lucent and is therefore a "negative" contrast agent; iodinized oils such as Lipiodol and, later, the popular Pantopaque (iophendylate) are dense and therefore "positive" contrast agents). Following Mixter and Barr's 1934 report on the syndrome of herniated intervertebral disk, myelography became a widely used test. In the 1980s, the wide availability of less toxic water-soluble agents and, finally, nonionic contrast agents such as iopamidol and iohexol made myelography a readily tolerated procedure.

Myelography is employed most commonly to evaluate for disk herniations and to rule out spinal cord compression caused by tumor or trauma. In many parts of the United States, CT and MRI have all but replaced myelography. However, in many locations, myelography is still com-

monly performed. A myelogram is often followed by a postmyelogram CT examination, which will be addressed later.

The technique for performing myelography is simple. The patient is placed prone on a fluoroscopy table. Under fluoroscopic guidance, a lumbar puncture (LP) is made with an 18- to 22-gauge spinal needle (a fluoroscopically guided LP is much easier than an LP performed on a sick patient on the ward in the decubitus position). Cerebrospinal fluid (CSF) is then drawn for laboratory tests, if needed, and contrast material is placed into the subarachnoid space. Once instillation of the contrast agent is fluoroscopically confirmed, the needle can be withdrawn and the patient studied. Depending on the spinal level to be examined, the patient can be standing, flat, or in Trendelenburg position. Typically, multiple views including lateral, AP, and oblique views are obtained. In the lumbar region, the cauda equina nerve roots are well visualized (Fig. 13-4*A*).

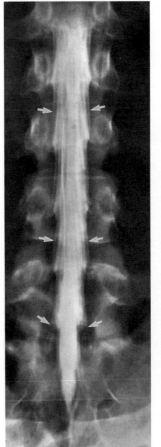

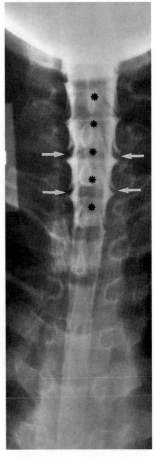

A   *B*

FIG. 13-4 (*A*) Normal lumbar myelogram, anteroposterior view. Note dense white contrast within the thecal sac. The nerve roots are readily identified as a "negative defect" within the dense contrast (*arrows*). (*B*) Cervical myelogram, anteroposterior view. The spinal cord (*asterisks*) can be seen as a lower-density "defect" within the contrast column. Exiting nerve roots also can be seen (*arrows*).

The conus medullaris, usually at L1–2, also can be seen. In the thoracic and cervical levels, the spinal cord can be seen as a "negative" shadow within the dense contrast, and its size and shape can therefore be evaluated (Fig. 13-4*B*). Cervical spinal nerves are also well seen (Fig. 13-4*B*). The presence of any lesions and their precise location relative to the dura usually can be determined on the basis of the myelographic appearance. For instance, lesions may be extradural, intradural but extramedullary (not in the spinal cord), or intramedullary.

Computed Tomography

CT utilizes x-rays to obtain images by means of multiple sources and detectors surrounding the patient in a radial fashion. This is why the patient appears to be entering a large doughnut-shaped device during the CT examination. The data obtained are processed by a computer, which then generates an image. Though sagittal reconstructions can be generated and are occasionally useful in spine imaging, the axial plane offers the highest image resolution. Once the raw data are obtained, images can be displayed with different *windows* and *level* values that take advantage of density (*attenuation* in CT lingo) differences between tissues. For instance, filming a set of soft-tissue windows allows differentiation of soft-tissue structures that are very similar in at-

tenuation to adjacent structures (e.g., muscle and fluid). This is one of the key features of CT: Whereas plain films usually cannot discriminate between different kinds of soft tissue, CT, with its superior resolution, can do just that. In the spine, CT makes it possible to discriminate between CSF, nerve roots, and ligaments, for instance. Without the administration of contrast agents, therefore, a CT examination can demonstrate the ligamentum flavum, nerve roots, epidural fat, and other structures that cannot be identified discretely on plain films (Fig. 13-5*A*). We also typically film a set of bone windows, whose window and level settings are adjusted to give detailed information on bony structures (Fig. 13-5*B*). On such images, little soft-tissue information is available.

CT is widely used to image the spine in the evaluation of almost all types of pathologic conditions. Most common indications include degenerative disk disease (i.e., to rule out disk herniation in patients with myelopathy or radiculopathy), suspected spinal tumors, and trauma. Assuming a normal appearance on plain films, CT is often the first study ordered in the evaluation of patients with back pain.

CT Myelography

As mentioned earlier, in patients who have undergone myelography, CT is often obtained immediately afterwards (Fig. 13-6). It has been shown that a postmyelogram CT is more sensitive in the detection of pathologic conditions than is either test alone. This is particularly true for lesions within the spinal canal, such as disk herniations or tumors

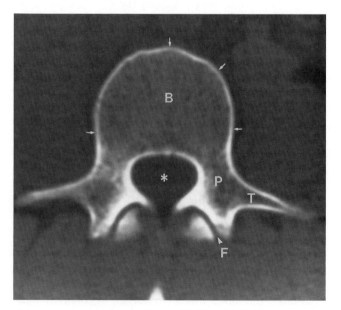

A   *B*

FIG. 13-5   CT of normal spine. (*A*) Soft-tissue windows (A = aorta; D = intervertebral disk; N = neural foramen; P = psoas muscles; *arrows* = ligamentum flavum; *asterisk* = thecal sac). (*B*) Bone window (* = spinal canal; P = pedicle; B = vertebral body; T = transverse process; F = facet joint). Notice the excellent bony detail and thin rim of normal dense cortical bone (*arrows*).

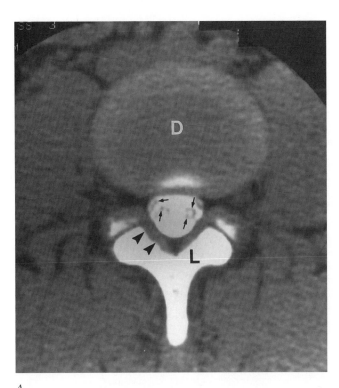

A

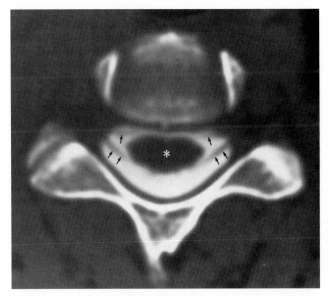

B

FIG. 13-6 Postmyelographic CT. (*A*) Lumbar spine soft-tissue window through L4–5 disk space. Dense contrast can be seen surrounding the small cauda equina nerve roots (*arrows*) (D = disk; L = lamina; *arrowheads* = ligamentum flavum). (*B*) Cervical spine bone window, disk space level. Spinal cord is easily seen (*). Dorsal and ventral nerve roots can be seen as they leave the cord and join to form spinal nerve (*arrows*).

unassociated with a bony component. The presence of subarachnoid contrast allows dramatic visualization of the cauda equina nerve roots and spinal cord in a way that cannot be achieved with regular CT. In our institution, the vast majority of myelograms are immediately followed by CT.

MR Imaging

Since the early 1980s MR imaging has gained widespread acceptance as the most sensitive imaging modality in the study of spine disease. Though not necessarily the first study performed, MR imaging undeniably allows visualization of intraspinal anatomy with much higher resolution than does any other modality. The ability to image directly in the sagittal plane contributes a great deal to the evaluation of the diseased spine. A description of the physics of MR imaging is beyond the scope of this chapter, and the reader is referred elsewhere for this information. Because dense cortical bone has few mobile protons (which are necessary to create an MR signal), MR imaging is sometimes limited in its ability to demonstrate either osteophytes that may be a source of clinical symptoms or calcific components of other lesions. In such cases, CT with its superb de-

piction of bony detail may be useful as an adjunct examination. On the other hand, MR imaging is very sensitive in its ability to detect abnormalities in bone marrow. The vertebral bodies normally contain a large amount of bone marrow, and an abnormal appearance may be seen in a variety of disorders, such as anemia, infection, and metastatic disease.

MR images can be obtained with a variety of *sequences.* Those most commonly utilized are called *spin-echo,* and these can be *weighted* for either T1 or T2. (A thorough explanation of these parameters can be found elsewhere). On a T1-weighted image, normal adult (yellow/fatty) bone marrow has a *high signal* (i.e., it is hyperintense, or whitish in color), and CSF has a *low signal* (i.e., it is hypointense, or black in color). Neural tissue, such as the spinal cord or nerve roots, is intermediate in signal intensity (Fig. 13-7A). Cortical bone, lacking mobile protons to produce a signal, is hypointense on all pulse sequences. On T2-weighted images, marrow becomes lower in signal intensity. CSF becomes hyperintense, and neural tissue maintains an intermediate signal intensity. However, the spinal cord *appears* relatively lower in signal intensity, surrounded as it is by CSF with its very high signal intensity (Fig. 13-7B). The intervertebral disks in normal individuals are typically of intermediate signal on T1-weighted images and, because of their water content, appear hyperintense on T2-weighted images. Any alterations in the expected normal signal intensity for an anatomic structure should prompt a search for either a technical or a pathologic explanation for the abnormal signal. In some clinical applications, scanning after administration of intravenous gadolinium (gadopentetate dimeglumine) or other paramagnetic contrast agents can add valuable information, which may either clarify questions raised by the precontrast imaging results or permit detection of lesions that were invisible

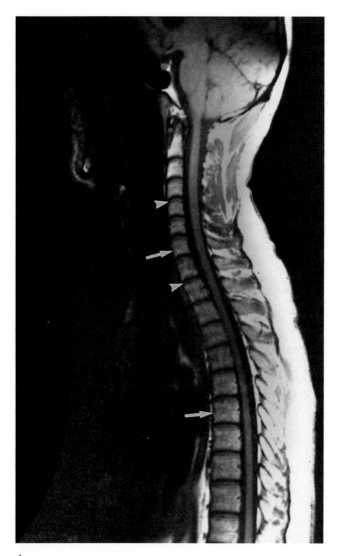

A

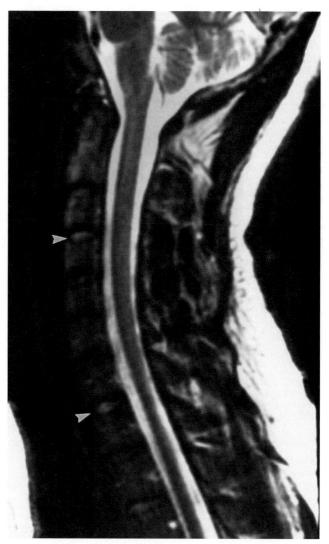

B

FIG. 13-7 Normal MR images. (*A*) T1-weighted sagittal, cervicothoracic spine. The spinal cord is very easily seen. Note that CSF anterior and posterior to the cord is hypointense, or of low signal intensity. The high signal arising from the vertebral body bone marrow (*arrows*) is due to the fat content. The disk spaces are readily visualized and are of lower signal intensity (*arrowheads*). This is the normal relative appearance of bone marrow and disk on T1-weighted images. Any reversal (i.e., disk is brighter or higher in signal intensity than marrow) should raise the suspicion of marrow disease. (*B*) T2-weighted sagittal cervical spine. CSF is now very hyperintense, and spinal cord appears to have relatively low signal intensity. The disks, because of their water content (when normal), appear higher in signal intensity when compared with the T1-weighted image (*arrowheads*). The bone marrow, on the other hand, is lower in signal intensity (*f*at *f*ades on T2).

without contrast. Despite its advantages, MR imaging is contraindicated in some patients, especially those with relentless claustrophobia, those who are unable to lie still, and those with certain medical prostheses (e.g., specific heart valves, certain aneurysm clips, and pacemakers).

TECHNIQUE SELECTION

A great many clinical circumstances may necessitate spine imaging. The purpose of this section is to convey a sense of which techniques would be most appropriate for the given clinical setting. In some instances, the choice is clear. In others, the test to be performed is determined by the technology available, and often the decision is influenced by the preferences of the person ordering the test. In some clinical settings, more than one imaging modality is acceptable as a first test. If the clinician consults with the radiologist before deciding on the initial test, unnecessary examinations may be avoided. Perhaps most important, however, if the clinician consults with the radiologist and conveys to him or her the clinical information, imaging often can be tailored to home in on the most likely site or type of abnormality. Still, general guidelines can be established to help decide which imaging test is appropriate. What follows is a brief outline providing general imaging recommendations for common clinical problems related to the spine. Only rarely is a particular test the *only* useful one for a suspected abnormality. In many cases, any of several tests would be useful as a baseline examination, with the understanding that additional imaging might be required to answer all clinical questions.

Trauma

Plain films are the best initial examination for the evaluation of spine trauma. In a potentially unstable patient, they are obtained readily and often yield an immediate diagnosis. For further characterization of complex fractures, for conditions in which plain films were inadequate (e.g., the cervical thoracic junction), or when additional information is required (e.g., to rule out canal compromise by a bone fragment), CT is frequently performed. CT is the best imaging study to evaluate complex spine fractures. In certain circumstances, such as suspected spinal cord contusion or transection, or hemorrhage within the spinal canal, MR imaging is indicated. It is also useful in evaluating the patient with delayed onset of neurologic dysfunction after trauma to rule out myelomalacia (softening) of the spinal cord or posttraumatic syrinx.

Back Pain

Back pain is one of the most common medical complaints. Though most cases are caused by muscle strains and the like, persistent severe pain, pain associated with sciatica (a shooting pain down the leg), or neurologic findings such as weakness, decreased sensation, or abnormal reflexes should prompt a search for an underlying structural abnormality. The most common pathologic conditions are related to bony degenerative disease (osteoarthritis) or intervertebral disk abnormalities. As with trauma, plain films are a good place to start. Though disk herniations (extrusion of the nucleus pulposus beyond the annulus fibrosus) are not visible on plain films, degenerative changes are generally quite apparent, and any unsuspected lesions such as compression fractures or metastatic disease (both of which are common in older patients) may be detected. For patients with a suspected herniated disk, MR imaging is generally considered the most sensitive examination. CT is still a good examination for the detection of disk herniation, and when combined with intrathecal contrast (CT myelography), it is still a widely used imaging modality. Although MR imaging is not essential for detecting disk

abnormalities, it is more sensitive and is especially useful for detecting other pathologic conditions that might clinically mimic disk herniation, such as lesions of the conus medullaris or metastatic disease. A possible exception to the use of MR imaging as a first-line cross-sectional imaging procedure in degenerative spine disease is for patients suspected of having foraminal nerve impingement by an osteophyte. Osteophytes are small, sharp projections of bone that occur in patients with osteoarthritis, and they may impinge on the spinal cord or nerve roots. Such osteophytes in the cervical spine may be difficult to detect with MR imaging. However, it is not always possible to differentiate clinically between patients who have disk herniations and those whose nerves are compressed by osteophytes. All in all, MR imaging is the best test to order for these patients. Occasionally, a CT examination may be needed in addition to answer specific questions.

Myelopathy

In patients who are suspected of having a myelopathy (a true cord syndrome as opposed to radicular symptoms), MR imaging is unequivocally the first study to be employed. MR imaging is the only imaging procedure that allows direct visualization of the spinal cord, and it is effective for diagnosing or excluding primary spinal cord lesions such as infarct, tumor, hemorrhage, or inflammatory conditions (e.g., multiple sclerosis or transverse myelitis).

Congenital Spine Lesions

A variety of congenital lesions may affect the spine. Plain films may be useful to survey the spine, but ultimately MR imaging is the modality of choice. Though bony defects may be imaged suboptimally, disorders of the spinal cord or nerve roots can be readily identified on MR images.

Metastatic Disease

If metastatic disease in the spine is suspected, plain films are an economical, easy way to rule out bony metastases. Unfortunately, plain films do not demonstrate such abnormalities until a significant amount of destruction has taken place. MR imaging, on the other hand, is quite sensitive to replacement of normal bone marrow by tumor and can establish the diagnosis much earlier. Gadolinium-enhanced MR imaging is also the best choice if spread of tumor to the subarachnoid space (carcinomatous meningitis or leptomeningeal carcinomatosis) is suspected clinically.

EXERCISE 13-1: DEGENERATIVE SPINE DISEASE

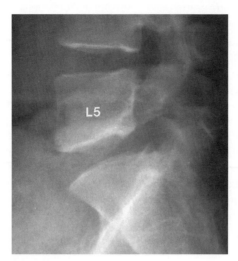

FIG. 13-E-1 *Panel A*

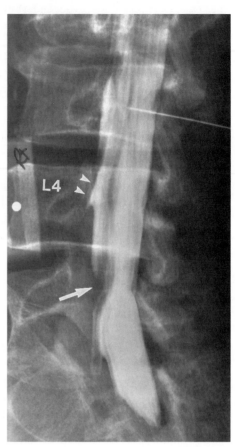

FIG. 13-E-2 *Panel A*

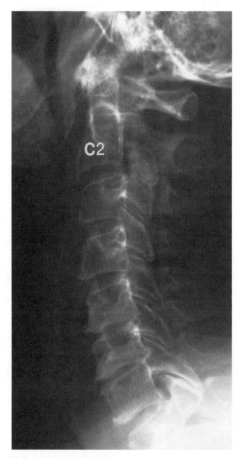

FIG. 13-E-3 *Panel A*

Clinical Histories:

CASE 13-1

A whiny 37-year-old neuroradiologist presents with low-back pain (Fig. 13-E-1A). A coned-down lateral plain film of the lumbar spine is shown.

CASE 13-2

A 58-year-old man presents with right-sided L5 radiculopathy (Fig. 13-E-2A). A myelogram was performed, and an oblique view demonstrating the right-sided nerve roots is displayed.

CASE 13-3

A 53-year-old woman presents with neck and right arm pain (Fig. 13-E-3A). Plain films of the cervical spine were ordered, and a lateral film is shown.

Questions:

13-1. In Case 13-1, what is the abnormality in Fig. 13-E-1A?
   A. The bones are too dense.
   B. The bones are not dense enough (osteopenia).
   C. There is a destructive bony lesion.
   D. There is an abnormality of alignment.
   E. There is a soft-tissue abnormality.

13-2. In Case 13-2, what is the lesion represented by the arrow most likely to be?
   A. A right-sided L4–5 herniated nucleus pulposus
   B. An extradural tumor
   C. An epidural abscess
   D. An intradural mass
   E. A bony lesion

13-3. In Case 13-3, the lateral cervical spine plain film suggests what as the *most* likely diagnosis?
   A. Degenerative disk disease at C2–3 and C3–4
   B. Neoplastic disease at C4
   C. Degenerative disk disease at C5–6 and C6–7
   D. Traumatic injury
   E. Disk space infection at C5–6 and C6–7

Radiologic Findings:

13-1. In this case, there is subtle anterior displacement of the L5 vertebral body relative to S1, known as *spondylolisthesis* (D is the correct answer to Question 13-1).

13-2. In this case, an extradural defect is seen at and below the L4–5 disk space, and the right L5 nerve root does not fill. These changes are most likely caused by a disk herniation (A is the correct answer to Question 13-2). Note the normal filling of the right L4 nerve root (*arrowheads*).

13-3. In this case, there is disk space narrowing and osteophytes are seen at the C5–6 and C6–7 disk spaces (C is the correct answer to Question 13-3).

Discussion:

Degenerative osteoarthropathy may affect different parts of the spine. When the facet joints are involved, the result is often bony osteophytes, which may project into the neural foramen or spinal canal and compress neural structures. When the disk space is affected, bony changes in the vertebral body endplate can occur. In addition, the intervertebral disk itself may be affected, and disk herniation can occur as a result. Differentiation between disk bulge (less clinically important, usually in the midline, with no significant compression of cord or thecal sac) and actual herniation (larger, off-midline, with possible compression of nerves or thecal sac) is not always possible. Treatment decisions must be based on clinical as well as radiologic data.

In Case 13-1 (author's spine), the spondylolisthesis of L5 over S1 is a result of a defect in the pars interarticularis. This is the place between the superior and inferior articular facet of a given vertebra (Figs. 13-3*C* and 13-E-1*B*). *Spondylolysis,* as this defect is known, is usually caused by a chronic stress fracture, though rarely it can be congenital or acute. If, as is commonly the case, the spondylolysis is bilateral, the vertebral body is essentially disconnected from the posterior elements, and this allows the anterior slipping, or spondylolisthesis, shown in Fig. 13-E-1*A*. This entity is included here because it is quite common, and because it predisposes to premature degenerative disease. In older patients, spondylolisthesis can be *secondary* to degenerative disease in the absence of a pars defect, and this "nonlytic" form is known as *pseudospondylolithesis,* or *degenerative spondylolisthesis.* When present, the spondylolysis defect is readily identified on oblique lumbar plain films as a "broken neck on the Scottie dog" (Fig. 13-E-1*C*). The lysis defect is also readily detected on CT (Fig. 13-E-1*D*) though it may superficially resemble a facet joint.

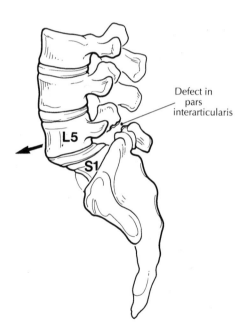

Defect in
pars
interarticularis

B

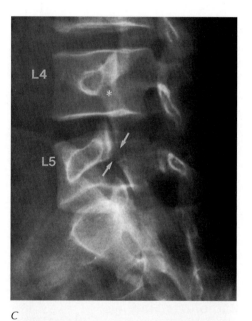

C

FIG. 13-E-1 (*Panel B*) Diagram of spondylolisthesis of L5 over S1 caused by spondylolysis of L5. (*Panel C*) Oblique plain film of lumbar spine (same patient) demonstrates a spondylolysis or pars defect on the right side of L5 (*arrows*). Note intact pars at L4 (*asterisk*). (*Panel D*) CT bone window of different patient shows spondylolysis defects (*arrows*). Though these resemble facet joints, they are more horizontal in orientation and more irregular, lacking a smooth cortical margin.

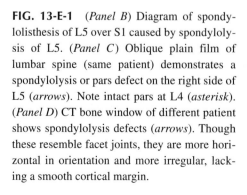

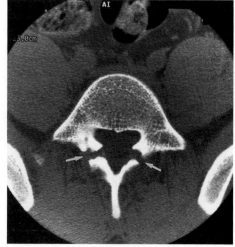

D

Disk herniations are a common medical problem. Though they can usually be diagnosed with noninvasive CT or MR imaging, myelography is still employed in some places to diagnose disk herniations. In Case 13-2, Fig. 13-E-2*A* shows an extradural defect, seen as an area of low density distorting the lateral aspect of the thecal sac and deviating the nerve roots. This is the typical appearance of a herniated nucleus pulposus (HNP) on myelography. We see the effect of the disk rather than the actual disk. On a CT study, the actual herniated disk can be visualized (Fig. 13-E-2*B*). Most of the myelographic filling defect can be seen to be below the L4–5 disk space, secondary to inferior migration of disk material. This helps explain why the patient had an L5 radiculopathy. The right L4 nerve root (*arrowheads* in Fig. 13-E-2*A*) had already exited and would be unaffected by an L4–5 HNP unless it was far lateral (Fig. 13-E-2*C*). As previously men-

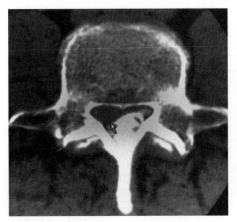

B

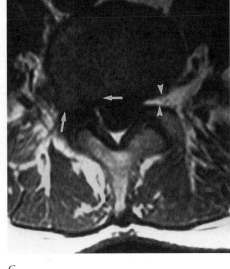

C

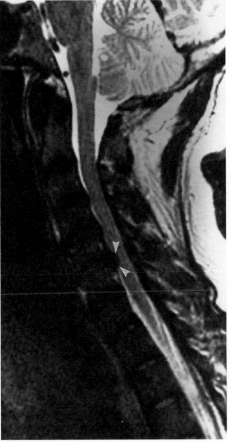

D

FIG. 13-E-2 (*Panel B*) Axial CT (same patient) just below the L4–5 disk space shows compression of the right anterolateral aspect of the thecal sac by the HNP (*arrow*). The image was obtained below the L4–5 disk space, indicating inferior migration of herniated disk material. (*Panel C*) Axial T1-weighted MR image of a different patient shows a far lateral right-sided HNP (*arrows*) with replacement of normal foraminal fat by intermediate signal representing the disk. Note normal perineural fat in the left neural foramen (*arrowheads*). A far lateral HNP such as this would probably be missed if only myelography were performed. (*Panel D*) Sagittal T2-weighted image shows a midline disk herniation at C5–6 which is compressing the spinal cord (*arrowheads*).

tioned, MR imaging is excellent in detecting disk herniations and eliminates the need for painful, invasive procedures such as myelography (Figs. 13-E-2*C,D*).

Osteophytic ridging is a common manifestation of degenerative bone disease and in the cervical spine may cause myelopathy (if the cord is compressed) or radiculopathy (if a nerve root is compressed). In Case 13-3, Fig. 13-E-3*A* shows marked narrowing and osteophyte formation at C5–6 and C6–7. An oblique radiograph is useful in demonstrating the foraminal compromise that can result if osteophytes occur in that location (Fig. 13-E-3*B*). Myelography can demonstrate effacement of nerve roots (Fig. 13-E-3*C*). CT, with or without intrathecal contrast material, is excellent in depicting foraminal stenosis caused by osteophytes (Fig. 13-E-3*D*). As mentioned earlier, MR imaging may be limited in its ability to depict subtle bony abnormalities such as foraminal compromise, though utilization of specialized techniques has resulted in improved detection with MR imaging.

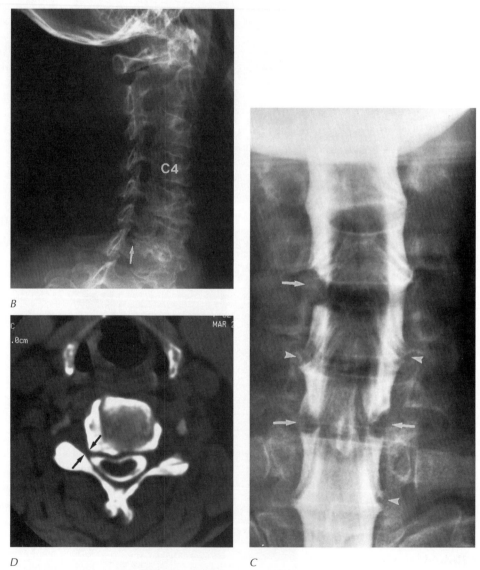

FIG. 13-E-3   (*Panel B*) Oblique radiograph shows compromise of the right C6–7 neural foramen by osteophytes (*arrow*). Note that the other foramina are patent. (*Panel C*) AP view cervical myelogram of a different patient. Effaced nerve roots (*arrows*) can be seen as defects larger than would be expected for a normal nerve root. Compare with normal nerve roots (*arrowheads*). (*Panel D*) Axial postmyelographic CT of same patient shows narrowing of the right neural foramen (*arrows*). The contralateral neural foramen is normal.

EXERCISE 13-2: NEOPLASTIC SPINE DISEASE

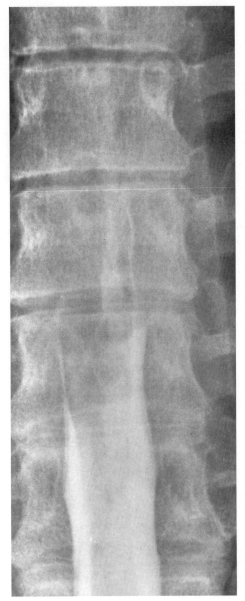

FIG. 13-E-4 *Panel A*

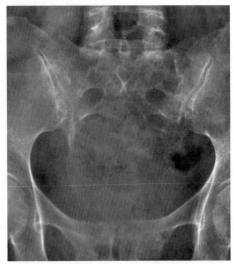

FIG. 13-E-5 *Panel A*

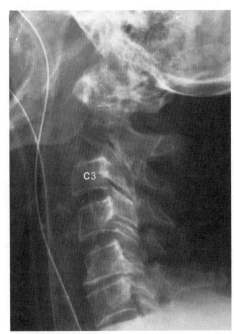

FIG. 13-E-6 *Panel A*

Clinical Histories:

CASE 13-4

A 39-year-old man presents with leg pain and weakness. A prior lumbar spine MR examination was normal. A thoracic myelogram is shown (Fig. 13-E-4A).

CASE 13-5

A 70-year-old woman presents with a 5-year history of back pain and recent onset of paresthesia in the groin and inner thighs (saddle distribution) (Fig. 13-E-5A).

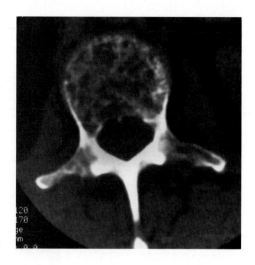

FIG. 13-E-7 *Panel A*

CASE 13-6
A 63-year-old man presents with severe upper neck pain not responding to anti-inflammatory medication (Fig. 13-E-6*A*).

CASE 13-7
A 65-year-old man presents with back pain. A CT bone window is shown (Fig. 13-E-7*A*).

Questions:

13-4. In Case 13-4, what does this AP view from a thoracic myelogram show?
  A. A bony abnormality
  B. An extradural mass
  C. An intradural-extramedullary mass
  D. An intramedullary mass
  E. A really big disk herniation

13-5. In Case 13-5, what is the most likely diagnosis?
  A. Sacroiliitis
  B. A sacral tumor
  C. Constipation
  D. Osteoporosis
  E. Uterine malignancy

13-6. In Case 13-6, what is the main radiologic finding?
  A. A lesion of the C7 spinous process
  B. An osteoblastic bony lesion
  C. An abnormality of alignment
  D. A destructive lesion at C2
  E. A fracture

13-7. In Case 13-7, what diagnostic possibilities should be most seriously considered?
  A. Congenital or traumatic lesions
  B. Metabolic or endocrine disease
  C. Myeloma or metastatic disease
  D. Infectious or inflammatory disease
  E. Degenerative or inflammatory disease

Radiologic Findings:

13-4. In this case, the patient has a lower thoracic primary spinal cord astrocytoma (*D* is the correct answer to Question 13-4). The cord is normal inferiorly but is seen to

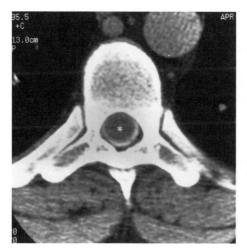

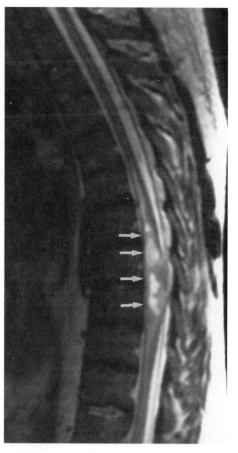

B

FIG. 13-E-4 (*Panel B*) Axial postmyelographic CT demonstrates enlargement of the spinal cord (*asterisk*), representing tumor, with narrowing of the subarachnoid/contrast space surrounding the cord. (*Panel C*) Sagittal T2-weighted MR image shows the tumor and resulting enlargement of the thoracic spinal cord, with areas of central hyperintense signal (*arrows*) probably representing necrosis.

C

get wider toward the middle of the image. The contrast column on either side of the lesion is narrowed, most noticeably on the patient's right. This lesion has caused a "block" to the flow of contrast. Subsequent postmyelography CT (Fig. 13-E-4*B*) confirmed the spinal cord enlargement. An MR image demonstrated the tumor (Fig. 13-E-4*C*) within the spinal cord.

13-5. In this case, the plain film shows a large destructive mass replacing most of the lower sacrum (*B* is the correct answer to Question 13-5). Notice how normal bone disappears below the midsacrum. A CT showed a large destructive mass with areas of calcification (Fig. 13-E-5*B*).

13-6. In this case, the plain film shows that the body of C2 has been destroyed (lytic destruction) (*D* is the correct answer to Question 13-6).

13-7. In this case, the CT image shows multiple small areas of lytic bony destruction. This is characteristic of either multiple myeloma or metastatic disease (*C* is the correct answer to Question 13-7).

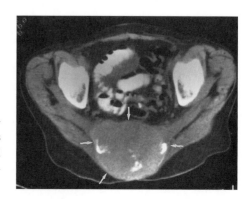

FIG. 13-E-5 (*Panel B*) CT study (without intravenous contrast material) shows a large mass replacing the lower sacrum (*arrows*). Internal areas of high density represent either tumor calcification or remnants of destroyed bone.

Discussion: Unfortunately, the spine is commonly involved by tumors of various types. In Case 13-4, the diagnosis was primary spinal cord glioma. Most of these are either astrocytomas or ependymomas. As with this patient, the diagnosis may be elusive for some time while other diseases such as disk herniation are ruled out. This patient even had a normal lumbar MR examination several months prior to the myelogram. While the thoracolumbar junction is usually visualized on a lumbar MR imaging study, this tumor (at T10) was just missed. A thoracic MR examination would certainly have made the diagnosis, but the patient's doctor ordered a myelogram. Spinal cord tumors are generally very difficult to treat and are associated with a poor prognosis, but more aggressive surgical approaches may offer greater hope to these patients.

Primary bony tumors also may affect the spine. A variety of benign bone tumors and cysts may be encountered. In the sacrum, giant cell tumor is the most common benign tumor. The most common primary sacral malignancy is chordoma. This is the diagnosis in Case 13-5. Chordomas develop from remnants of the embryonic notochord and represent 2 to 4 percent of primary malignant bone tumors. The sacrum is the most common site for chordoma, accounting for 50 percent of these lesions. The skull base accounts for 35 percent and other vertebrae account for 15 percent. Typical presentation of sacral chordoma is low-back pain, paresthesias, or rectal dysfunction. Figure 13-E-5*A* shows the typical radiographic appearance of expansile, lytic destruction. On CT (Fig. 13-E-5*B*), a large soft-tissue mass with internal calcifications is characteristic.

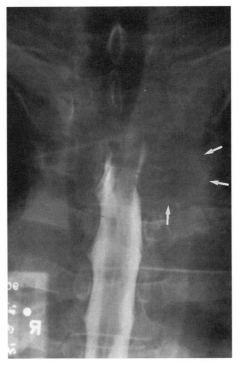

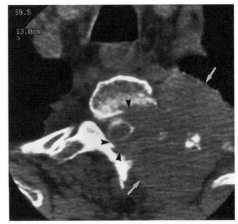

B   *C*

FIG. 13-E-6   (*Panel B*) A 49-year-old man with lung carcinoma and direct contiguous spread into the spine. AP view thoracic myelogram shows a mass in the left upper lung with bone destruction (*arrows*). The contrast column was blocked, and there was no flow cephalad to the lesion despite steep Trendelenburg positioning. The appearance of this block is typical for an extradural process. (*Panel C*) Postmyelographic CT of same patient at the level of the block demonstrates the large lung mass (*arrows*) extending into the spine, destroying bone, and involving the epidural space (*arrowheads*). (*Panel D*) Sagittal T1-weighted MR image of a different patient after intravenous administration of Gd-DTPA. The patient has known lung carcinoma. Enhancing masses (*arrows*) indicate subarachnoid tumor deposits. Contrast-enhanced MR imaging may be the only way to confirm this diagnosis, since CSF cytology is often falsely negative.

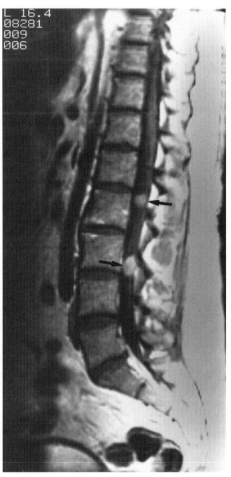

FIG. 13-E-6 (*Continued*)

D

By far the most common type of spinal tumor is metastatic disease, with lung and breast being the most frequent primary sites. Virtually any tumor may metastasize to the spine. In general, certain tumors tend to result in osteoblastic or dense metastases, and prostate adenocarcinoma falls in this category. Other primary malignancies, such as those in the lung and breast, tend to have osteolytic, destructive spine metastases. The patient in Case 13-6 had lung carcinoma, and Fig. 13-E-6*A* represents a hematogenous spread of tumor to the C2 vertebral body. Metastatic disease may affect the spine by other mechanisms. Tumors adjacent to the spine may grow directly into it (Fig. 13-E-6*B,C*). This may occur in lung carcinoma and lesions such as neuroblastoma or lymphoma (with retroperitoneal/paraspinal lymphadenopathy). Finally, the spinal cord may be affected by spread of malignant neoplasm. Rarely, a metastatic lesion may occur in the spinal cord itself, usually as a terminal event. Metastatic disease may occur in the subarachnoid space by two methods. First, an intracranial malignancy (i.e., glioma, medulloblastoma) can seed the subarachnoid space and "fall" into the spine. These are known as "drop" metastases. Hematogenous spread to the subarachnoid space may occur in non-CNS primary tumors. Such involvement is known as *leptomeningeal carcinomatosis,* or *carcinomatous meningitis* (Fig. 13-E-6*D*), and is associated with a very poor prognosis.

Multiple myeloma is a disseminated malignancy caused by a proliferation of plasmacytes, typically occurring in the middle-aged and elderly, with a slight male predominance. The spine may be affected primarily or secondarily, and bone pain caused by pathologic compression factors is the most common symptom. Plain films may be normal early in the course of the disease or show only mild osteopenia. Later, multiple,

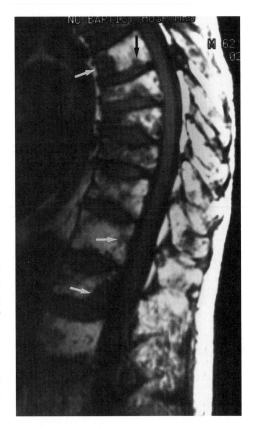

FIG. 13-E-7 (*Panel B*) Sagittal T1-weighted MR image of the thoracic spine shows multiple small hypointense foci of myeloma (*arrows*) replacing normal bone marrow. Compression fractures are also seen, indicated by loss of height of several upper thoracic vertebral bodies. The spinal cord is intact, but spread of tumor or retropulsion of fractured bone could result in cord compression. Note that metastatic tumor other than myeloma could have an identical appearance.

small, lytic, "punched out" lesions may be seen. CT is very sensitive, and Fig. 13-E-7*A* shows the typical CT appearance of multiple myeloma. The findings, however, would be indistinguishable from those of small lytic metastases of other origin, and for this reason, metastases and myeloma are often mentioned together in the context of multiple small lytic bony lesions. MR imaging of multiple myeloma may have different appearances, but the typical pattern would be multiple, small foci of decreased signal intensity replacing the normal hyperintense bone marrow on T1-weighted images (Fig. 13-E-7*B*).

EXERCISE 13-3: SPINE TRAUMA

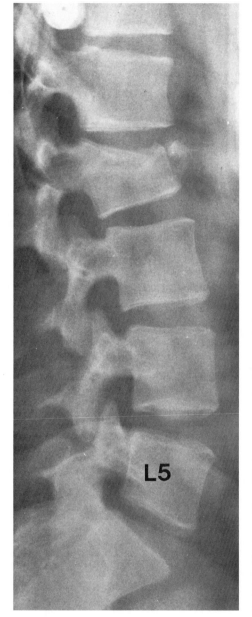

FIG. 13-E-8 *Panel A*

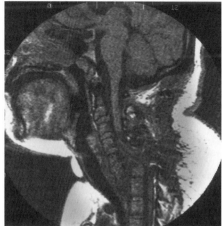

FIG. 13-E-9

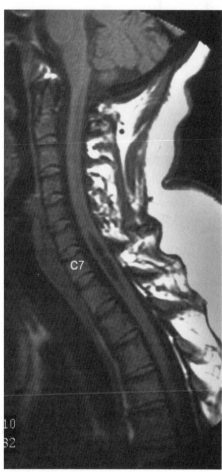

FIG. 13-E-10

Clinical Histories:

CASE 13-8

A 23-year-old woman is seen who was involved in a motor vehicle accident (Fig. 13-E-8*A*).

CASE 13-9
A 21-year-old quadriplegic woman presents 4 weeks after a motor vehicle accident (Fig. 13-E-9).

CASE 13-10
A 38-year-old woman presents who is now experiencing slowly progressive upper extremity and upper trunk sensory deficits 3 years after a motor vehicle accident (Fig. 13-E-10).

Questions:

13-8. In Case 13-8, what is the most likely diagnosis?
    A. Spinal tumor aggravated by trauma
    B. Abnormality of bone density
    C. Disruption of facet joints at multiple levels
    D. Subluxation of L4 over L5
    E. L2 compression fracture with kyphotic angulation

13-9. Regarding the patient in Case 13-9, which of the following is true?
    A. The condition probably predated the trauma.
    B. The prospects for a full recovery are good.
    C. Surgical repair will likely be successful.
    D. The patient will probably never have normal neurologic function below C6.
    E. The spinal cord is intact.

13-10. In Case 13-10, what is the most likely diagnosis?
    A. Delayed posttraumatic syrinx
    B. Subluxation
    C. Spinal cord tumor
    D. Abnormal bone marrow
    E. Disk abnormality

Radiologic Findings:

13-8. In this case, there is a compression fracture of the L2 vertebral body with kyphotic angulation (*E* is the correct answer to Question 13-8).

13-9. In this case, the sagittal T1-weighted MR image shows a complete subluxation of C6 on C7 and a complete transection of the cervical spinal cord at that level. In all likelihood this patient will never regain use of her legs or have any normal neurologic function below C6 (*D* is the correct answer to Question 13-9).

13-10. In this case, the sagittal T1-weighted MR image shows a low signal abnormality within the cervical spinal cord from C6 to T1. This is a typical appearance of syringomyelia or syrinx (*A* is the correct answer to Question 13-10).

Discussion:

Spinal trauma is a major medical problem, usually caused by motor vehicle and occupational accidents. Accurate and complete diagnosis is essential to maintain spine stability and ensure preservation of neurologic function. As mentioned previously, plain films should be obtained initially, and this often makes the diagnosis. However, additional imaging tests are often necessary to fully evaluate a case of spine trauma. For instance, in Case 13-8, there was clinical concern that the spinal canal was compromised. Small bony fragments within the spinal canal may not be visible with plain film alone. For this reason, CT was performed (Fig. 13-E-8*B,C*). This allowed a better appreciation of the extent of the fractures and ruled out neural compression. An example of spinal canal compromise is shown in Fig. 13-E-8*D*.

In severe trauma, the spinal cord may be affected. Contusions may occur with or without fracture/subluxation, and MR imaging would be required for diagnosis. In a severe fracture/subluxation, the spinal cord can be completely transected. In Case 13-9, the

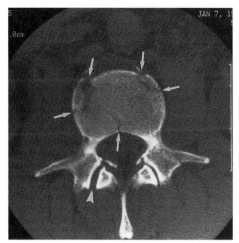

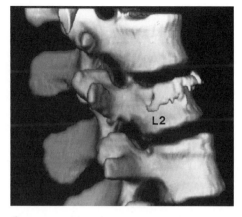

C

B

FIG. 13-E-8 (*Panel B*) Axial CT bone window shows different components of the fracture (*arrows*). The spinal canal was intact. Note the separation of the facet joint on the right (*arrowhead*). (*Panel C*) Three-dimensional reconstruction shows compression of L2 and fracture sites. Such reconstructions are sometimes useful in cases of spine trauma. (*Panel D*) Axial CT bone window of a different patient demonstrates multiple fractures and retropulsion of a bone fragment causing narrowing of the spinal canal (*arrows*).

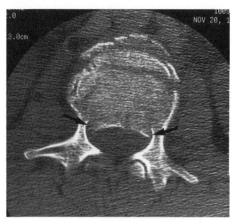

D

patient was known to have a severe C6–7 subluxation, but because of obesity, plain film and CT imaging were very limited. In this case, only MR imaging was able to demonstrate the full extent of her spinal cord injury.

Rarely, patients who have recovered from an acute spinal injury experience a delayed onset of neurologic symptoms, occurring 1 to 15 years after the trauma. This suggests the possibility of delayed posttraumatic syrinx (Case 13-10). Symptoms include pain on coughing or exertion, sensory disturbances, or motor deficits. MR imaging is essential for diagnosis. The condition is sometimes amenable to surgical shunting. Syringomyelia also can be idiopathic or can be secondary to certain congenital or inflammatory conditions. Imaging often cannot distinguish among different possible etiologies, and history is important.

BIBLIOGRAPHY

Atlas SW (ed): *Magnetic Resonance Imaging of the Brain and Spine.* New York, Raven Press, 1991.

Epstein BS: *The Spine: A Radiological Test and Atlas,* 3d ed. Philadelphia, Lea & Febiger, 1969.

Greenspan A, Montesano P: *Imaging of the Spine in Clinical Practice.* London, Mosby Europe, 1993.

Harris JH Jr, Edeiken-Monroe B: *The Radiology of Acute Cervical Spine Trauma,* 2d ed. Baltimore, Williams & Wilkins, 1987.

Manelfe C (ed): *Imaging of the Spine and Spinal Cord,* rev. ed. New York, Raven Press, 1992.

INDEX

Note: Page numbers in italics refer to figures; page numbers followed by t indicate tables.